Infection Prevention in the Intensive Care Setting

Misti Ellsworth • Luis Ostrosky-Zeichner
Editors

Infection Prevention in the Intensive Care Setting

Springer

Editors
Misti Ellsworth
Division of Pediatric Infectious Diseases
McGovern Medical School at
UTHealth Houston
Houston, TX, USA

Luis Ostrosky-Zeichner
Division of Infectious Diseases
McGovern Medical School at
UTHealth Houston
Houston, TX, USA

ISBN 978-3-031-67061-9 ISBN 978-3-031-67062-6 (eBook)
https://doi.org/10.1007/978-3-031-67062-6

This Springer imprint is published by the registered company Springer Nature Switzerland AG
The registered company address is: Gewerbestrasse 11, 6330 Cham, Switzerland

Acknowledgment

This book is dedicated to the healthcare staff who stand on the front lines of infection control. Thank you for your diligence, skill, and commitment to the prevention of hospital acquired infections. From the infection prevention practitioners who work tirelessly to educate and support infection prevention best practices within their facilities, to the healthcare workers who diligently wash their hands and don protective equipment, to the cleaning staff who ensure that every surface is disinfected—your roles are critical. You are the backbone of the hospital's defense system against the spread of infections.

The pages of this book are filled with knowledge, evidence-based practices, and innovative strategies aimed at preventing infections in the intensive care setting. We hope it becomes a valuable resource in your continuous efforts to improve patient safety and prevent infections.

Contents

1 Introduction to Infection Prevention in the ICU Setting 1
Misti Ellsworth and Luis Ostrosky-Zeichner
Introduction 1
References 2

2 Device-Associated Infections 5
Jose A. Cadena
Device-Associated Infections, Background, and Epidemiology 5
Device-Associated Infections: Specific Infections and Surveillance Definitions 8
CLABSI Overview, Cost, and Surveillance Definition 8
CAUTI Overview and Definitions 9
VAP and VAE Overview and Definitions 10
References 13

3 Strategies to Prevent Central Line-Associated Bloodstream Infections (CLABSIs) 15
Gautam Sikka, Saad Farooq, Bela Patel, and Robier Aguillon Prada
Introduction 15
Risk Factors for CLABSIs 17
Pathogenesis 18
Microbiology 18
History of CLABSI Prevention 18
Must Dos 20
Should Dos 23
Don'ts 24
NOVEL Practices 24
Conundrum 24
Framework to Reduce CLABSIs in Health Care Settings 25
References 26

4 **Current and Emerging Practices for Preventing CAUTI in the ICU** 33
Bilal Zafar and Mark T. Warner
Introduction 33
Incidence and Mortality Associated with CAUTI 34
Practices for Preventing CAUTI in the ICU 35
Appropriate Indications for Urinary Catheterization 35
Aseptic Catheter Insertion and Maintenance 35
Regular Catheter Care and Hygiene 36
Urinary Catheter Removal Protocols 36
Alternative Methods of Urine Collection 36
Antimicrobial Catheters and Coatings 36
Education and Training 37
Surveillance and Data Analysis 37
Hospital Management of CAUTIs 37
Future Research and Innovation 38
Conclusion 38
References 39

5 **VAP Prevention in the ICU** 41
Ruckshanda Majid
Introduction 41
VAP Prevention Strategies 45
High-Flow Nasal Oxygen and Noninvasive Ventilation 45
Elevation of the Head of the Bed 47
Methods of Enteral Feeding 48
Monitoring Gastric Residuals 48
Early Versus Late Initiation of Enteral Nutrition 48
Gastric Versus Post-pyloric Nutrition 49
Stress Ulcer Prophylaxis 50
Oral Antiseptics and Antibiotics 51
Topical Oral Antiseptics 51
Enteral and Parenteral Antibiotics 53
Inhaled Antibiotics 55
Probiotics 55
Avoidance of Sedation and Paralytic Agents 56
Endotracheal Tubes with Subglottic Secretion Aspiration Ports 56
Silver-Coated Endotracheal Tubes 58
Ventilator Weaning and Extubation Protocols 59
Early Tracheostomy 60
Ventilator Circuit Management Strategies 61
Avoiding Routine Changes of Ventilator Circuits 61
Heat and Moisture Exchangers or Heated Humidifiers 62
Suctioning Systems: Closed Versus Open Tracheal Suctioning System 62

Monitoring Endotracheal Tube Cuff Pressure 63
VAP Prevention Bundles.................................. 63
References... 65

6 **Infection Prevention Challenges in the Medical Intensive Care Unit (MICU)** 77
Brandy McKelvy, Jennifer Cortes, and Anabelle Keene
Introduction... 77
Mechanical Ventilation and the MICU 78
MICU in the Time of COVID-19 78
COVID-19 and Secondary Infections........................ 79
Decreasing Opportunistic Infections in MICU Patients 80
Ventilator-Associated Pneumonia (VAP) 81
Ventilator-Associated Pneumonia Pathogens 82
Prolonged Mechanical Ventilation (PMV) and Tracheostomy 82
Benefits and Risk of Tracheostomy 83
Tracheostomy and Tracheostomy in COVID-19 Patients.......... 84
Prevention of Tracheostomy-Associated Infections 85
Prevention of VAP and Tracheostomy-Associated Infections 86
IDSA Guidelines Recommended Multiple Ways to Help Prevent VAP 86
Hand Washing... 86
Using Gloves While Handling Respiratory Secretions.......... 86
Staff Education 86
ICU Staffing Levels: Limited Staff/Staffing Rations/New Staff....................................... 86
Oral Hygiene... 87
Avoiding Unnecessary Intubation.......................... 87
Minimalizing Sedation and Paralytic Agents 88
Avoiding Naso-Tracheal Intubation and Naso-Grastic Tubes....................................... 88
Adequate Endotracheal Tube Cuff Pressure 88
Aspiration of Subglottic Secretions 89
Use of Silver-Coated Endotracheal Tubes 89
Enteral Nutrition Versus Parenteral Nutrition................ 89
Restricted Transfusion 90
Selective Oropharyngeal Decontamination and Selective Digestive Decontamination....................... 91
Keeping Head of the Bed >30°........................... 91
Only Changing Ventilator Circuits When Soiled or at 7 Days 92
Use of Heated Moisture Exchangers........................ 92
Cleaning of Respiratory Equipment 92
Additional Methods Not Covered in This Chapter............. 93
Use of Bundles to prevent VAP............................ 93

The Use of Extracorporeal Membrane Oxygenation in MICU and Antimicrobial Prophylaxis . . . 93
The Use of Proton Pump Inhibitors for Stress Ulcer Prophylaxis (SUP) in the MICU . . . 97
Conclusion . . . 99
References . . . 100

7 Infection Prevention in the Surgical ICU . . . 105
Chelsea Guy-Frank, Ryan Rihani, and Lillian S. Kao
Introduction . . . 105
Overview of Prevention Strategies . . . 106
General Hygiene and Bathing . . . 106
Oral Hygiene and Care . . . 106
Glycemic Control . . . 107
General . . . 107
Burn . . . 108
Nutritional Optimization . . . 108
General . . . 108
Burn . . . 109
Antimicrobial Prophylaxis . . . 109
General . . . 109
Trauma . . . 110
Burn . . . 110
Antifungal Prophylaxis . . . 111
Avoiding Deconditioning: Mobilization and Respiratory Training . . . 111
MRSA Screening and Decolonization . . . 112
Prevention Strategies for Specific Surgical Infections . . . 112
Surgical Site Infections . . . 112
Hospital-Associated Pneumonia (HAP) and Ventilator-Associated Pneumonia (VAP) . . . 114
Infections Due to Skin and Pressure Injuries . . . 115
Line and Tube-Related Infections . . . 117
Conclusion . . . 119
References . . . 119

8 Infection Control in Neonatal and Pediatric Intensive Care Units . . . 125
David McMann, Peter Scully, and Chiamaka Aneji
Central Line-Associated Bloodstream Infections . . . 125
Catheter-Associated Urinary Tract infections . . . 126
Multidrug-Resistant Organisms . . . 127
MRSA . . . 127
VRE . . . 128
MDR-GNB . . . 129

Ventilator-Associated Pneumonias and Ventilator-Associated Events 129
Hospital-Acquired Respiratory Infections 130
Healthcare-Associated Diarrheal Infections 131
Clostridioides difficile 132
Rotavirus 132
The Cardiovascular ICU (CVICU) 133
References 134

9 Infection Control in the Immunocompromised Host 141
Febres-Aldana Anthony and Al Mohajer Mayar
Introduction 141
Standard Precautions and the Protective Environment 143
Standard Precautions 143
The Protective Environment 144
The Oncologic Patient and Recipients of Cellular Therapies 146
Bloodstream Infections in HCT Recipients 146
Other HAI in HCT Recipients and Neutropenic Patients 148
Fungal Etiologies of HAI in HCT Recipients 148
Viral Reactivations in HCT Recipients 148
Chimeric Antigen Receptor T-Cell Therapy Recipients 149
Antimicrobial Prophylaxis Regimens 149
Prevention of Hospital-Acquired Infections in the Oncologic Patient and the Recipient of Cellular Therapies 150
Solid Organ Transplant Recipients 150
Microbiology of Hospital-Acquired Infections in the Solid Organ Transplant Recipient 151
Distribution of HAI According to the Transplanted Organ 151
Viral Reactivations and In-Hospital Transmission in SOT Recipients 152
Antimicrobial Prophylaxis 152
Prevention of Hospital-Acquired Infections in the Solid Organ Transplant Recipient 153
MDRO Decolonization Protocols 153
Other Hospital-Acquired Infections 155
Tuberculosis 155
Invasive Mold Infections 156
Pneumocystis jirovecii 156
Legionellae 157
Clostridioides difficile 157
Viral Respiratory Infections 158
Coronavirus Disease 2019 159
Conclusion 160
References 160

10 Preventing Fungal Infections in the ICU Setting . . . 169
Dallas J. Smith, Janet Glowicz, Meghan Lyman, Jeremy A. W. Gold, and Tom Chiller
Introduction . . . 169
Candidiasis . . . 170
Epidemiology of Healthcare-Associated Candidiasis . . . 170
Pathogenesis of *Candida* spp. . . . 171
Emerging Infections . . . 171
Prevention of Invasive Candidiasis . . . 172
Healthcare-Associated Invasive Mold Infections . . . 174
Epidemiology of Healthcare-Associated Aspergillosis . . . 174
Epidemiology of Healthcare-Associated Mucormycosis . . . 175
Prevention of Healthcare-Associated Invasive Mold Infections . . . 176
Prevention of Healthcare-Associated Mucormycosis . . . 177
Conclusion . . . 178
References . . . 178

11 Healthcare-Associated Infections Outbreak Detection in the ICU Setting . . . 181
Alicia Lopez-Romo and Estefania Sienra-Iracheta
Introduction . . . 181
Economic Burden of an Outbreak . . . 182
Outbreak Mechanisms and Source of Transmission . . . 182
Direct and Indirect Contact . . . 183
Environmental Surface Contamination . . . 184
Water Contamination . . . 184
Droplet and Airborne Spread . . . 184
Evaluation of the ICU Outbreaks . . . 184
Epidemiological Surveillance and Analysis Tools . . . 187
Laboratory Tools . . . 188
Pseudo-Outbreaks . . . 190
Infection Control and Prevention Strategies . . . 190
Improve Hand Hygiene Compliance . . . 190
Active Patient and Environmental Screening . . . 191
Isolation . . . 191
Cleaning and Disinfection of Environment and Devices . . . 192
Closing ICU . . . 192
Specific Pathogen ICU Outbreaks . . . 192
Clostridiodes difficile . . . 192
Acinetobacter baumannii . . . 193
Carbapenem-Resistant Enterobacteriaceae (CRE) . . . 193
Fungal Infections . . . 194
SARS-CoV-2 . . . 194
Norovirus . . . 195
Conclusions . . . 197
References . . . 198

Index . . . 201

Chapter 1
Introduction to Infection Prevention in the ICU Setting

Misti Ellsworth and Luis Ostrosky-Zeichner

Introduction

Hospitals are supposed to be places of healing, where patients can receive the best possible medical care in a clean and safe environment. However, despite the best efforts of healthcare professionals, hospitals can also be breeding grounds for dangerous infections that are acquired during the course of treatment. These infections, known as hospital-acquired infections (HAIs), are a serious problem that affects millions of patients around the world every year. HAIs are caused by a variety of microorganisms, including bacteria, viruses, and fungi. They can range from mild infections to life-threatening illnesses such as bloodstream infections, pneumonia, and sepsis. HAIs not only prolong hospital stays and increase healthcare costs but also cause significant morbidity and mortality. The National Healthcare Safety Network (NHSN) system reports that approximately 1 in every 31 hospitalized patients develop at least one hospital-acquired infection. Deaths associated with these infections are estimated to be up to 99,000 per year [1]. In 2015 alone, there were an estimated 687,000 HAIs linked to the acute care hospital setting [1]. According to the WHO, in high-income countries, 30% of these infections occur in the Intensive Care Unit (ICU) [2]. ICUs have infection prevention and control protocols in place, such as hand hygiene, isolation precautions, and environmental cleaning. However, these measures can be challenging to implement and maintain

M. Ellsworth (✉)
Division of Pediatric Infectious Diseases, McGovern Medical School at UTHealth Houston, Houston, TX, USA
e-mail: Misti.Ellsworth@uth.tmc.edu

L. Ostrosky-Zeichner
Division of Infectious Diseases, McGovern Medical School at UTHealth Houston, Houston, TX, USA
e-mail: luis.ostrosky-zeichner@uth.tmc.edu

M. Ellsworth, L. Ostrosky-Zeichner (eds.), *Infection Prevention in the Intensive Care Setting*, https://doi.org/10.1007/978-3-031-67062-6_1

in the fast-paced and often chaotic environment of the ICU. Patients in the ICU often have multiple risk factors that increase the risk of developing a HAI. These risk factors include the need for indwelling catheters and other medical devices, patient-related factors such as underlying comorbidities, immunosuppression, and the need for recurrent hospitalizations [3].

Medical devices play a crucial role in the treatment of critically ill patients in the ICU. However, the use of medical devices also carries the risk of device-associated infections. These infections can occur when microorganisms colonize the surface of a medical device and form a biofilm, which can then lead to an infection in the patient. The three most common infections acquired in the ICU include bloodstream infections (BSI), pneumonia, and urinary tract infections (UTIs). These infections are often linked to medical devices with 83% of pneumonias occurring in ventilated patients, 97% of UTIs occurring in catheterized patients, and 87% of BSIs occurring in patients with central line [4]. Preventing device-associated infections in the ICU requires a multi-faceted approach that includes proper insertion and maintenance of medical devices, regular monitoring for signs of infection, and prompt removal once no longer required. However, the implementation of these measures can be challenging, and healthcare workers in the ICU may face competing priorities and time constraints.

Nosocomial infections lead to significant morbidity and mortality. Patients in the ICU are already critically ill and vulnerable to infections, and the additional burden of an HAI can further complicate their condition and delay their recovery. Vincent et al. found that patients who develop infections in the ICU have double the mortality and morbidity when compared to noninfected patients [5]. In addition to the increased morbidity and mortality, cost of care and length of stay is also significantly higher [6]. HAIs in the ICU can also have an impact on healthcare workers and the healthcare system as a whole. They can lead to increased use of resources, such as isolation rooms and personal protective equipment, and can increase the workload and stress on healthcare workers. In addition, the spread of HAIs can also increase the risk of transmission to other patients in the ICU and beyond. Despite widespread adoption of infection prevention practices in the ICU setting, preventable infections still occur daily in ICUs across the country. The purpose of this book will be to present the current recommendations for infection prevention in the ICU including the basics of infection prevention, prevention of the most commonly acquired device associated with nosocomial infections, fungal infections, and how to identify unit HAI outbreaks. In addition, we will address unique aspects of infection prevention in special populations such as neonates, pediatric patients, and immunocompromised hosts, as well as explore unique infection risks in trauma, surgical, and burn units. By increasing awareness and understanding of this critical issue, we hope to contribute to the development of effective solutions that will reduce the incidence of HAIs in the ICU and improve patient outcomes.

References

1. https://www.cdc.gov/hai/data/index.html.
2. https://www.who.int/gpsc/country_work/gpsc_ccisc_fact_sheet_en.pdf.

3. Osman MF, Askari R. Infection control in the intensive care unit. Surg Clin North Am. 2014;94(6):1175–94. https://doi.org/10.1016/j.suc.2014.08.011. Epub 2014 Oct 30.
4. Richards MJ, Edwards JR, Culver DH, Gaynes RP. Nosocomial infections in combined medical-surgical intensive care units in the United States. Infect Control Hosp Epidemiol. 2000;21(8):510–5. https://doi.org/10.1086/501795.
5. Vincent JL, Rello J, Marshall J, Silva E, Anzueto A, Martin CD, Moreno R, Lipman J, Gomersall C, Sakr Y, Reinhart K, EPIC II Group of Investigators. International study of the prevalence and outcomes of infection in intensive care units. JAMA. 2009;302(21):2323–9. https://doi.org/10.1001/jama.2009.1754.
6. Warren DK, Quadir WW, Hollenbeak CS, Elward AM, Cox MJ, Fraser VJ. Attributable cost of catheter-associated bloodstream infections among intensive care patients in a nonteaching hospital. Crit Care Med. 2006;34(8):2084–9. https://doi.org/10.1097/01.CCM.0000227648.15804.2D.

Chapter 2
Device-Associated Infections

Jose A. Cadena

Device-Associated Infections, Background, and Epidemiology

Since the 1950, there has been a growing concern regarding the emergence of healthcare-associated infections (HAI), at least in part due to the "staphylococcal pandemic" of the 1950s and 1960s. In 1958, the American Hospital Association's Advisory Committee on Infections within Hospitals recommended hospitals to do surveillance for HAI [1, 2]. Subsequent studies in Boston, and the CDC established the Comprehensive Hospital Infection Project (CHIP), implementing standardized surveillance in eight hospitals and finding that patients with some device-associated infections and bacteremia had higher mortality than those without bacteremia [2]. In 1974, the CDC engaged on a project (Study on the Efficacy of Nosocomial Infection Control–SENIC Project) to evaluate infection control practices in US hospitals, including the effect of surveillance and infection control interventions on HAI [3].

Device-associated infections are some of the most important sources of morbidity despite the fact that a significant proportion of these HAI are preventable [2]. The degree to which they are preventable has changed over time, given potential improvement on the science behind preventive measures and implementation methods (i.e., through evidence-based interventions and bundles) [4].

Early reports from the SENIC project estimated that when a HAI surveillance and control program was implemented, about 31% of healthcare-associated urinary tract infections (most were catheter-associated urinary tract infections—CAUTI), and about 35% of nosocomial bacteremia were preventable [1]. Subsequent analysis

J. A. Cadena (✉)
South Texas Veterans Healthcare System, San Antonio, TX, USA

University of Texas Health San Antonio, San Antonio, TX, USA
e-mail: cadenazuluag@uthscsa.edu

M. Ellsworth, L. Ostrosky-Zeichner (eds.), *Infection Prevention in the Intensive Care Setting*, https://doi.org/10.1007/978-3-031-67062-6_2

aggregating the effectiveness of multi-modal interventions in studies published between 1990 and 2002 to decrease the rate of central line-associated bloodstream infections (CLABSI) among critically ill patients was 56%, and there was also a more modest but significant effect decreasing ventilator-associated pneumonia (VAP) [5]. This was confirmed by a meta-analysis performed by Schreiber et al. which reviewed the effect of multifaceted interventions to prevent CLABSI, CAUTI, VAP in studies published between 2005 and 2016 [4]. They found that multifaceted interventions were effective in decreasing CAUTI (IRR of 0.543—95% CI, 0.445–0.662), CLABSI (IRR 0.459—95% CI, 0.381–0.554), and VAP (IRR 0.553—95% CI, 0.465–0.657) [4].

Device-associated infections are a common cause of morbidity and mortality in the US. The CDC performed a survey including 11,282 patients from 183 hospitals and found that about 4% had a HAI. Device-associated infections accounted for 25.6% of those infections. They estimated that in the year 2011, there were 35,600 CAUTIS, 15,600 CLABSI, and 49,900 VAP [6].

The burden of device-associated infections is felt at many institutions throughout the world. A report that included device-associated HAI from a diverse group of 523 ICU in 42 countries from January 1, 2012 to December 31, 2017 found that the rates of device-associated infections were higher in facilities outside the US when compared with NHSN rates (i.e., the rate of CLABSI in the medical ICUs was 4.47 per 1000 catheter days in the cohort vs. 1.1 per 1000 catheter days in the US; the VAP rate was 12.7 per 1000 device days vs. 0.9 device days in the US; CAUTI was 4.4 per 1000 catheter days vs. 2 in the US). Findings were similar for medical/surgical ICUs, pediatric, and other types of ICU [7].

Currently, most hospitals in the US report device-associated infections to the CDC through the National Healthcare Safety Network (NHSN). This is an internet-based system that allows facilities to track HAI, adherence to practices to prevent HAI, and compare them to other US facilities [8]. Data is usually collected by a local trained infection preventionist through patient-based, prospective surveillance and uploaded to the site [8].

Initially, the reporting was commonly standardized as cases per 1000 device days. More recently the CDC implemented the Standardized Infection Ratio (SIR), which is useful to track HAI. The SIR compares the number of HAI at an individual facility with the expected number of HAI, adjusted by several risk factors that are significantly associated with infection incidence. A SIR >1 means there is a higher number of infections than expected and a SIR <1 means there is a lower number of infections that expected [8]. Similarly, since most preventive bundles recommend decreasing the device utilization, the CDC provides a Standardized Utilization Ratio (SUR) that compares the actual number of device days with what would be predicted when adjusted by factors associated with device utilization [8].

During the year 2019, there was a decrease in the number of CLABSI (7%) with a 3% decline in device utilization, CAUTI (8%) with a 7% decline in utilization, and there was a modest increase in the rate of VAE of 2%, with a 3% increment in the rate of device utilization. Of note, in 2019, 51 states showed improvement in two or more HAI compared with 2015. Among acute care hospitals, there was a significant number of states that performed better in device-associated infections than compared with 2015 in CLABSIs (48 states), CAUTIs (42 states), and VAEs (14 states) [9].

In December 2019, the cases of pneumonia of unknown cause were reported in Wuhan, China. They were initially linked to the Huanan seafood market and shared some clinical features with Sars-CoV-1 [10]. The number of cases continued to grow through the month and the potential cluster was reported to the World Health Organization (WHO). In January 2020, a novel coronavirus was identified as a novel coronavirus, later called SARS-CoV-2 and started spreading outside China, and later a pandemic was declared [11]. As the pandemic progressed, it became a serious challenge to the public health establishment, healthcare systems, and infection prevention programs in the US. Significant resources from infection control programs were redirected to the pandemic response, testing capacity was limited, and there was a significant shortage in personal protective equipment and personnel. In addition, non-conventional care sites were implemented, and potentially less trained personnel had to participate in patient care, especially during COVID-19 surges [12, 13].

The effects of the pandemic on HAI and device-associated infections were profound. It put a significant burden on healthcare settings and altered practices. Before the pandemic, from 2015 to 2019, there were significant improvement in the SIR for CLABSI and CAUTI in the US, with a relatively stable rate of VAE. Weiner-Lastinger et al. performed a comparison of SIR for CLABSI, CAUTI, and VAE between 2019 and 2020, comparing quarters in 2019 with the same quarter in 2020. For CLABSI, they found that there was a drop in CLABSI in Q1 2020, followed by a significant increase in Q3 and Q4, when the SARS-CoV-2 cases increased in the US. In Q3, there was a 53% increment in the number of cases compared to 2019. The increment in CLABSI SIR was more pronounced in certain states such as Arizona (149% higher than 2019 in Q2) and Massachusetts (doubled) Louisiana and Michigan (both had significant CLABSI SIR increments >70%). Other states that did not have significant increments in CLABSI SIR reported a significant drop in the number of reporting institutions (i.e., New York had a 40% decrease in reporting hospitals in Q2 2020 compared to Q2 2021) [14]. The CAUTI SIR increased through 2020 and compared to similar quarters of 2019 (i.e., there was an increment in Q4 2020 compared to Q4 2019 of about 19%, driven by a 36% increment in the number of infections). The SIR for VAE increased significantly in 2020 as well, with a SIR of 1.31 for Q2, 1.29 for Q3, and 1.39 for Q4 2020; the largest increment compared to similar quarters of 2019 was in Q4, with an estimated increment of 45% [14].

Device-Associated Infections: Specific Infections and Surveillance Definitions

CLABSI Overview, Cost, and Surveillance Definition

Central lines are necessary for the care of certain patients, in particular critically ill individuals, and those requiring infusions of medications that cannot be administered peripherally and can be used for hemodynamic monitoring. Catheter-related bloodstream infections are very common in the US, and it has been estimated that between 84,000 and 204,000 infections a year with an estimate of 25,000 preventable deaths and a cost of 21 billion dollars a year [15].

Catheter-related bloodstream infection (CRBSI) is utilized more as a clinical definition/diagnosis and central line-associated bloodstream infection (CLABSI) is utilized as a surveillance definition (CLABSI can lack clinical specificity for catheter infection so over the years it has been modified to exclude certain infections that may originate in other areas such as the GI tract of immunosuppressed patients, see below). A CRBSI is usually defined as bacteremia in a patient with symptoms of sepsis in with no other identifiable source in a patient with a CVC, and >15 CFU on the tip of the catheter of the same organism, simultaneous peripheral and CVC cultures with a quantitative ratio of $\geq 3 \times 1$ (CVC vs. peripheral) or time to positivity of 2 h of more faster from CVC culture than peripheral culture [15].

In general, the CDC defines CLABSI (laboratory-confirmed bloodstream infection, LCBSI 1) as a positive blood culture or an organism identified in blood to the genus or species level by non-culture based microbiologic testing, and the organism is not related to an infection at another site, with the exception of organisms included on the NHSN common commensal list. This must occur in the presence of a central venous catheter that has been present for at least 2 consecutive days (CVC, i.e., tunneled catheters, implanted catheters, non-tunneled, non-implanted catheter, and any umbilical catheter). Alternative, CLABSI can be diagnosed in a patient with a central line, fever ($T > 38$ °C) or hypotension or chills (in adults LCBI 2; or fever, hypothermia (<36.0 °C), apnea, or bradycardia in patients <1 year old LCBI 3) and an organism in the blood stream that is not related to an infection in another site, and is a commensal organism identified in two or more blood cultures (i.e., *Corynebacterium* spp., *Bacillus* spp. (non-*B. anthracis*, *Propionibacterium* spp., coagulase-negative staphylococci, *S. viridans*, Aerococcus, among others) [8].

Not all the bacteremias meeting CLABSI criteria originate in the central venous catheter. This is particularly important among patients with neutropenia or with injury to the mucous membranes like that seen among patients with bone marrow transplantation and graft vs. host disease. The CDC created a new category for these patients called Mucosal Barrier Injury Laboratory-Confirmed Bloodstream Infection (MBI-LCBI). If the origin is another site, it is considered a secondary bloodstream infection.

The MBI-LCBSI has to be caused by a defined NHSN MBI intestinal organism—see appendix A on Ref. 6—(among patients with LCBI 1) or by viridans Group Streptococcus and/or *Rothia* spp. alone (among patients with LCBI 2 or 3). In addition, they have to meet one of the following: is an allogeneic hematopoietic stem cell transplant recipient within the past year with grade II or IV gastrointestinal graft vs. host disease or ≥1-L diarrhea in a 24-h period (or ≥20 mL/kg in a 24-h period for patients <18 years of age); within 7 days of the positive blood specimen collection. Alternatively, they meet criteria if they are neutropenic with ANC or WBC <500 cells/mm^3 the day of blood collection, 3 days before or 3 days after (7 days window) [8].

CLABSI are preventable in most instances. This was illustrated by the Keystone ICU project. This was a collaborative cohort study to decrease CLABSI over an 18-month period that implemented a bundle of simple and inexpensive measures to decrease CLABSI in several US hospitals, mostly located in Michigan [16]. A group of 103 hospitals provided data. They assigned a nurse and a physician champion at each site and implemented a daily goal sheet to improve communication, VAP prevention, and a unit-based safety program. Interventions to prevent CLABSI included hand washing, use of full barrier precautions during insertion, utilization of chlorhexidine-based skin preparation before insertion, avoiding femoral lines when possible, and removing unnecessary catheters. The median rate of CLABSI decreased from 2.7 (mean 7.7) per 1000 catheter days to 0 (mean 2.3) at 3 months, and it was sustained through 18 months [16].

CAUTI Overview and Definitions

Urinary tract infections are very common in US healthcare settings, accounting for an estimated 9.5–12.9% of HAI in acute care hospitals with an estimated number of 62,700 cases per year [8, 17]. CAUTI are very common in the critical care unit, accounting for 23% of HAI in the ICU [17]. Approximately, 12–16% of adult inpatients will have a urinary catheter during the hospitalization, and risk of CAUTI increases by 3–7% per day of catheterization. CAUTI can be associated with serious complications such as pyelonephritis, prostatitis, gram-negative bacteremia among others. It is estimated that more than 13,000 deaths associated with UTI occur in the US [8, 18].

A significant proportion of CAUTI is preventable (65–70%), and the Center for Medicare and Medicaid does not reimburse hospitals for the cost of CAUTI. The etiological agents of CAUTI are diverse, and most infections are caused by gram negatives, Enterobacteriaceae, and Pseudomonas. Many of these isolates are antimicrobial resistant, and the resistance has continued to increase through the years (for example, carbapenem resistance has been reported to be as high as 10% among Klebsiella isolates) [17].

Risk factors for CAUTI include prolonged catheterization (long-term catheterization defined as 1 month or more), lack of training from the inserter, catheter insertion outside the operating room and after the sixth day of admission, lack of aseptic technique/bundle compliance, female sex, age >50, severe underlying illness, diabetes mellitus, and elevated serum creatinine (>2 mg/dL) [17].

The CDC defines CAUTI as a symptomatic UTI on a patient who has had an indwelling urinary catheter in place for more than 2 consecutive days and was present for any portion of the day of the event, or removed the day of the event. In addition, the patient must have one or more of the following symptoms fever >38 °C, supra pubic tenderness, costovertebral angle pain, or tenderness (if the catheter was removed then urinary urgency, frequency, or dysuria, but they don't count if the catheter is still in place). The fever counts as part of the criteria regardless if there are other potential causes, but the costovertebral angle or supra pubic tenderness cannot have other identifiable cause. Finally, if the patient meets the time and symptoms criteria above, they must have a urine culture with ≤2 species of organisms, at least one of which is a bacterium of $\geq 10^5$ CFU/mL. Candida, yeast, mold, dimorphic fungi, or parasites are excluded from the CAUTI definition [8]. The CAUTI rate is usually presented as number of CAUTI cases divided by the number of catheter days and multiplied by 1000 (rate in cases per 1000 catheter days) [18].

The cost of CAUTI depends on the setting where it occurs. Hollenbeak et al. performed a systematic review of the cost of CAUTI between 2000 and 2017 and adjusted the costs by inflation to 2016 dollars. They found that costs were variable, between 875$ for inpatients from the perspective of the hospital costs (diagnostic tests and treatment) and 8.398$ for pediatric inpatients. From the perspective of insurers, the cost can be even higher, with Medicare costs of $1764 for non-ICU patients and $10,197 for ICU patients [19].

VAP and VAE Overview and Definitions

Ventilator-associated pneumonia (VAP) prevention has been an important aspect of infection prevention in the ICU for years. It has been estimated that about 300,000 patients receive mechanical ventilation a year in the US and mortality of acute lung injury is between 24% and 60%, higher with older age [8]. However, the diagnosis of VAP is not always easy, and previous surveillance definitions created by the CDC lacked interobserver reliability and reproducibility, it had multiple subjective criteria, was very complex and had limited correlation with mortality [20]. The criteria utilized were highly subjective (i.e., "changes in quality or quantity of sputum"), and multiple studies show a significant interobserver variability [20]. The previous

VAP definition required evaluation of chest films. Furthermore, the bundles utilized to prevent VAP were not associated necessarily with better patient outcomes [21]. Due to these limitations, in 2013, the CDC developed the surveillance concept of VAE (ventilator-associated event), based on objective criteria, but encompassing much more than the infectious complications of mechanical ventilation and VAP. The VAE is a surveillance concept (not a clinical diagnosis), its objective and reproducible, but may have multiple causes (besides VAP), VAE causes significant morbidity and may be associated with mortality, and previously utilized VAP prevention bundles may not be enough to prevent all VAE [20].

VAE can be caused by respiratory infection, pulmonary edema, ARDS, atelectasis, volume overload, pulmonary embolism, transfusion-associated acute lung injury, extrapulmonary infections, neurological events among many others [21]. In line with the multiple potential etiologies for VAE, precipitating or predisposing factors are diverse, including volume overload, need for renal replacement therapy, positive volume balance, transfusions, sedation, and use of paralytics (i.e., benzodiazepines and propofol), high tidal volume mechanical ventilation (increases with each mL above 6 mL/kg), mandatory modes of ventilation (this last two likely due to increased barotrauma), aspiration among others [21].

VAP has decreased over the past 20 years, but it is not clear how much the subjective nature of the definition contributed to this decrease. The morbidity, mortality, and cost of VAP are significant, with an estimated attributable mortality of 10%. VAP and VAE increased ICU and hospital length of stay, as well as duration of mechanical ventilation. Patients with VAE are at even higher risk of mortality than those with VAP [22].

VAE encompasses three different surveillance definitions including ventilator-associated condition (VAC), infection-related ventilator-associated complication (IVAC), and possible ventilator-associated pneumonia (PVAP) (see Table 2.1) [22].

VAC is defined as worsening of oxygenation after a period of stable or improving oxygenation during 2 calendar days. Worsening oxygenation is defined as one of the following: Increase in daily minimum FiO_2 of ≥ 0.20 over baseline, and sustained for ≥ 2 calendar days OR increase in daily minimum PEEP of ≥ 3 cmH_2O over the daily minimum PEEP over the baseline period. (Daily minimal PEEP/FiO_2 is defined by the lowest value during the first day of stable oxygenation, lasting for at least 1 h) [22].

If a patient with VAC has fever, leukopenia, or leukocytosis and requires systemic antimicrobials that are continued for 4 calendar days, they may meet IVAC criteria. If in addition, patients meet certain laboratory criteria, they are classified as having PVAP (see Table 2.1). It is important to note that these are only surveillance definitions, not clinical diagnosis [22].

Table 2.1 Summary of criteria to diagnose ventilator-associated event [22]

<table>
<tr><td colspan="3">Baseline period of stability or improvement on the ventilator, defined by ≥2 calendar days of stable or decreasing daily minimum FiO_2/PEEP values
Followed by:
Worsening oxygenation as defined by:
1. Increase in daily minimum FiO_2 of ≥0.20, during 2 or more calendar days OR
2. Increase in daily minimum PEEP values of ≥3 cmH_2O, during 2 or more calendar days</td><td>Ventilator-associated condition (VAC)</td></tr>
<tr><td colspan="3">During or after calendar day 3 of MV, within ±2 calendar days before or after worsening oxygenation, both of the following occur:
1. Temperature >38 °C or <36 °C, OR WBC ≥12,000 cells/mm^3 or ≤4000 cells/mm^3
AND
2. A qualifying new antimicrobial agent(s)[a] is started and is continued for ≥4 qualifying antimicrobial days</td><td>Infection-related ventilator-associated complication (IVAC)</td></tr>
<tr><td colspan="3">Meets one of the following criteria, without any excluded organisms[b]</td><td rowspan="2">Possible ventilator-associated pneumonia (PVAP)</td></tr>
<tr><td>Criterion 1:
Culture (+)
• ET aspirate, ≥10^5 CFU/mL[c]
• BAL, ≥10^4 CFU/mL[c]
• Lung tissue, ≥10^4 CFU/g[c]
• Protected specimen brush, ≥10^3 CFU/mL[c]</td><td>Criterion 2:
Purulent respiratory secretions[d]
AND
Organism isolated in culture (even if they don't meet criterion 1) from: Sputum, ET aspirate, BAL, lung tissue or protected specimen brush</td><td>Criterion 3:
One of the following positive tests:
• Organism identified from pleural fluid
• Lung histopathology, showing: abscess formation/foci of consolidation with intense neutrophil accumulation in bronchioles and alveoli OR evidence of lung parenchyma invasion by fungi OR evidence of infection with the viral pathogens based on of lung tissue (immunohistochemical stains, cytology, or microscopy)
• Positive test for Legionella spp.
• Test on respiratory secretions for respiratory viruses[e]</td></tr>
</table>

Adapted from NHSN Ventilator-Associated Event (VAE), January 2022 [22]
BAL bronchoalveolar lavage, *ET* endotracheal
[a] Systemic antimicrobials available on appendix "List of Antimicrobial Agents Eligible for IVAC, PVAP". Pages 10–26 and 10–27. Ventilator-associated Event (VAE) (cdc.gov)
[b] i.e., "Mixed or Normal respiratory/oral flora," "normal oral flora," "mixed respiratory flora," "mixed oral flora," or similar results indicating isolation of commensal flora; *Candida* spp. or yeast not specified; coagulase-negative *Staphylococcus* spp.; and any *Enterococcus* spp.
[c] Or corresponding semi-quantitative result
[d] Secretions from lungs, bronchi, or trachea containing ≥25 neutrophils and ≤10 squamous epithelial cells per low power field
[e] Influenza, respiratory syncytial virus, adenovirus, parainfluenza, rhinovirus, human metapneumovirus, coronavirus

Acknowledgements This material is the result of work supported with resources at the South Texas Veterans Health Care System. The contents do not represent the views of the U.S. Department of Veterans Affairs or the United States Government.

References

1. Haley RW, Culver DH, White JW, Morgan WM, Emori TG, Munn VP, et al. The efficacy of infection surveillance and control programs in preventing nosocomial infections in US hospitals. Am J Epidemiol. 1985;121(2):182–205.
2. Hughes JM. Nosocomial infection surveillance in the United States: historical perspective. Infect Control. 1987;8(11):450–3.
3. Haley RW, Quade D, Freeman HE, Bennett JV. Study on the efficacy of nosocomial infection control (SENIC project): summary of study design. Am J Epidemiol. 1980;111(5):472–85.
4. Schreiber PW, Sax H, Wolfensberger A, Clack L, Kuster SP, Swissnoso. The preventable proportion of healthcare-associated infections 2005–2016: systematic review and meta-analysis. Infect Control Hosp Epidemiol. 2018;39(11):1277–95.
5. Harbarth S, Sax H, Gastmeier P. The preventable proportion of nosocomial infections: an overview of published reports. J Hosp Infect. 2003;54(4):258–66; quiz 321.
6. Magill SS, Edwards JR, Bamberg W, Beldavs ZG, Dumyati G, Kainer MA, et al. Multistate point-prevalence survey of health care-associated infections. N Engl J Med. 2014;370(13):1198–208.
7. Rosenthal VD, Bat-Erdene I, Gupta D, Belkebir S, Rajhans P, Zand F, et al. International Nosocomial Infection Control Consortium (INICC) report, data summary of 45 countries for 2012–2017: device-associated module. Am J Infect Control. 2020;48(4):423–32.
8. Center for Disease Control and Prevention. Bloodstream infection event (Central line-associated bloodstream infection and non-central line associated bloodstream infection) [updated Jan 2024]. Available at: https://www.cdc.gov/nhsn/pdfs/pscmanual/4psc_clabscurrent.pdf. Accessed 8/9/24.
9. Center for Disease Control and Prevention. National and state healthcare-associated infections progress report. Center for Disease Control and Prevention; 2019.
10. Huang C, Wang Y, Li X, Ren L, Zhao J, Hu Y, et al. Clinical features of patients infected with 2019 novel coronavirus in Wuhan, China. Lancet. 2020;395(10223):497–506.
11. To KK, Sridhar S, Chiu KH, Hung DL, Li X, Hung IF, et al. Lessons learned 1 year after SARS-CoV-2 emergence leading to COVID-19 pandemic. Emerg Microbes Infect. 2021;10(1):507–35.
12. Henderson DK, Haessler S, Weber DJ. The coronavirus disease 2019 (COVID-19) pandemic—looking back and looking forward. Infect Control Hosp Epidemiol. 2021;42(10):1245–50.
13. Thompson CN, Baumgartner J, Pichardo C, Toro B, Li L, Arciuolo R, et al. COVID-19 outbreak—New York City, February 29–June 1, 2020. MMWR Morb Mortal Wkly Rep. 2020;69(46):1725–9.
14. Weiner-Lastinger LM, Pattabiraman V, Konnor RY, Patel PR, Wong E, Xu SY, et al. The impact of coronavirus disease 2019 (COVID-19) on healthcare-associated infections in 2020: a summary of data reported to the National Healthcare Safety Network. Infect Control Hosp Epidemiol. 2022;43(1):12–25.
15. Bell T, O'Grady NP. Prevention of central line-associated bloodstream infections. Infect Dis Clin N Am. 2017;31(3):551–9.
16. Pronovost P, Needham D, Berenholtz S, Sinopoli D, Chu H, Cosgrove S, et al. An intervention to decrease catheter-related bloodstream infections in the ICU. N Engl J Med. 2006;355(26):2725–32.
17. Shuman EK, Chenoweth CE. Urinary catheter-associated infections. Infect Dis Clin N Am. 2018;32(4):885–97.
18. CDC. Urinary tract infection (Catheter-associated urinary tract infection [CAUTI] and non-catheter-associated urinary tract infection [UTI]) events [Jan 2024]. Available at https://www.cdc.gov/nhsn/pdfs/pscmanual/7psccauticurrent.pdf. Accessed 8/9/2024.
19. Hollenbeak CS, Schilling AL. The attributable cost of catheter-associated urinary tract infections in the United States: a systematic review. Am J Infect Control. 2018;46(7):751–7.

20. Klompas M. Ventilator-associated events: what they are and what they are not. Respir Care. 2019;64(8):953–61.
21. Weinberger J, Cocoros N, Klompas M. Ventilator-associated events: epidemiology, risk factors, and prevention. Infect Dis Clin N Am. 2021;35(4):871–99.
22. Center for Disease Control and Prevention. Ventilator-associated event (VAE) [updated Jan 2024]. https://www.cdc.gov/nhsn/pdfs/pscmanual/10-vae_final.pdf. Accessed 8/9/24.

Chapter 3
Strategies to Prevent Central Line-Associated Bloodstream Infections (CLABSIs)

Gautam Sikka, Saad Farooq, Bela Patel, and Robier Aguillon Prada

Introduction

Central venous catheters (CVCs) are commonly used in health care settings globally. They are used for intravenous access in patients who require vasoactive or phlebosclerotic medications such as vasopressors, in patients with limited peripheral access, in patients who require dialysis or plasmapheresis and even to introduce Swan-Ganz catheters to monitor hemodynamics or to pass temporary pacemakers in high degree heart blocks [1]. Central line insertion is a commonly performed procedure, most often done at bedside using the Seldinger technique and using an ultrasound machine if available [2]. This technique is used for inserting a catheter into a vein or artery. It begins with the puncture of the target vessel using a sharp needle. Once the vessel is accessed, a thin, flexible guide wire is inserted through the needle and into the vessel, the needle is then removed, and the insertion site is enlarged with a dilator to accommodate the catheter. Finally, the catheter is threaded over the guidewire and the guidewire is removed. This technique is highly valued in medicine for its precision and reduced risk of complications compared to other methods of catheter insertion.

Currently, an estimated 27 million central lines are inserted annually in the world, whereas in the US alone, approximately 5 million are placed annually, accounting for 15 million central line days per annum [3]. There are several types of CVCs divided by the number and size of the lumen, length of the catheter, antimicrobial-impregnated catheters, tunneled and non-tunneled catheters, etc. They can be inserted for either short or long term and most often go into three large veins in the body, i.e., internal jugular, subclavian, or femoral on either side of the

G. Sikka (✉) · S. Farooq · B. Patel · R. A. Prada
University of Texas Health Science Center at Houston, Houston, TX, USA
e-mail: gautam.sikka@uth.tmc.edu; saad.farooq@uth.tmc.edu; bela.patel@uth.tmc.edu; robier.a.aguillonprada@uth.tmc.edu

M. Ellsworth, L. Ostrosky-Zeichner (eds.), *Infection Prevention in the Intensive Care Setting*, https://doi.org/10.1007/978-3-031-67062-6_3

body. Temporary venous catheters are often inserted for a duration of less than 2 weeks at a time, whereas long-term catheters are intended to be used for durations more than 6 weeks and include peripherally inserted central catheters (PICC line), tunneled central lines (often used for dialysis), and totally implanted ports (often used for chemotherapy) [4].

While there are several advantages to these lines; there are also several complications that may arise from the use of CVCs. Immediate complications include pneumothorax, vascular injury, misplacement, and air embolism, whereas long-term complications include thrombosis and blood stream infections. Central Line-Associated Bloodstream Infections (CLABSIs) have long been a significant concern in the healthcare industry, particularly in the intensive care unit (ICU) setting. The first awareness of CLABSIs emerged approximately 50 years ago when the Centers for Disease Control and Prevention (CDC) started collecting data on ICU-CLABSIs and established standards for their prevention nationwide. Over time, a paradigm shift occurred as clinicians and observers recognized that these infections were preventable, leading to a substantial reduction in CLABSI rates in the early 2000s compared to the 1990s [5, 6]. Today, every CLABSI is considered preventable, and healthcare institutions are committed to implementing strategies that foster patient safety and reduce the occurrence of CLABSIs. This evolution in healthcare practice is, in part, influenced by a system of incentives designed to encourage the adoption of effective preventative measures. Institutions may be rewarded with accolades, financial incentives, or superior quality ratings for successfully mitigating CLABSIs. Conversely, a framework of penalties is in place to underscore the criticality of safety adherence, with repercussions for non-compliance including diminished quality scores, or curtailed reimbursements from health insurance entities. Such mechanisms serve a dual purpose: they emphasize the paramount importance of rigorous safety protocols, and they motivate healthcare facilities to continuously strive toward exemplary patient care standards to avert the occurrence of CLABSIs. According to the CDC, in 2017 there were approximately 24,000 CLABSIs reported and this represented a 19% decline compared to 2015 [7]. Furthermore, between 2008 and 2016, there was roughly a 50% decrease in the rates of CLABSI in the US (Fig. 3.1) [8]. This represents an enormous collaborative multidisciplinary effort between different agencies, researchers, insurance companies, and hospitals [8]. Ongoing collaboration is pivotal for the continued decrease seen in CLABSI rates. This is evidenced by the fact that during the COVID-19 pandemic, mandatory reporting was halted according to an extraordinary circumstance exception policy and data collection resumed in 2021. The results were astonishing; among acute-care hospitals, there was an overall increase in health care-associated infection, including a 7% increase in CLABSIs. The largest increase was observed in ICUs at around 10%, thus proving that sustained efforts by all stakeholders are needed to continue the downward trend of CLABSIs [9].

CLABSIs are among the top three causes of nosocomial infections and often prolong hospital admissions by a mean of 7 days [10, 11].They are associated with increased mortality of up to 20% [11]. CLABSIs are not only detrimental to patient care and safety but also expensive for hospitals. One report estimated CLABSIs to

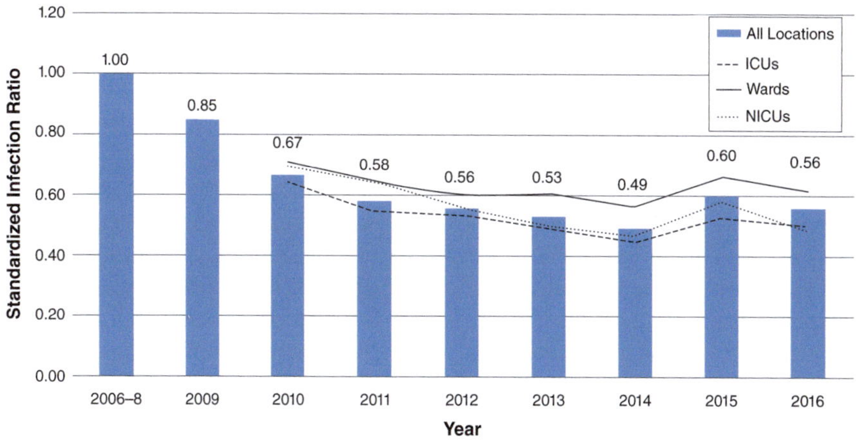

Fig. 3.1 Changes over time in CLABSI SIR in US hospitals using 2006–2008 baseline, NHSN 2006–2016

be the most costly health care-associated infection with a median cost of almost 46,000 dollars per infection [12], whereas a European study found the cost to increase by almost 7000 pounds [13]. It is therefore imperative that we continue to invest in strategies that help prevent CLABSIs, improve patient safety, and help conserve health care resources.

Risk Factors for CLABSIs

There are several risk factors that are associated with an increased risk of CLABSIs. These include immunodeficiency, either being a bone marrow transplant recipient, HIV infection, total parenteral nutrition (TPN) administration, previous blood stream infection, neutropenia, hematologic malignancies, extremes of age, BMI > 40, reduced nurse-to-patient ratio in the ICU, heavy microbial colonization at insertion site or catheter hub, multiple catheters, prolonged hospitalization before CVC insertion, loss of skin integrity, for example, in burn patients, and transfusion of blood in children [14–16].

Catheter-related factors such as type of catheter material, duration of insertion, site of insertion, and insertion conditions are also important for prevention of CLABSIs. Cuffed and tunneled catheters are associated with lower rates of blood stream infection compared to uncuffed and non-tunneled catheters. Central venous ports are also related to lower rates of infection compared with short-term CVCs. Multi-lumen catheters are more commonly associated with CLABSIs than single lumen catheters [17, 18].

Pathogenesis

It is important to understand the pathogenesis of CLABSIS to formulate strategies most effective for their prevention. Most commonly, the skin around the insertion site is the portal of entry. Microorganisms from the patient's skin or health care staff can enter through the wound and travel along the catheter to the fibrin sheath that surrounds the catheter. A biofilm develops around the catheter which helps pathogens to attach on to the catheter and evade host immune response. Microorganisms can then travel around the external site of the catheter to the distal tip and ultimately cause bloodstream infections. Furthermore, a distal infectious source can also colonize the CVC. In longer term catheters (more than 2 weeks), hub and intraluminal contamination is an important cause of bloodstream infections [10, 14].

Microbiology

Among data reported by the CDC, from 2011 to 2014, the most common cause of CLABSI in the US was coagulase negative staphylococcus (16.4%) followed by *Staphylococcus aureus* (13.2%), *Klebsiella pneumoniae/oxytoca* (8.4%), *Enterococcus faecalis* (8.4%), *Enterococcus faecium* (6.8%), *Candida albicans* (6%), *E. coli* (5.4%), *Enterobacter* (4.4%), *Pseudomonas aeruginosa* (4%), *Candida glabrata* (3.4%), etc. Fifteen pathogen groups accounted for 87% of reported pathogens. Interestingly, more than half of *Staphylococcus aureus* was resistant to methicillin (MRSA). More than 80% of *E. faecium* was resistant to vancomycin, whereas half of Acinetobacter was multi-drug resistant [19].

Of note, there are special populations such as burn patients, hemodialysis patients, and patients with hematological malignancies in which the epidemiology is different as compared to the general population. Among burn patients, for example, *Pseudomonas aeruginosa* is the most common cause of bloodstream infection [20].

History of CLABSI Prevention

1. Evolution of Awareness and Prevention Efforts: The history of CLABSI prevention is marked by the evolution of awareness and attitudes among healthcare professionals. First and foremost, it involves the recognition that CLABSIs are preventable harm and there are strategies that can be implemented to prevent their occurrence. The CDC began collecting data on CLABSI in the 1970s and then started publishing it which helped establish national benchmarks for comparison. The publication of the first guidelines for the prevention of intravascular catheter-related infections by the CDC in 1991 played a crucial role in initiating

preventive efforts [21]. However, it required a collective change in attitudes and implementation of evidence-based science can help reduce rates of CLABSI. Today, CLABSIs are considered avoidable but it has taken decades of hard work to change the perception and raise awareness among hospitals and clinicians.

2. Core Elements of Change: The transformation in CLABSI prevention can be attributed to several core elements, including:

   (a) Reliable and Valid Measurement Systems: The development of transparent and scalable measurement systems allowed healthcare facilities to collect and report performance data, thus facilitating targeted interventions. In a 1999 report "To err is human," a recommendation had been put forward to establish a nationwide reporting system about adverse events resulting in harm or death [22]. The CDC created this measure which helped hospitals track their rates of CLABSIs and compare themselves to other facilities. This holds health care systems and clinicians accountable, thus evidence-based strategies can be implemented to reduce CLABSI rates.
   (b) Adoption of Evidence-Based Care Practices: Embracing evidence-based care practices, such as catheter insertion best practices and infection prevention protocols, contributed to reducing CLABSIs. These evidence-based practices are constantly updated and all stakeholders including clinicians and hospitals should regularly review current data to ensure they are using best practices [23]. Most recent guidelines to reduce CLABSI rates are discussed further on in this article.
   (c) Investment in Implementation Sciences: Understanding the implementation science behind CLABSI prevention strategies allowed for their effective integration into healthcare practices. This was proven by the Michigan Collaborative and CDC collaborative which significantly reduced ICU infection rates [24, 25].
   (d) Creation of Peer Learning Communities: Establishing peer learning communities facilitates knowledge exchange and encourages continuous improvement.
   (e) Synchronous and Synergistic Collaboration: Collaborative efforts between researchers, clinicians, coordinators, and policymakers with shared goals and measures led to more effective CLABSI prevention initiatives [21].

3. Collaborative Efforts in CLABSI Prevention: The prevention of CLABSIs now falls under the umbrella of healthcare-associated infections, and various professional societies have played a critical role in formulating strategies for acute-care hospitals. Notably, a collaborative effort led by the Society for Healthcare Epidemiology of America (SHEA), the Infectious Diseases Society of America (IDSA), the Association for Professionals in Infection Control and Epidemiology (APIC), the American Hospital Association (AHA), and The Joint Commission (JC) all have been instrumental in driving CLABSI prevention efforts forward.

Must Dos

Guidelines for prevention of CLABSIs are updated every few years to reflect any advances made in infection prevention. The 2022 guidelines from Buetti et al. reflect a collaborative effort between several different health care agencies and offer a framework to help avoid CLABSIs [16].

1. Education and Competency Assessment: Healthcare providers involved in the insertion, care, and maintenance of central venous catheters (CVCs) must undergo education and competency assessments on CLABSI prevention protocols. This includes indications and risks of insertion, maintenance guidelines, infection prevention strategies, etc. This step ensures that all staff members are well-informed and adhere to best practices. Only trained and credentialed personnel should be involved in the insertion and care of CVCs. Periodic knowledge assessment and adherence to guidelines should be done to ensure compliance [26]. If available, simulations may be used to provide further education and training.
2. Daily Bathing with Chlorhexidine: Bathe ICU patients aged >2 months with a chlorhexidine preparation daily, as this has been shown to reduce the risk of CLABSIs [27–31]. In a randomized control trial, patients in the chlorhexidine intervention arm were significantly less likely to acquire a bloodstream infection than in the non-intervention arm (4.1 vs. 10.4/1000 patient days) [32]. The benefit of this practice remains unclear in non-ICU patients, and further studies are needed to see if it is beneficial in non-ICU patients as well.
3. Alcoholic Chlorhexidine Skin Preparation: Use an alcoholic chlorhexidine antiseptic for skin preparation before CVC insertion, as it has been shown to be effective in reducing infections [33–38]. This antiseptic should dry completely before puncturing the skin. In the CLEAN trial, chlorhexidine-alcohol was associated with lower risk of catheter-related infection compared to povidone-iodine alcohol solution (0.28 vs. 1.77 per 1000 catheter-days). Severe skin reactions were more common in chlorhexidine-alcohol group, thus povidone-iodine alcohol solution remains a viable options in such patients [36].
4. Chlorhexidine-Containing Dressings: In addition to being physical barriers, these dressings provide a continuous antimicrobial effect, maintaining a reduced risk of infection or colonization over time [39–47]. It reduces skin flora at the insertion site, which is a common source of pathogens causing CLABSIs.
5. Adherence to Infection Prevention Practices: Both ICU and non-ICU settings should have a process in place, such as a checklist, to ensure strict adherence to infection prevention practices during CVC insertion [48]. The checklist may serve several functions. The checklist ensures that all necessary procedural steps are consistently executed across different cases, thereby minimizing the likelihood of procedural discrepancies and potential errors. It encompasses critical measures founded on research and best practices, such as rigorous hand hygiene, the application of maximal sterile barriers, meticulous skin antisepsis, and the strategic selection of the catheter insertion site. Facilitation of Team

Communication: The checklist enhances communication among healthcare professionals. It provides a clear framework of the steps undertaken and those pending, ensuring a cohesive and coordinated approach to catheter insertion. The checklist serves as an educational resource for training new healthcare personnel and acts as a reminder for all staff about the criticality of infection control practices. It also fosters a sense of accountability, ensuring that each step in the process is diligently followed. Regular review and updating of the checklist, based on evolving evidence and institutional experiences, promote a culture of continuous improvement, driving advancements in patient safety and care quality.

6. Hand Hygiene: This remains the cornerstone for prevention of CLABSIs [49–54]. Healthcare providers must perform hand hygiene before catheter insertion or manipulation to prevent the introduction of pathogens into the bloodstream. This practice is pivotal due to its effectiveness in eradicating pathogens from the hands, thus significantly lowering the risk of pathogen transmission during catheter-related procedures. Acting as a crucial link breaker in the infection chain, hand hygiene is a straightforward yet profoundly impactful strategy. It is a practice backed by extensive research and endorsed by health authorities, such as the CDC and WHO, as a fundamental component of infection control. The simplicity of hand hygiene, coupled with its substantial efficacy, renders it an indispensable part of any infection prevention protocol, particularly in the context of averting CLABSIs.
7. Site Preference: In the ICU setting, the subclavian and internal jugular site is often preferred for CVC placement, as it reduces the risk of infectious complications. Many studies have revealed that subclavian and internal jugular catheter insertion were associated with the lowest risk of bloodstream infection, but did have a higher chance of mechanical complications such as pneumothorax when compared to femoral catheter insertion. On the other hand, femoral line insertion was associated with the highest risk of bloodstream infection; therefore, it should be avoided except in emergent cases [55–59].
8. Use of all-inclusive catheter cart kit containing all necessary supplies for CVC insertion in one cart streamlines the catheter insertion process, minimizing the chance of contamination that could occur when gathering items from multiple locations [16, 60].
9. Ultrasound Guidance for Catheter Insertion: Utilize ultrasound guidance during catheter insertion to improve accuracy and reduce insertion-related complications. Fewer attempts may mean less manipulation of the catheter and skin, which decreases the risk of introducing pathogens. It may reduce the risk of complications like hematoma or inadvertent arterial puncture, facilitate targeted insertion in patients with difficult venous access, and reduce the time and manipulation, thereby lowering the infection risk [61, 62].
10. Maximum Sterile Barrier Precautions: Use maximum sterile barrier precautions such as masks, cap, sterile gown, and gloves along with a full body drape on patients during CVC insertion should be used to create a sterile environment and minimize the risk of infection [63–68].

11. Nurse-to-Patient Ratio and Float Nurses: Hospitals should ensure an appropriate nurse-to-patient ratio in ICUs and limit the use of float nurses to maintain the quality of care and reduce the risk of errors [69, 70].
12. Dressing Change and Site Care: For non-tunneled CVCs in adults and children, change transparent dressings and perform site care with a chlorhexidine-based antiseptic at least every 7 days or immediately if the dressing is soiled, loose, or damp. Change gauze dressings every 2 days or earlier if the dressing is soiled, loose, or damp. In a study done at Emory, among pediatric patients undergoing hematopoietic cell transplant, a non-randomized parallel assignment trial to compare CLABSI rates in two groups was done; one arm received the parafilm over the CVC hub or around the CBC hub and the second arm contained the retrospective historic cohort receiving hematopoietic cell treatment. The published results demonstrated that application of parafilm as a protective CVC barrier was feasible and suggested it could reduce CLABSI rates from 4.37 per 1000 lines placed to 3.69 per 1000 lines placed. Subgroup analysis from this study is still expected [71].
13. Disinfection of Catheter Hubs and Connectors: Disinfecting catheter hubs, needleless connectors, and injection ports before accessing the catheter prevents contamination. Moreover, disinfection removes or kills pathogens that may accumulate on these components and within the grooves, which can be a significant source of infection [72–76].
14. Removal of Nonessential Catheters: Promptly remove nonessential catheters to minimize the risk of infection associated with their prolonged use. One recent study found that both the CLABSI incidence and multi drug-resistant organism blood stream infection increased as the number of days of catheter duration increased [77].
15. Routine Replacement of Administration Sets: Routine replacement of administration sets not used for blood, blood products, or lipid formulations can be performed at intervals up to 7 days to maintain catheter patency and reduce infection risk [16].
16. Surveillance for CLABSI: Regularly performing surveillance for CLABSI in both ICU and non-ICU settings helps identify any potential outbreaks or clusters [78–80]. It also allows for the comparison of infection rates across different units or institutions, facilitating the sharing of best practices, and promotes accountability.
17. Evidence-Based List of CVC Indications: Provide easy access to an evidence-based list of indications for CVC use to minimize unnecessary CVC placement, which can be a risk factor for CLABSIs.
18. It is recommended to utilize a CVC with the fewest number of lumens or ports necessary for the patient's treatment. This practice is guided by evidence indicating that each additional lumen increases the risk of CLABSI. By minimizing the number of ports, providers can reduce potential infection entry points and simplify the line management, thereby decreasing the patient's infection risk [26].

19. Routine assessment of a catheter insertion site through palpation for tenderness, while an important aspect of catheter care, does not directly contribute to the reduction of CLABSI incidence. Nevertheless, regular monitoring of the catheter site, including checking for tenderness, remains a vital component of comprehensive catheter management. This practice aids in early detection of potential complications like local infections or thrombophlebitis, which, if left unaddressed, could escalate into bloodstream infections. Therefore, while palpation of the insertion site is not a primary measure for CLABSI prevention, it is an integral part of the overall strategy for maintaining catheter integrity and preventing complications that could lead to bloodstream infections.
20. Emergently inserted central line catheters (crash lines) should be removed as soon as possible, ideally within 24–48 h.

Should Dos

1. Use of Antiseptic- or Antimicrobial-Impregnated CVCs: Consider using antiseptic- or antimicrobial-impregnated CVCs to further reduce the risk of CLABSIs. This may be especially important in patients who are at high risk of CLABSIs or where sequelae of a CLABSI could be potentially catastrophic, for example, in patients with recently implanted valves or grafts.
2. Antimicrobial Lock Therapy (ALT) for Long-Term CVCs: Consider implementing antimicrobial lock therapy for long-term CVCs to prevent infections and maintain catheter patency. In a meta-analysis of 23 studies, ALT led to a 69% reduction in CLABSI rates along with a 32% reduction in site infections although further prospective studies are needed to determine utility [81].
3. Utilization of Infusion or Vascular Access Teams: Create infusion or vascular access teams that specialize in catheter insertion and maintenance to reduce CLABSI rates. A randomized control trial done in 1998 found that catheters started and maintained by a dedicated IV team had less signs and symptoms of inflammation compared to catheters inserted and maintained by ward teams [82]. Further studies are needed to see if this difference translates to central lines as well.
4. Antimicrobial Ointments for Hemodialysis Catheter Insertion Sites: Use antimicrobial ointments for hemodialysis catheter insertion sites to prevent infections in patients undergoing hemodialysis.
5. Use of Antiseptic-Containing Hub/Connector Cap/Port Protector: Utilize an antiseptic-containing hub/connector cap/port protector to cover connectors and further minimize infection risk.

Don’ts

1. Avoid Routine Antimicrobial Prophylaxis: Do not use antimicrobial prophylaxis for short-term or tunneled catheter insertion or while catheters are in situ, as this may contribute to antimicrobial resistance.
2. Avoid Routine Catheter Replacement: Do not routinely replace CVCs or arterial catheters unless clinically indicated, as unnecessary catheter manipulation increases infection risk.

NOVEL Practices

This section highlights emerging strategies that have shown promise in CLABSI prevention but may require further research and validation. Some of these practices include:

- Routine use of needleless connectors as a CLABSI prevention strategy before an assessment of risks, benefits, and education regarding proper use.
- Surveillance of other types of catheters to assess their CLABSI risk is yet to demonstrate significance. Most current surveillance systems do not encompass peripheral arterial catheters, short-term peripheral venous catheters, and midline catheters, despite their association with the risk of bloodstream infections. To enhance the comprehensiveness and effectiveness of future surveillance, it may be advisable to include bloodstream infections related to these catheter types. Concerned systems may consider expanding their surveillance programs to cover all catheter types, which will provide a more accurate assessment of the scope of the issue and inform targeted infection prevention strategies [83, 84].
- The extensive application of chlorhexidine-based products, including chlorhexidine bathing, antisepsis, and dressings, may lead to decreased chlorhexidine susceptibility. However, the methods for testing chlorhexidine susceptibility lack standardization, leaving the clinical implications of reduced susceptibility largely undetermined [85].
- Sutureless securement methods to minimize complications related to catheter securement. A study by Yamamoto et al. suggested that sutureless securement devices such as StatLock had a quicker securement time and had significantly lower PICC line-related bloodstream infections [26].

Conundrum

This section outlines areas where the evidence or consensus on CLABSI prevention strategies remains unclear. Some of the practices include:

- Silver zeolite-impregnated umbilical catheters have been used, and in a randomized study, umbilical catheters treated with this antimicrobial agent were considered safe and effective for use in neonatal intensive care unit patients [86].
- The effectiveness of using an antiseptic-containing cap in comparison to manual disinfection for reducing the risk of CLABSI remains unclear.
- Routine pre-insertion hair removal. Data extrapolated for a Cochrane review of surgical site infections suggests that there is no evidence that routine preoperative hair removal reduces the risk of surgical site infections. It is unclear if this will apply to central lines as well [87].
- The adoption of sutureless methods for catheter securement can potentially help in reducing complications associated with catheter fixation including reduction in infection risk and potential needle stick injuries, however device failure can be a major problem especially in patients requiring early mobilization. In small studies conducted by Yamamoto et al. [88] and Karpanen et al. respectively, it was noted that sutureless securement devices, like StatLock, offer a faster method of securement and are associated with a significant reduction in line-related bloodstream infections as noted with PICC lines, and both methods were non inferior to each other comparing catheter migration and unplanned removal, there is conflicting data in post cardiac surgery patient suggesting tissue adhesive with simple polyurethane dressing without suture had a higher degree of jugular central venous device failure when compared to the cohort that additionally received sutures [89, 90].

Framework to Reduce CLABSIs in Health Care Settings

To effectively minimize CLABSIs, healthcare facilities must establish a robust infection prevention and control unit. This specialized team, equipped with appropriate resources, is crucial for educating staff involved in the insertion and upkeep of CVCs. Prompt and efficient laboratory support is essential for the timely collection and analysis of samples from patients suspected of having CLABSI. Additionally, information technology support plays a vital role in tracking CVC utilization by accurately calculating total CVC days.

Regular internal reporting is vital, encompassing hospital and nursing leadership, clinicians, and all relevant stakeholders. This reporting should focus on adherence to checklists, hand hygiene practices, daily patient assessments, and aseptic techniques in catheter handling, thereby identifying areas for improvement. External report to state and local health authorities is also crucial for setting benchmarks and ensuring greater accountability. Mandatory reporting requirements for CLABSI in some institutions necessitate the systematic collection and dissemination of data to the appropriate bodies.

To implement CLABSI prevention strategies effectively, the Plan, Do, Study, Act model, also called PDSA model can be employed. For instance, one study demonstrated how 14 interventions, executed through this model, reduced CLABSI rates from 4.2 to 1.8 per 1000 CVC days [91]. Another effective framework is the 4Es model (Engage, Educate, Execute, Evaluate), which aids in the implementation of recommended CLABSI prevention interventions and fosters continuous improvement.

Strategies to prevent CLABSIs have come a long way, driven by increased awareness, evidence-based practices, and collaborative efforts between healthcare professionals and organizations. By implementing essential practices, additional strategies, and staying vigilant about emerging research, healthcare institutions can continue to reduce CLABSI rates, ensuring better patient outcomes and improved overall patient safety in ICU and non-ICU settings while also decreasing healthcare resource utilization. Continued investment in research and implementation science will further enhance CLABSI prevention efforts, making these infections increasingly rare and preventable.

References

1. Leib AD, England BS, Kiel J. Central line. In: StatPearls. StatPearls Publishing; 2023. http://www.ncbi.nlm.nih.gov/books/NBK519511/. Accessed 27 Aug 2023.
2. Seldinger SI. Catheter replacement of the needle in percutaneous arteriography; a new technique. Acta Radiol. 1953;39(5):368–76. https://doi.org/10.3109/00016925309136722.
3. Mer M. Central venous catheter-related infection—back to basics. Afr J Thorac Crit Care Med. 2022;28(1) https://doi.org/10.7196/AJTCCM.2022.v28i1.244.
4. Moir D, Bodenham A. A narrative review of long-term central venous access devices for the intensivist. J Intensive Care Soc. 2018;19(3):236–46. https://doi.org/10.1177/1751143717741249.
5. Dudeck MA, Edwards JR, Allen-Bridson K, et al. National Healthcare Safety Network (NHSN) Report, Data Summary for 2013, device-associated module. Am J Infect Control. 2015;43(3):206–21. https://doi.org/10.1016/j.ajic.2014.11.014.
6. NNIS System. National Nosocomial Infections Surveillance (NNIS) System Report, Data Summary from January 1990–May 1999, issued June 1999. A report from the NNIS System. Am J Infect Control. 1999;27(6):520–32. https://doi.org/10.1016/s0196-6553(99)70031-3.
7. CDC. Current HAI progress report. HAI. CDC. 2022. https://www.cdc.gov/hai/data/portal/progress-report.html. Accessed 27 Aug 2023.
8. Data summary 2006–2016. HAI. CDC. 2019. https://www.cdc.gov/hai/data/archive/data-summary-assessing-progress.html. Accessed 13 Aug 2023.
9. 2021 National and State Healthcare-Associated Infections Progress Report.
10. Intravascular catheter-related infection: up date and overview. https://doi.org/10.10520/EJC63422.
11. Appendix 3. Guidelines to prevent central line-associated blood stream infections. https://www.ahrq.gov/hai/clabsi-tools/appendix-3.html. Accessed 28 Aug 2023.
12. Zimlichman E, Henderson D, Tamir O, et al. Health care-associated infections: a meta-analysis of costs and financial impact on the US health care system. JAMA Intern Med. 2013;173(22):2039–46. https://doi.org/10.1001/jamainternmed.2013.9763.
13. Tarricone R, Torbica A, Franzetti F, Rosenthal VD. Hospital costs of central line-associated bloodstream infections and cost-effectiveness of closed vs. open infusion containers. The case of Intensive Care Units in Italy. Cost Eff Resour Alloc. 2010;8(1):8. https://doi.org/10.1186/1478-7547-8-8.

14. Intravascular catheter-related infection: epidemiology, pathogenesis, and microbiology. UpToDate. https://www.uptodate.com/contents/intravascular-catheter-related-infection-epidemiology-pathogenesis-and-microbiology?search=clabsi&source=search_result&selectedTitle=5~90&usage_type=default&display_rank=5. Accessed 27 Aug 2023.
15. Tokars JI, Cookson ST, McArthur MA, Boyer CL, McGeer AJ, Jarvis WR. Prospective evaluation of risk factors for bloodstream infection in patients receiving home infusion therapy. Ann Intern Med. 1999;131(5):340–7. https://doi.org/10.7326/0003-4819-131-5-199909070-00004.
16. Buetti N, Marschall J, Drees M, et al. Strategies to prevent central line-associated bloodstream infections in acute-care hospitals: 2022 update. Infect Control Hosp Epidemiol. 2022;43(5):553–69. https://doi.org/10.1017/ice.2022.87.
17. Maki DG, Kluger DM, Crnich CJ. The risk of bloodstream infection in adults with different intravascular devices: a systematic review of 200 published prospective studies. Mayo Clin Proc. 2006;81(9):1159–71. https://doi.org/10.4065/81.9.1159.
18. Mollee P, Jones M, Stackelroth J, et al. Catheter-associated bloodstream infection incidence and risk factors in adults with cancer: a prospective cohort study. J Hosp Infect. 2011;78(1):26–30. https://doi.org/10.1016/j.jhin.2011.01.018.
19. Weiner LM, Webb AK, Limbago B, et al. Antimicrobial-resistant pathogens associated with healthcare-associated infections: summary of data reported to the National Healthcare Safety Network at the Centers for Disease Control and Prevention, 2011–2014. Infect Control Hosp Epidemiol. 2016;37(11):1288–301. https://doi.org/10.1017/ice.2016.174.
20. Brusselaers N, Monstrey S, Snoeij T, et al. Morbidity and mortality of bloodstream infections in patients with severe burn injury. Am J Crit Care. 2010;19(6):e81–7. https://doi.org/10.4037/ajcc2010341.
21. Pronovost PJ, Cleeman JI, Wright D, Srinivasan A. Fifteen years after To Err is Human: a success story to learn from. BMJ Qual Saf. 2016;25(6):396–9. https://doi.org/10.1136/bmjqs-2015-004720.
22. Institute of Medicine (US) Committee on Quality of Health Care in America. To err is human: building a safer health system. National Academies Press; 2000.
23. SHEA. New guidance for preventing healthcare-associated bloodstream infections. SHEA. https://shea-online.org/new-guidance-for-preventing-healthcare-associated-bloodstream-infections/. Accessed 13 Aug 2023.
24. Reduction in central line-associated bloodstream infections among patients in intensive care units—Pennsylvania, April 2001–March 2005. https://www.cdc.gov/mmwr/preview/mmwrhtml/mm5440a2.htm. Accessed 13 Aug 2023.
25. Bryan Sexton J, Berenholtz SM, Goeschel CA, et al. Assessing and improving safety climate in a large cohort of intensive care units. Crit Care Med. 2011;39(5):934. https://doi.org/10.1097/CCM.0b013e318206d26c.
26. O'Grady NP, Alexander M, Burns LA, et al. Guidelines for the prevention of intravascular catheter-related infections. Clin Infect Dis. 2011;52(9):e162–93. https://doi.org/10.1093/cid/cir257.
27. Noto MJ, Domenico HJ, Byrne DW, et al. Chlorhexidine bathing and healthcare-associated infections: a randomized clinical trial. JAMA. 2015;313(4):369–78. https://doi.org/10.1001/jama.2014.18400.
28. Zerr DM, Milstone AM, Dvorak CC, et al. Chlorhexidine gluconate bathing in children with cancer or those undergoing hematopoietic stem cell transplantation: a double-blinded randomized controlled trial from the Children's Oncology Group. Cancer. 2021;127(1):56–66. https://doi.org/10.1002/cncr.33271.
29. Milstone AM, Elward A, Song X, et al. Daily chlorhexidine bathing to reduce bacteremia in critically ill children: a multicenter, cluster-randomized, two-period crossover trial. Lancet. 2013;381(9872):1099–106. https://doi.org/10.1016/S0140-6736(12)61687-0.
30. Climo MW, Yokoe DS, Warren DK, et al. Daily chlorhexidine bathing-effect on healthcare-associated BSI and MDRO acquisition. N Engl J Med. 2013;368(6):533–42. https://doi.org/10.1056/NEJMoa1113849.

31. Afonso E, Blot K, Blot S. Prevention of hospital-acquired bloodstream infections through chlorhexidine gluconate-impregnated washcloth bathing in intensive care units: a systematic review and meta-analysis of randomised crossover trials. Eurosurveillance. 2016;21(46):30400. https://doi.org/10.2807/1560-7917.ES.2016.21.46.30400.
32. Bleasdale SC, Trick WE, Gonzalez IM, Lyles RD, Hayden MK, Weinstein RA. Effectiveness of chlorhexidine bathing to reduce catheter-associated bloodstream infections in medical intensive care unit patients. Arch Intern Med. 2007;167(19):2073–9. https://doi.org/10.1001/archinte.167.19.2073.
33. Masuyama T, Yasuda H, Sanui M, Lefor AK. Effect of skin antiseptic solutions on the incidence of catheter-related bloodstream infection: a systematic review and network meta-analysis. J Hosp Infect. 2021;110:156–64. https://doi.org/10.1016/j.jhin.2021.01.017.
34. Pages J, Hazera P, Mégarbane B, et al. Comparison of alcoholic chlorhexidine and povidone-iodine cutaneous antiseptics for the prevention of central venous catheter-related infection: a cohort and quasi-experimental multicenter study. Intensive Care Med. 2016;42(9):1418–26. https://doi.org/10.1007/s00134-016-4406-4.
35. Chaiyakunapruk N, Veenstra DL, Lipsky BA, Saint S. Chlorhexidine compared with povidone-iodine solution for vascular catheter-site care: a meta-analysis. Ann Intern Med. 2002;136(11):792–801. https://doi.org/10.7326/0003-4819-136-11-200206040-00007.
36. Mimoz O, Lucet JC, Kerforne T, et al. Skin antisepsis with chlorhexidine-alcohol versus povidone iodine-alcohol, with and without skin scrubbing, for prevention of intravascular-catheter-related infection (CLEAN): an open-label, multicentre, randomised, controlled, two-by-two factorial trial. Lancet. 2015;386(10008):2069–77. https://doi.org/10.1016/S0140-6736(15)00244-5.
37. Garland JS, Buck RK, Maloney P, et al. Comparison of 10% povidone-iodine and 0.5% chlorhexidine gluconate for the prevention of peripheral intravenous catheter colonization in neonates: a prospective trial. Pediatr Infect Dis J. 1995;14(6):510–6. https://doi.org/10.1097/00006454-199506000-00008.
38. Humar A, Ostromecki A, Direnfeld J, et al. Prospective randomized trial of 10% povidone-iodine versus 0.5% tincture of chlorhexidine as cutaneous antisepsis for prevention of central venous catheter infection. Clin Infect Dis. 2000;31(4):1001–7. https://doi.org/10.1086/318145.
39. Timsit JF, Mimoz O, Mourvillier B, et al. Randomized controlled trial of chlorhexidine dressing and highly adhesive dressing for preventing catheter-related infections in critically ill adults. Am J Respir Crit Care Med. 2012;186(12):1272–8. https://doi.org/10.1164/rccm.201206-1038OC.
40. Ullman AJ, Cooke ML, Mitchell M, et al. Dressing and securement for central venous access devices (CVADs): a Cochrane systematic review. Int J Nurs Stud. 2016;59:177–96. https://doi.org/10.1016/j.ijnurstu.2016.04.003.
41. Camins BC, Richmond AM, Dyer KL, et al. A crossover intervention trial evaluating the efficacy of a chlorhexidine-impregnated sponge (BIOPATCH®) to reduce catheter-related bloodstream infections in hemodialysis patients. Infect Control Hosp Epidemiol. 2010;31(11):1118–23. https://doi.org/10.1086/657075.
42. Ruschulte H, Franke M, Gastmeier P, et al. Prevention of central venous catheter related infections with chlorhexidine gluconate impregnated wound dressings: a randomized controlled trial. Ann Hematol. 2009;88(3):267–72. https://doi.org/10.1007/s00277-008-0568-7.
43. Levy I, Katz J, Solter E, et al. Chlorhexidine-impregnated dressing for prevention of colonization of central venous catheters in infants and children: a randomized controlled study. Pediatr Infect Dis J. 2005;24(8):676–9. https://doi.org/10.1097/01.inf.0000172934.98865.14.
44. Timsit JF, Schwebel C, Bouadma L, et al. Chlorhexidine-impregnated sponges and less frequent dressing changes for prevention of catheter-related infections in critically ill adults: a randomized controlled trial. JAMA. 2009;301(12):1231–41. https://doi.org/10.1001/jama.2009.376.
45. Ho KM, Litton E. Use of chlorhexidine-impregnated dressing to prevent vascular and epidural catheter colonization and infection: a meta-analysis. J Antimicrob Chemother. 2006;58(2):281–7. https://doi.org/10.1093/jac/dkl234.

46. Garland JS, Alex CP, Mueller CD, et al. A randomized trial comparing povidone-iodine to a chlorhexidine gluconate-impregnated dressing for prevention of central venous catheter infections in neonates. Pediatrics. 2001;107(6):1431–6. https://doi.org/10.1542/peds.107.6.1431.
47. Puig-Asensio M, Marra AR, Childs CA, Kukla ME, Perencevich EN, Schweizer ML. Effectiveness of chlorhexidine dressings to prevent catheter-related bloodstream infections. Does one size fit all? A systematic literature review and meta-analysis. Infect Control Hosp Epidemiol. 2020;41(12):1388–95. https://doi.org/10.1017/ice.2020.356.
48. Wichmann D, Belmar Campos CE, Ehrhardt S, et al. Efficacy of introducing a checklist to reduce central venous line associated bloodstream infections in the ICU caring for adult patients. BMC Infect Dis. 2018;18(1):267. https://doi.org/10.1186/s12879-018-3178-6.
49. Elgohari S, Wilson J, Saei A, Sheridan EA, Lamagni T. Impact of national policies on the microbial aetiology of surgical site infections in acute NHS hospitals in England: analysis of trends between 2000 and 2013 using multi-centre prospective cohort data. Epidemiol Infect. 2017;145(5):957–69. https://doi.org/10.1017/S0950268816003058.
50. Yilmaz G, Koksal I, Aydin K, Caylan R, Sucu N, Aksoy F. Risk factors of catheter-related bloodstream infections in parenteral nutrition catheterization. JPEN J Parenter Enteral Nutr. 2007;31(4):284–7. https://doi.org/10.1177/0148607107031004284.
51. Boyce JM, Pittet D, Healthcare Infection Control Practices Advisory Committee, HICPAC/SHEA/APIC/IDSA Hand Hygiene Task Force. Guideline for hand hygiene in health-care settings. Recommendations of the Healthcare Infection Control Practices Advisory Committee and the HICPAC/SHEA/APIC/IDSA Hand Hygiene Task Force Society for Healthcare Epidemiology of America/Association for Professionals in Infection Control/Infectious Diseases Society of America. MMWR Recomm Rep. 2002;51(RR-16):1–45, quiz CE1–4.
52. Rosenthal VD, Guzman S, Safdar N. Reduction in nosocomial infection with improved hand hygiene in intensive care units of a tertiary care hospital in Argentina. Am J Infect Control. 2005;33(7):392–7. https://doi.org/10.1016/j.ajic.2004.08.009.
53. Capretti MG, Sandri F, Tridapalli E, Galletti S, Petracci E, Faldella G. Impact of a standardized hand hygiene program on the incidence of nosocomial infection in very low birth weight infants. Am J Infect Control. 2008;36(6):430–5. https://doi.org/10.1016/j.ajic.2007.10.018.
54. van der Kooi T, Sax H, Pittet D, et al. Prevention of hospital infections by intervention and training (PROHIBIT): results of a pan-European cluster-randomized multicentre study to reduce central venous catheter-related bloodstream infections. Intensive Care Med. 2018;44(1):48–60. https://doi.org/10.1007/s00134-017-5007-6.
55. Timsit JF, Bouadma L, Mimoz O, et al. Jugular versus femoral short-term catheterization and risk of infection in intensive care unit patients. Causal analysis of two randomized trials. Am J Respir Crit Care Med. 2013;188(10):1232–9. https://doi.org/10.1164/rccm.201303-0460OC.
56. Parienti JJ. Catheter-related bloodstream infection in jugular versus subclavian central catheterization. Crit Care Med. 2017;45(7):e734–5. https://doi.org/10.1097/CCM.0000000000002400.
57. Arvaniti K, Lathyris D, Blot S, Apostolidou-Kiouti F, Koulenti D, Haidich AB. Cumulative evidence of randomized controlled and observational studies on catheter-related infection risk of central venous catheter insertion site in ICU patients: a pairwise and network meta-analysis. Crit Care Med. 2017;45(4):e437–48. https://doi.org/10.1097/CCM.0000000000002092.
58. Merrer J, De Jonghe B, Golliot F, et al. Complications of femoral and subclavian venous catheterization in critically ill patients: a randomized controlled trial. JAMA. 2001;286(6):700–7. https://doi.org/10.1001/jama.286.6.700.
59. Parienti JJ, Mongardon N, Mégarbane B, et al. Intravascular complications of central venous catheterization by insertion site. N Engl J Med. 2015;373(13):1220–9. https://doi.org/10.1056/NEJMoa1500964.
60. Berenholtz SM, Pronovost PJ, Lipsett PA, et al. Eliminating catheter-related bloodstream infections in the intensive care unit. Crit Care Med. 2004;32(10):2014–20. https://doi.org/10.1097/01.ccm.0000142399.70913.2f.
61. Brass P, Hellmich M, Kolodziej L, Schick G, Smith AF. Ultrasound guidance versus anatomical landmarks for internal jugular vein catheterization. Cochrane Database Syst Rev. 2015;2015(1):CD006962. https://doi.org/10.1002/14651858.CD006962.pub2.

62. Karakitsos D, Labropoulos N, De Groot E, et al. Real-time ultrasound-guided catheterisation of the internal jugular vein: a prospective comparison with the landmark technique in critical care patients. Crit Care. 2006;10(6):R162. https://doi.org/10.1186/cc5101.
63. Lee D-h, Jung KY, Choi YH. Use of maximal sterile barrier precautions and/or antimicrobial-coated catheters to reduce the risk of central venous catheter-related bloodstream infection. Infect Control Hosp Epidemiol. 2008;29(10):947–50. https://doi.org/10.1086/590356.
64. Central Line Associated Bacteraemia in NSW Intensive Care Units (CLAB ICU) Collaborative, Burrell AR, McLaws ML, et al. Aseptic insertion of central venous lines to reduce bacteraemia. Med J Aust. 2011;194(11):583–7. https://doi.org/10.5694/j.1326-5377.2011.tb03109.x.
65. Ishikawa Y, Kiyama T, Haga Y, et al. Maximal sterile barrier precautions do not reduce catheter-related bloodstream infections in general surgery units: a multi-institutional randomized controlled trial. Ann Surg. 2010;251(4):620–3. https://doi.org/10.1097/SLA.0b013e3181d48a6a.
66. Hu KK, Lipsky BA, Veenstra DL, Saint S. Using maximal sterile barriers to prevent central venous catheter-related infection: a systematic evidence-based review. Am J Infect Control. 2004;32(3):142–6. https://doi.org/10.1016/j.ajic.2003.10.006.
67. Raad II, Hohn DC, Gilbreath BJ, et al. Prevention of central venous catheter-related infections by using maximal sterile barrier precautions during insertion. Infect Control Hosp Epidemiol. 1994;15(4 Pt 1):231–8.
68. Mermel LA, McCormick RD, Springman SR, Maki DG. The pathogenesis and epidemiology of catheter-related infection with pulmonary artery Swan-Ganz catheters: a prospective study utilizing molecular subtyping. Am J Med. 1991;91(3B):197S–205S. https://doi.org/10.1016/0002-9343(91)90369-9.
69. Fridkin SK, Pear SM, Williamson TH, Galgiani JN, Jarvis WR. The role of understaffing in central venous catheter-associated bloodstream infections. Infect Control Hosp Epidemiol. 1996;17(3):150–8. https://doi.org/10.1086/647262.
70. Cimiotti JP, Haas J, Saiman L, Larson EL. Impact of staffing on bloodstream infections in the neonatal intensive care unit. Arch Pediatr Adolesc Med. 2006;160(8):832–6. https://doi.org/10.1001/archpedi.160.8.832.
71. Stenger EO, Newton JG, Leong T, et al. Application of parafilm as a physical barrier on CVC connections is feasible and may reduce Clabsi among pediatric HCT patients. Biol Blood Marrow Transplant. 2019;25(3):S131. https://doi.org/10.1016/j.bbmt.2018.12.416.
72. Salzman MB, Isenberg HD, Rubin LG. Use of disinfectants to reduce microbial contamination of hubs of vascular catheters. J Clin Microbiol. 1993;31(3):475–9.
73. Luebke MA, Arduino MJ, Duda DL, et al. Comparison of the microbial barrier properties of a needleless and a conventional needle-based intravenous access system. Am J Infect Control. 1998;26(4):437–41. https://doi.org/10.1016/s0196-6553(98)70042-2.
74. Casey AL, Worthington T, Lambert PA, Quinn D, Faroqui MH, Elliott TSJ. A randomized, prospective clinical trial to assess the potential infection risk associated with the PosiFlow needleless connector. J Hosp Infect. 2003;54(4):288–93. https://doi.org/10.1016/s0195-6701(03)00130-0.
75. Munoz-Price LS, Dezfulian C, Wyckoff M, et al. Effectiveness of stepwise interventions targeted to decrease central catheter-associated bloodstream infections. Crit Care Med. 2012;40(5):1464–9. https://doi.org/10.1097/CCM.0b013e31823e9f5b.
76. Soothill JS, Bravery K, Ho A, Macqueen S, Collins J, Lock P. A fall in bloodstream infections followed a change to 2% chlorhexidine in 70% isopropanol for catheter connection antisepsis: a pediatric single center before/after study on a hemopoietic stem cell transplant ward. Am J Infect Control. 2009;37(8):626–30. https://doi.org/10.1016/j.ajic.2009.03.014.
77. Pitiriga V, Bakalis J, Kampos E, Kanellopoulos P, Saroglou G, Tsakris A. Duration of central venous catheter placement and central line-associated bloodstream infections after the adoption of prevention bundles: a two-year retrospective study. Antimicrob Resist Infect Control. 2022;11(1):96. https://doi.org/10.1186/s13756-022-01131-w.

78. Marschall J, Leone C, Jones M, Nihill D, Fraser VJ, Warren DK. Catheter-associated bloodstream infections in general medical patients outside the intensive care unit: a surveillance study. Infect Control Hosp Epidemiol. 2007;28(8):905–9. https://doi.org/10.1086/519206.
79. Zingg W, Sax H, Inan C, et al. Hospital-wide surveillance of catheter-related bloodstream infection: from the expected to the unexpected. J Hosp Infect. 2009;73(1):41–6. https://doi.org/10.1016/j.jhin.2009.05.015.
80. Gastmeier P, Geffers C, Brandt C, et al. Effectiveness of a nationwide nosocomial infection surveillance system for reducing nosocomial infections. J Hosp Infect. 2006;64(1):16–22. https://doi.org/10.1016/j.jhin.2006.04.017.
81. Zacharioudakis IM, Zervou FN, Arvanitis M, Ziakas PD, Mermel LA, Mylonakis E. Antimicrobial lock solutions as a method to prevent central line-associated bloodstream infections: a meta-analysis of randomized controlled trials. Clin Infect Dis. 2014;59(12):1741–9. https://doi.org/10.1093/cid/ciu671.
82. Soifer NE, Borzak S, Edlin BR, Weinstein RA. Prevention of peripheral venous catheter complications with an intravenous therapy team: a randomized controlled trial. Arch Intern Med. 1998;158(5):473–7. https://doi.org/10.1001/archinte.158.5.473.
83. O'Horo JC, Maki DG, Krupp AE, Safdar N. Arterial catheters as a source of bloodstream infection: a systematic review and meta-analysis. Crit Care Med. 2014;42(6):1334–9. https://doi.org/10.1097/CCM.0000000000000166.
84. Mermel LA. Short-term peripheral venous catheter-related bloodstream infections: a systematic review. Clin Infect Dis. 2017;65(10):1757–62. https://doi.org/10.1093/cid/cix562.
85. Batra R, Cooper BS, Whiteley C, Patel AK, Wyncoll D, Edgeworth JD. Efficacy and limitation of a chlorhexidine-based decolonization strategy in preventing transmission of methicillin-resistant Staphylococcus aureus in an intensive care unit. Clin Infect Dis. 2010;50(2):210–7. https://doi.org/10.1086/648717.
86. Bertini G, Elia S, Ceciarini F, Dani C. Reduction of catheter-related bloodstream infections in preterm infants by the use of catheters with the AgION antimicrobial system. Early Hum Dev. 2013;89(1):21–5. https://doi.org/10.1016/j.earlhumdev.2012.07.003.
87. Tanner J, Woodings D, Moncaster K. Preoperative hair removal to reduce surgical site infection. Cochrane Database Syst Rev. 2006;(3):CD004122. https://doi.org/10.1002/14651858.CD004122.pub3.
88. https://pubmed.ncbi.nlm.nih.gov/11788698/.
89. Rickard CM, Edwards M, Spooner AJ, et al. A 4-arm randomized controlled pilot trial of innovative solutions for jugular central venous access device securement in 221 cardiac surgical patients. J Crit Care. 2016;36:35–42. https://doi.org/10.1016/j.jcrc.2016.06.006.
90. Karpanen TJ, Casey AL, Whitehouse T, et al. A clinical evaluation of two central venous catheter stabilization systems. Ann Intensive Care. 2019;9(1):49. https://doi.org/10.1186/s13613-019-0519-6.
91. Russell TA, Fritschel E, Do J, et al. Minimizing central line-associated bloodstream infections in a high-acuity liver transplant intensive care unit. Am J Infect Control. 2019;47(3):305–12. https://doi.org/10.1016/j.ajic.2018.08.006.

Chapter 4
Current and Emerging Practices for Preventing CAUTI in the ICU

Bilal Zafar and Mark T. Warner

Introduction

A urinary catheter is a carefully designed rubber tube which is placed into the bladder, either through the urethral externally or surgically directly through the abdominal wall and held in place by a balloon inflated with sterile saline connected to a drainage and collection bag. While the patient's experience with an external catheter with a drainage bag is not always comfortable or pleasant for the patient, urinary catheters are commonly used in healthcare facilities, generally well tolerated, and frequently used in the intensive care unit (ICU) for many reasons. They help drain urine from the bladder passively when the patients require bed rest continuously for critical illness and are not able to mobilize back and forth to the toilet to void. Urinary catheters also allow accurate measurement of urine production and even allow for invasive continuous body temperature measurement and rarely, measurement of intra-abdominal pressure. Utilization of urinary catheters helps clinicians guide therapies and monitor for complications by assessing urine production along with laboratory changes. Like many other medical devices, urinary catheters are also prone to complications which commonly include infection. Catheterization of the bladder with a rubber tube bypasses normal defenses present in the urethra and presents an ongoing risk of infection while present, and shortly after, use. Additional complications of urinary catheters include urethral irritation and/or trauma, hemorrhage, and complications of misplacement, which only serve to increase the possibility of infection and need for prolonged catheter dwell time or repeated placement.

Urinary catheters increase the risk of bacteriuria. Bacteriuria can be clinically benign as it may represent contamination by bacteria colonizing the periurethral

B. Zafar · M. T. Warner (✉)
Division of Critical Care, Department of Internal Medicine, McGovern Medical School at the University of Texas Health Science Center Houston, Houston, TX, USA
e-mail: bilal.zafar@uth.tmc.edu; mark.t.warner@uth.tmc.edu

M. Ellsworth, L. Ostrosky-Zeichner (eds.), *Infection Prevention in the Intensive Care Setting*, https://doi.org/10.1007/978-3-031-67062-6_4

area or present as a serious infection. The Infectious Diseases Society of America (IDSA) guidelines [1] define catheter-associated bacteriuria as follows:

- Symptomatic bacteriuria (urinary tract infection [UTI])—Culture growth of $\geq 10^3$ colony forming units (cfu)/mL of uropathogenic bacteria in the presence of symptoms or signs compatible with UTI without other identifiable source in a patient with indwelling urethral, indwelling suprapubic, or intermittent catheterization. Compatible symptoms include fever, suprapubic or costovertebral angle tenderness, and otherwise unexplained systemic symptoms such as altered mental status, hypotension, or evidence of a systemic inflammatory response syndrome or progression to sepsis.
- Asymptomatic bacteriuria—Culture growth of $\geq 10^5$ cfu/mL of uropathogenic bacteria in the absence of symptoms compatible with UTI in a patient with indwelling urethral, indwelling suprapubic, or intermittent catheterization.

Patients who are no longer catheterized but had a urinary catheter that was removed within the past 48 h are also considered to have catheter-associated UTI or asymptomatic bacteriuria if they meet these definitions.

Catheter-associated urinary tract infections (CAUTIs) pose a significant challenge in the intensive care unit setting. These infections can lead to increased patient morbidity, extended hospital stays, and additional healthcare costs. To address this issue, healthcare professionals have been continuously working on refining and adopting various strategies to prevent CAUTIs.

Incidence and Mortality Associated with CAUTI

CAUTIs are among the most common healthcare-associated infections, accounting for approximately 15–25% of all hospital-acquired infections. In the ICU, where patients are often critically ill and more susceptible to infections, the incidence of CAUTIs tends to be higher. Studies have shown that the risk of developing CAUTI increases with the duration of catheterization. Bacteriuria in patients with indwelling bladder catheters occurs at a rate of approximately 3–10% per day of catheterization. Of those with bacteriuria, 10–25% develop symptoms of urinary tract infection. CDC data reports that approximately 75% of UTIs in the hospital are associated with a urinary catheter. The consequences of CAUTIs extend beyond the immediate infection. Research indicates that patients who develop CAUTIs have longer hospital stays, leading to increased healthcare costs. Moreover, CAUTIs are associated with additional complications, such as bloodstream infections and sepsis, further exacerbating patient outcomes. Mortality rates among ICU patients with CAUTIs can range from 10% to 20%, emphasizing the severity of the issue [2, 3].

Practices for Preventing CAUTI in the ICU

Appropriate Indications for Urinary Catheterization

One of the fundamental steps in preventing CAUTIs is ensuring that urinary catheters are only used when necessary. Common indications for use of a urinary catheter include reasons for continuous bed rest, which include application of non-invasive or invasive mechanical ventilation, critical hemodynamic compromise or neurologic, orthopedic, cardiovascular, or other maladies that prevent mobilization and ambulation to the restroom. Patients may also have genitourinary or perineal wounds, infections, or structural abnormalities that require continued presence of a urinary catheter. Avoiding unnecessary catheterizations reduces the overall risk of infection. It is noted that some patients will have reasons for temporary or permanent urinary retention. Repeated placement of the urinary catheter following removal may be clinically indicated, but this should prompt additional discussion to ensure maintenance and infection prevention practices with this patient subpopulation are optimal, as it is observed that these patients are most susceptible to CAUTI development with repeated insertions.

Medical professionals should follow evidence-based guidelines to determine the appropriate indications for catheterization and assess the need for its continued use daily. Most hospital units have a standardized process to evaluate patients daily for progress in their care plan. We suggest that best practice in the ICU includes utilization of a checklist, bundle, or other standardized process to assess daily the need for continued use of the urinary catheter. This discussion should be multidisciplinary including nursing, allied health providers, and the physician team. When it is determined that the urinary catheter is no longer indicated, it should be removed promptly [4].

Aseptic Catheter Insertion and Maintenance

Proper insertion and maintenance techniques are crucial for preventing CAUTIs. Healthcare providers must adhere to strict aseptic procedures during catheter insertion to minimize the introduction of pathogens. Most often nurses insert urinary catheters and hospitals often develop a standardized approach where nurses are instructed and continually assessed, at least annually, for proper performance of this skill. This standard should be maintained regardless of the unit of insertion (including the emergency department or operating room) and regardless of whether the catheter is placed by a trained nurse or a physician, in cases where there are anatomical or other challenges to safe and sterile urinary catheter placement. Additionally, maintaining a closed drainage system and using sterile techniques during catheter maintenance can further reduce the risk of infection [5–8].

Regular Catheter Care and Hygiene

Frequent cleaning of the perineal area and the catheter insertion site, often daily, using mild soap and water or antibacterial wipes or similar processes are essential to prevent CAUTIs. Keeping the area clean helps prevent the migration of nearby bacteria residing on the surrounding skin into the urinary tract. This can be a challenging task for nursing when patients are immobile, sedated or critically ill and have prolonged immobility. Furthermore, ensuring that the catheter is positioned correctly and securely taped can prevent unnecessary movement and friction that could lead to infection.

Urinary Catheter Removal Protocols

Prompt removal of urinary catheters is crucial to prevent CAUTIs. ICU staff should establish protocols for assessing the ongoing need for catheterization and removing the catheter as soon as it is no longer required. Prolonged catheterization increases the risk of infection, and a proactive approach to removal can significantly reduce this risk. As stated above, many organizations have standardized daily processes for evaluation of continuing necessity and a shared decision for prompt removal. Many other processes are possible, including a nursing-driven discussion for removal or other protocols that prompt early removal discussions [9].

Alternative Methods of Urine Collection

In recent years, alternatives to indwelling urinary catheters have gained traction to prevent CAUTIs. External collection devices, such as condom catheters for male patients and periurethral collection systems for both male and female patients, offer options for urine collection without the need for invasive catheterization [10]. These alternatives may be considered based on patient suitability and medical requirements. Also, as patients improve from illness and become more mobile, strict measurement of hourly urine production can be obtained using urinal devices, bedside commodes, and other devices with measurement capability.

Antimicrobial Catheters and Coatings

Emerging technologies in catheter design include the use of antimicrobial materials and coatings. These innovations are aimed at reducing bacterial colonization on the catheter surface, thus lowering the risk of CAUTIs. While research is ongoing to assess their long-term effectiveness, these approaches hold promise in preventing infections associated with urinary catheters. Given the positioning of the urinary catheter through the urethral meatus, there will always be some movement of the catheter in the urethra with the possibility of infection from bacterial migration. Removal of urinary catheters will always be the most effective method of decreasing possibility of infection, but antimicrobial coating or impregnation brings promise for situations that require prolonged indwelling catheters and other situations where risk of infection can be minimized but not reduced to zero.

Education and Training

Proper education and training of healthcare staff play a pivotal role in CAUTI prevention. Keeping medical professionals updated on the latest guidelines, best practices, and emerging technologies empowers them to make informed decisions regarding catheter use, insertion, maintenance, and removal. Training in communication among the multidisciplinary team with use of checklists, bundles, and protocols can also be of value, most notably in creating a streamlined and repeatable process for urinary catheter insertion, maintenance, and speedy removal.

Surveillance and Data Analysis

Regular surveillance of CAUTI rates within the ICU helps identify trends, potential risk factors, and areas for improvement. The data can be helpful to note specific opportunities with individual staff members, patient populations or identify process issues at the unit or institution level. Active surveillance will also allow review of patient-level data to determine unique characteristics that increase the possibility of infection of urinary catheters. By analyzing data on infection rates, healthcare facilities can implement targeted interventions and monitor the impact of their prevention strategies. Daily reports and dashboards are options of visual data display that can be useful to bring awareness to the team and prompt discussion of urinary catheter necessity.

Hospital Management of CAUTIs

Effective management of CAUTIs requires a multidisciplinary approach that involves not only healthcare providers but also hospital administrators and quality improvement teams. Hospitals can implement infection prevention programs that focus on CAUTI reduction, including regular staff training, audit and feedback mechanisms, and real-time surveillance of infection rates. Collaborative efforts between clinicians, infection control practitioners, and hospital leadership can drive the adoption of evidence-based guidelines and best practices. Additionally, hospitals should establish clear protocols for addressing CAUTI cases, including timely diagnosis, appropriate antimicrobial treatment, and continuous monitoring of patient progress. Investing in advanced catheter technologies, such as antimicrobial-coated catheters, may also be a part of the hospital's strategy to reduce CAUTI rates. By fostering a culture of infection prevention and providing the necessary resources, hospitals can effectively manage CAUTIs and work toward the common goal of improving patient outcomes and safety.

Future Research and Innovation

In the realm of CAUTI prevention and management, ongoing research is paving the way for innovative approaches to enhance patient safety and outcomes. Current efforts extend beyond established practices, with researchers delving into various uncharted territories. Novel catheter technologies, including advanced materials and coatings, are being investigated to deter bacterial adherence and biofilm formation. Innovative catheter designs are also on the horizon, aiming to minimize risks associated with indwelling catheters [11]. Biomarkers for early infection detection may hold the potential to revolutionize diagnosis and treatment timelines [12]. Additionally, the exploration of alternative urine collection methods offers promise for reducing reliance on traditional catheterization. As telemedicine gains traction, research is examining ways to remotely monitor catheterized patients, while patient centered studies aim to better understand the human experience with urinary catheters [13]. Cost effectiveness analyses are underway, providing valuable insights into healthcare institutions. The collective efforts in these diverse areas of research underscore the commitment to preventing CAUTIs and improving patient care in the years to come [14].

Conclusion

Preventing CAUTIs in the ICU is a multifaceted challenge that requires a comprehensive and proactive approach. By focusing on evidence-based practices such as appropriate catheterization indications, aseptic techniques, catheter care, and timely removal, healthcare providers can significantly reduce the incidence of CAUTIs. Additionally, exploring emerging strategies like alternative collection methods and antimicrobial technologies further enhances the arsenal of tools available for CAUTI prevention. Through continuous education, vigilant surveillance, and the integration of innovative solutions, the ICU community can work together to safeguard patient health and improve overall outcomes. The data underscores the urgency of these efforts, as reducing CAUTI incidence directly contributes to improved patient safety and reduced healthcare costs. The ongoing and diverse research endeavors also point toward a promising future, where CAUTIs are further mitigated through groundbreaking advancements in prevention and management practices.

References

1. Hooton TM, Bradley SF, Cardenas DD, Colgan R, Geerlings SE, Rice JC, Saint S, Schaeffer AJ, Tambayh PA, Tenke P, Nicolle LE, Infectious Diseases Society of America. Diagnosis, prevention, and treatment of catheter-associated urinary tract infection in adults: 2009 International Clinical Practice Guidelines from the Infectious Diseases Society of America. Clin Infect Dis. 2010;50(5):625–63. https://doi.org/10.1086/650482.
2. Nicolle LE. Catheter associated urinary tract infections. Antimicrob Resist Infect Control. 2014;3:23.
3. Sabih A, Leslie SW. Complicated urinary tract infections. 2023 Nov 12. In: StatPearls [Internet]. Treasure Island (FL): StatPearls Publishing; 2024 Jan–. PMID: 28613784.
4. Gould CV, Umscheid CA, Agarwal RK, Kuntz G, Pegues DA, Healthcare Infection Control Practices Advisory Committee. Guideline for prevention of catheter-associated urinary tract infections 2009. Infect Control Hosp Epidemiol. 2010;31(4):319–26.
5. Warren JW, Platt R, Thomas RJ, Rosner B, Kass EH. Antibiotic irrigation and catheter-associated urinary-tract infections. N Engl J Med. 1978;299(11):570–3. https://doi.org/10.1056/NEJM197809142991103.
6. Haley RW, Hooton TM, Culver DH, Stanley RC, Emori TG, Hardison CD, Quade D, Shachtman RH, Schaberg DR, Shah BV, Schatz GD. Nosocomial infections in U.S. hospitals, 1975–1976: estimated frequency by selected characteristics of patients. Am J Med. 1981;70(4):947–59. https://doi.org/10.1016/0002-9343(81)90561-1.
7. Tambyah PA, Maki DG. Catheter-associated urinary tract infection is rarely symptomatic: a prospective study of 1,497 catheterized patients. Arch Intern Med. 2000;160(5):678–82. https://doi.org/10.1001/archinte.160.5.678.
8. Saint S. Clinical and economic consequences of nosocomial catheter-related bacteriuria. Am J Infect Control. 2000;28(1):68–75. https://doi.org/10.1016/s0196-6553(00)90015-4.
9. Van Decker SG, Bosch N, Murphy J. Catheter-associated urinary tract infection reduction in critical care units: a bundled care model. BMJ Open Qual. 2021;10:e001534. https://doi.org/10.1136/bmjoq-2021-001534.
10. Beeson T, Davis C. Urinary management with an external female collection device. J Wound Ostomy Continence Nurs. 2018;45:187–9. https://doi.org/10.1097/WON.0000000000000417.
11. Kanti SPY, Csóka I, Jójárt-Laczkovich O, Adalbert L. Recent advances in antimicrobial coatings and material modification strategies for preventing urinary catheter-associated complications. Biomedicines. 2022;10(10):2580. https://doi.org/10.3390/biomedicines10102580.
12. Horváth J, Wullt B, Naber KG, Köves B. Biomarkers in urinary tract infections—which ones are suitable for diagnostics and follow-up? GMS Infect Dis. 2020;8:Doc24. https://doi.org/10.3205/id000068.
13. Daumeyer NM, Kreitzberg D, Gavin KM, Bauer TA. Real-world evidence: telemedicine for complicated cases of urinary tract infection. PLoS One. 2023;18(2):e0280386. https://doi.org/10.1371/journal.pone.0280386.
14. Gray M, Skinner C, Kaler W. External collection devices as an alternative to the indwelling urinary catheter: evidence-based review and expert clinical panel deliberations. J Wound Ostomy Continence Nurs. 2016;43(3):301–7. https://doi.org/10.1097/WON.0000000000000220. PMID: 26974963; PMCID: PMC4870965.

Chapter 5
VAP Prevention in the ICU

Ruckshanda Majid

Introduction

Ventilator-associated pneumonias (VAPs) are hospital-acquired infections which (by definition) develop after 48 h of mechanical ventilation [1]. Reported incidences vary widely from 5% to 40%. VAPs can present with purulent tracheal secretions, fevers, and a worsening in the respiratory condition in the setting of positive respiratory cultures. Diagnosing VAPs requires a high level of clinical suspicion on bedside evaluation with consistent findings on radiographic examination and confirmation on microbiologic analysis of respiratory secretions [2]. The lower respiratory tract infection is thought to result from the infection of the lung parenchyma by microorganisms that colonize the oral and gastric secretions. The translocation and subsequent invasion of the lower airways can occur due to a compromise in the host protective mechanism of the respiratory tract secondary to the placement of the endotracheal tube [3].

The duration of intubation is one of most important (and potentially modifiable) risks associated with nosocomial pneumonia. Intubation for more than 48 h substantially increases that risk although VAPs may also occur sooner. Langer et al. reported on the incidence of acquired pneumonias in the intensive care unit (21.3%) over 3 months. About 54.2% of these infections were acquired during the first 4 days in the ICU (early-onset VAP) [4]. It is important to distinguish this from late-onset VAPs, which develop after 4 days after initiation of MV as the culprit microbiology of the infection if often different. The outcomes are also more favorable in early-onset versus late-onset VAPs [5, 6]. A review of the microbial flora implicated

R. Majid (✉)
Division of Pulmonary, Critical Care and Sleep Medicine, Department of Internal Medicine, The University of Texas Health Sciences Center at Houston, UT Health, McGovern Medical School, Houston, TX, USA
e-mail: Ruckshanda.Majid@uth.tmc.edu

M. Ellsworth, L. Ostrosky-Zeichner (eds.), *Infection Prevention in the Intensive Care Setting*, https://doi.org/10.1007/978-3-031-67062-6_5

in causing VAPs reveals that only a handful on organisms are responsible for the majority of infections [7] with certain factors related to the host which favor certain pathogens (Table 5.1).

The specific causative organisms are further modified depending on preexisting comorbid pulmonary (or non-pulmonary) disease, pattern of prior antibiotic use (type and duration), and the time since intubation [8, 9]. VAPs are predominantly caused by Methicillin-sensitive *Staphylococcus aureus*, *Streptococcus pneumoniae*, and unencapsulated *Haemophilus influenzae* within the first week of intubation [10–13]. Later, VAPs are more likely to be caused by multiresistant flora, such as *Pseudomonas aeruginosa*, methicillin-resistant staphylococci, or *Acinetobacter baumannii* [7, 14–16] (Figs. 5.1 and 5.2). Fungi may also be considered in the setting of a severely immunocompromised host. All of these multiresistant pathogens

Table 5.1 Risk factors for specific VAP pathogens[a]

Pathogen	Risk factor(s)
Streptococcus pneumoniae	Smoking
	COPD
	Absence of antibiotic therapy
Haemophilus influenzae	Smoking
	COPD
	Absence of antibiotic therapy
Staphylococcus aureus (MSSA)	Younger age
	Traumatic coma
	Neurosurgery
Staphylococcus aureus (MRSA)	COPD
	Steroid therapy
	Longer duration of mechanical
	Ventilation
	Prior antibiotic therapy
	Prior bronchoscopy
Pseudomonas aeruginosa	COPD
	Steroid therapy
	Longer duration of mechanical ventilation
Acinetobacter species	ARDS
	Head trauma
	Neurosurgery
	Gross aspiration
	Prior cephalosporin therapy

David R Park. The Microbiology of Ventilator-Associated Pneumonia. Respiratory Care Jun 2005, 50(6): 742–765 [7]

VAP ventilator-associated pneumonia, *COPD* chronic obstructive pulmonary disease, *MSSA* methicillin-sensitive *Staphylococcus aureus*, *MRSA* methicillin-resistant *Staphylococcus aureus*, *ARDS* acute respiratory distress syndrome

See text for explanation and references

[a] Associations shown in case-control studies of patients with ventilator-associated pneumonia

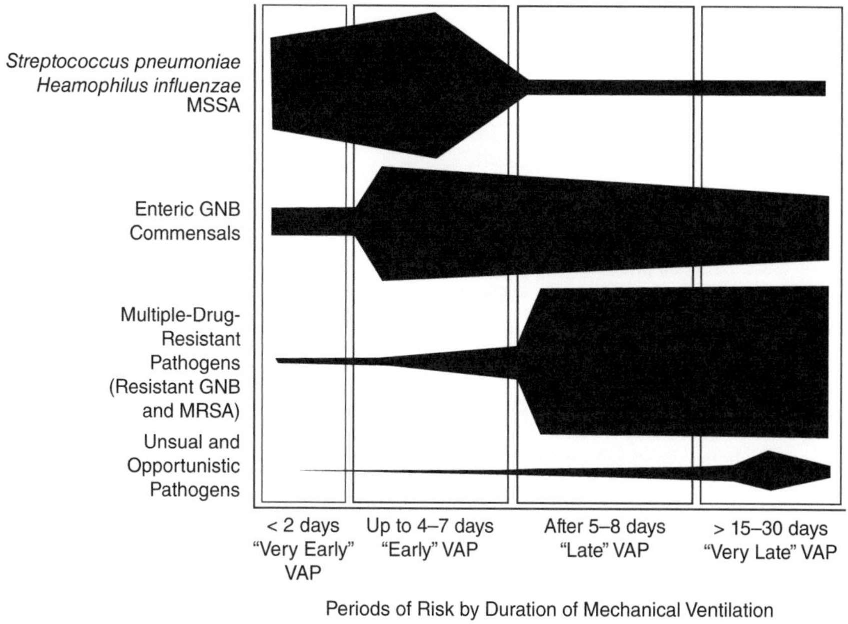

Fig. 5.1 Pathogen risk based on duration of mechanical ventilation. Periods of risk for various microbial causes of ventilatorassociated pneumonia (VAP), according to the duration of mechanical ventilation. Stages of increasing duration of mechanical ventilation are listed in sequence across the horizontal axis. The relative importance of the common bacterial pathogens on the left is indicated by the thickness of the bars as they progress through each stage from left to right. *MSSA* methicillin-sensitive *Staphylococcus aureus*, *GNB* gram-negative bacilli, *MRSA* methicillin-resistant *Staphylococcus aureus*. (David R Park. The Microbiology of Ventilator-Associated Pneumonia. Respiratory Care Jun 2005, 50 (6):742–765 [7])

(particularly *P. aeruginosa*) are responsible for most of the deaths directly related to pneumonia [17, 18]. In certain populations (e.g., chronic obstructive pulmonary disease patients who may be colonized by *P. aeruginosa*), the causative organisms are likely to be different.

VAPs are one of the most commonly encountered hospital-acquired infections in the intensive care unit (ICU) and can be associated with significant morbidity, prolonged duration of mechanical ventilation, and ICU stay, in addition to the increased cost of ICU care [19]. VAP prevention strategies have hence been the focus of many clinical trials. This has included the avoidance of intubation in certain clinical situations. For example, the use of noninvasive positive pressure ventilation (NIPPV) in the management of acute respiratory failure secondary to chronic obstructive pulmonary disease (COPD) exacerbations and pulmonary edema has also been investigated with favorable outcomes [20]. Electing NIPPV and avoiding intubation allow for the protective upper airway mechanisms to remain intact. The use of NIPPV has in addition been shown to reduce the number of VAPs in immunocompromised patients [21]. Other VAP prevention strategies have included daily sedation holidays

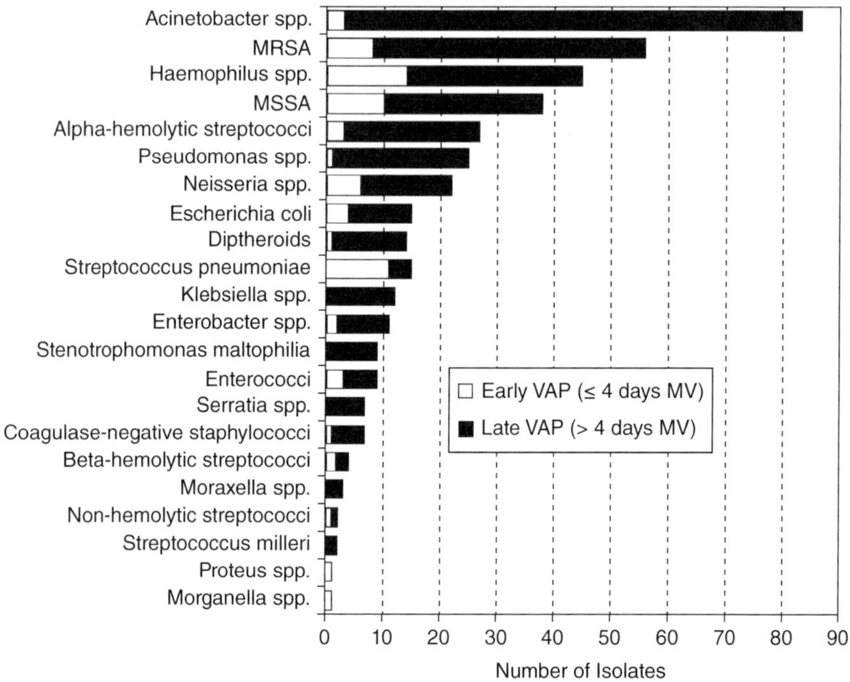

Fig. 5.2 Bacterial causes of early-onset and late-onset ventilator-associated pneumonia (VAP). The bars show the frequency of bacterial causes of VAP from 267 bronchoscopically-confirmed cases seen at Harborview Medical Center, in Seattle, Washington. Isolates from early-onset VAP cases (occurring within 4 days of beginning mechanical ventilation) are represented by the white portions of the bars. Isolates from late-onset cases (occurring after 4 days of mechanical ventilation) are represented by the black portions of the bars. All of the 11 early-onset cases with multipledrug-resistant isolates had other risk factors for these infections (see text for explanation). *MRSA* methicillin-resistant *Staphylococcus aureus*, *MSSA* methicillin-sensitive *Staphylococcus aureus*, *MV* mechanical ventilation. (Data courtesy of Timothy Dellit MD and Jeannie Chan PharmD, Harborview Medical Center, Seattle, Washington. Dellit TH, Chan JD, Nathens AB, Skerrett SJ, Hooton TM. Development of ventilator-associated pneumonia guidelines based on local microbiology and resistance patterns. Proceedings of the 42nd Annual Meeting of the Infectious Diseases Society of America, 2004 Sept 30–Oct 3, Boston, Massachusetts. A216 [16])

and early ventilator and weaning protocols. These interventions have been shown to facilitate a decrease in the number of ventilator days by optimizing timely extubations, hence preventing additional ventilator days [22]. Minimizing aspiration or colonization of respiratory secretions by elevating the head end of the bed above 30°, scheduled oral care with removal of subglottic secretions, selective digestive and oropharyngeal decontamination, and antimicrobial-coated endotracheal tubes have also been investigated with variable results. Implementation of bundled interventions into a "VAP prevention protocol" has also been investigated with some success in reducing VAP rates.

In this review, we will discuss in detail the current literature relating to evidence-based VAP prevention strategies and the clinically relevant interventions that have resulted in the decrease in this hospital-acquired infection.

VAP Prevention Strategies

1. Noninvasive ventilation
2. Elevation of the head of the bed
3. Methods of enteral feeding
4. Stress ulcer prophylaxis
5. Oral antiseptics and antibiotics
6. Avoidance of sedation and paralytic agents
7. Endotracheal tubes with subglottic secretion aspiration ports
8. Silver-coated endotracheal tubes
9. Ventilator weaning and extubation protocols
10. Early tracheostomy
11. Ventilator circuit management strategies
12. Ventilator-associated pneumonia prevention bundles

High-Flow Nasal Oxygen and Noninvasive Ventilation

High-flow nasal oxygen can be used in patients with hypoxemic respiratory failure to avoid initial intubation and also to prevent reintubation of critically ill patients and postoperative patients who have been extubated but still require significant amounts of oxygen [23–26]. High-flow nasal oxygen has been associated with less nosocomial pneumonia in patients with hypoxemic respiratory failure by virtue of avoiding mechanical ventilation and hence the development of a VAP [27].

Noninvasive ventilation (NIV) refers to the administration of ventilatory support without the use of an invasive artificial airway. NIV has become an important tool in the management of both acute and chronic respiratory failure, and in some circumstances, it can be also used to either avoid intubation or shorten the mechanical ventilation days.

Instituting NIV as an initial respiratory support strategy has resulted in fewer episodes of ventilator-associated pneumonia. This has been most widely investigated in patients with chronic obstructive lung disease (COPD) with acute hypercapnic respiratory failure. In one such study, 26 patients were randomized to NIV with a resulting trend demonstrated toward a lower rate of ventilator-associated pneumonias (3 vs. 9; $p = 0.07$) and severe sepsis or septic shock (6 vs. 13; $p = 0.07$) [28]. Intubation was however required in 52% patients initially randomized to NIV either due to mask intolerance, hemodynamic instability, worsening hypercapnia, and deterioration in mental status or copious secretions which would be of concern in an unprotected airway. Patient selection, reevaluation, and follow-up are important if NIV is going to be used. Additional complications in the NIV group developed only after intubation (six patients developed severe sepsis or septic shock). Jurjevik et al. also concluded that invasive ventilation was associated with a longer total duration of ventilation and ICU stay [29]. Mortality was similar in the NIV and the invasive groups; however, the patients receiving bilevel NIV had fewer episodes of ventilator-associated pneumonia and less requirement for tracheostomy.

Early ventilator liberation to NIV has also been introduced as a strategy to reduce ventilator days, reestablish patient respiratory protective mechanisms, and potentially reduce the VAP incidence, without increasing re-intubations or mortality. One study looked at difficult to wean patients who were intubated for acute on chronic respiratory failure. They were randomized either to continued conventional weaning of the invasive mechanical ventilation or to the intervention group in which the patients were electively extubated to NIV as the weaning strategy, hence shortening the time of intubation [30]. The number of days on the ventilator were reduced in the NIV group as compared to the control group (4.56 ± 1.85 days vs. 7.69 ± 3.79 days, $p = 0.004$) with no difference in the reintubation rates, demonstrating that this a potentially safe strategy. In another multicenter, randomized controlled trial involving 50 COPD patients, NIV was again used as an early liberation tool and weaning technique [31]. This group of patients included those that initially failed NIV and required intubation based on pre-established criteria [32]. When patients demonstrated improved neurologic status, were afebrile (temperature less than 37 °C), and hemodynamically stable with improved respiratory parameters (SpO_2 greater than 88% on an FiO_2 of 40%), they were liberated to NIV for 20–22 h a day with brief periods allowed on supplemental oxygen without NIV support (to allow eating and expectoration). There was a reduced duration of mechanical ventilation for the noninvasive ventilation group (16.6 ± 11.8 days vs. 10.2 ± 6.8 days $p = 0.021$). The ICU stay was also reduced, with an improved 2-month survival rate in the NIV group (72% vs. 95%; $p = 0.009$). Seven of the 25 patients (28%) weaned invasively developed a nosocomial pneumonia, whereas none of the patients weaned noninvasively did. A meta-analysis reviewed five relevant studies with 171 patient's data analyzed [33]. Two studies only included COPD patients, and the other three studies included a mixed patient population. The COPD patients were liberated to NIV after 36–48 h of mechanical ventilation. Burns et al. concluded that weaning to NIV was associated with a decrease in VAPs (relative risk 0.28, 95% CI: 0.09–0.85), and in mortality (relative risk 0.41, 95% CI: 0.22–0.76).

NIV can hence be considered as an effective alternative respiratory support tool and weaning strategy to effect early liberation from mechanical ventilation in a select group of patients with respiratory failure to minimize VAP risk. Chronic obstructive pulmonary disease exacerbation with hypercapnia has the highest level of evidence, with cardiogenic pulmonary edema, immunocompromised patients, and trauma patients also demonstrated to benefit from NIV [20].

Elevation of the Head of the Bed

Aspiration of upper airway secretions can be avoided by maintaining an elevated head end of the bed on patients who are mechanically ventilated. Aspiration of gastric contents and oropharyngeal secretions colonized with potentially pathogenic microorganisms likely contribute to the development of VAPs [34, 35]. Supine body positioning which prevents an effective protective cough and mucociliary clearance has also been shown to be independently associated with the development of ventilator-associated pneumonias [36]. Consequently, intentional elevation of the head end of the bed has been investigated as a potential VAP preventative measure [37].

In a multivariate analysis of a prospective cohort of 277 intubated patients, supine positioning in the first 24 h after initiation of mechanical ventilation had a stronger association toward the development of a VAP (odds ratio [OR] 2.9; 95% CI: 1.3–6.8) in addition to an increase in mortality (OR: 3.1; 95% CI: 1.2–7.8) [36]. Drakulovic et al. also found a statistically significant reduction in both clinical and microbiological diagnoses of VAPs with the head end of the bed elevated to 45° vs. 0° although the study was not adequately powered to conclude that the semi-recumbent position also decreased the duration of mechanical ventilation, ICU length of stay, or mortality [38]. The supine position was especially associated with an increased risk of developing a VAP if the patient was concurrently receiving enteral nutrition (adjusted OR: 5.7; 95% CI: 1.5–22.8). In a larger multicenter trial, Van Nieuwenhoven et al. did not find any decrease in VAP rates, or duration of ventilation, intensive care length of stay, and mortality in the semi-recumbent patients versus the supine patients (45° elevation of the backrest vs. 10° in the control group) [39]. The conflicting findings however were likely a function of not achieving the intended intervention, with a resulting lower elevation of the head end of the bed (22.6°) in the intervention group and the higher elevation in the control group (16.1°). This likely negated any effective difference in potential VAP prevention from the intervention. This study outcome emphasizes the practical challenges of keeping the head end of the bed elevated and the resulting loss of the potential benefit if the intubated patient is not kept at the intended elevation. Loss of optimal head elevation is often observed during transportation and repeated repositioning or cleaning of the mechanically ventilated patient where the patient is maintained in a lower position for that period of time. Patient transportation has been found to be an independent risk factor for the development of a VAP likely by facilitating the aspiration of contaminated secretions from the upper airway and the ventilator circuits when kept in the supine position for the duration of this event. In a study by Bercault et al. also found that intra-hospital transport was one of two factors independently associated with ventilator-associated pneumonia (odds ratio, 3.1; 95% CI, 1.4–6.7), the second factor being the need for reintubation [40].

Semi-recumbent patient positioning is a low-cost, low risk approach to prevent ventilator-associated pneumonias that should be considered in all eligible patients. Head elevation however must be maintained for maximum effectiveness. Education of all ICU personnel should routinely include the benefits of head elevation in intubated patients with potential frequent audits (and corrections when needed) while the patient is intubated.

Methods of Enteral Feeding

Enteral alimentation is a commonly used modality for providing nutritional support in the ICU while intubated. Infectious complications and aspiration risk however may be associated with placement and maintenance of orogastric and nasogastric tubes used for the delivery of enteral nutrition and hence may not be of benefit to all patients [41–43].

Monitoring Gastric Residuals

A randomized control trial looked at comparing two groups on mechanical ventilation receiving early enteral nutrition via a nasogastric tube (within 36 h of intubation) [44]. The intervention group did not undergo routine monitoring of their residual gastric volumes (intolerance was based on regurgitation and vomiting) while the control group continued routine monitoring (a residual gastric volume greater than 250 mL at six hourly measurements as an additional measurement of intolerance). The incidence of VAPs did not differ significantly between the two groups (16.7% vs. 15.8%). Despite an observed higher vomiting rate in the intervention group without routine residual gastric content monitoring (39.6% vs. 27%), the prokinetic drug use was lower and the calories delivered were higher in that group. Not monitoring residual gastric volume was concluded not to be inferior to residual gastric volume monitoring in regard to affecting VAP incidence.

Early Versus Late Initiation of Enteral Nutrition

Nutrition supplies vital cell substrates, antioxidants, vitamins, and minerals that optimize recovery from illness. The optimal time to start nutritional support has been a topic of much debate. In a systematic review of the literature, Marik and Zaloga looked at 15 studies, with a total of 753 patients and concluded that early initiation of enteral nutrition (within 36 h) post-surgery or after admission, reduced overall infections (relative risk reduction, 0.45; 95% CI, 0.30–0.66; $p = 0.00006$), and hospital length of stay (mean reduction of 2.2 days; 95% CI, 0.81–3.63 days; $p = 0.004$) [45]. Infectious complications occurred in 19% of the early nutritional group as compared with 41% in the delayed group. No demonstrable difference in mortality however was found, and all of the studies included in the analysis were performed in surgical patients.

Medical ICU patients were prospectively looked at by Ibrahim et al. [46]. About 150 patients were randomized to either early feeding (day 1) or late feeding (day 5) of mechanical ventilation. Patients in the early feeding group were found to have statistically greater incidences of ventilator-associated pneumonia (49.3% vs. 30.7%; $p = 0.020$) and prolonged lengths of stay in the hospital. Artinian et al. also looked at medical ICU patients and admitted predominantly for respiratory failure, requiring mechanical ventilation for more than 2 days. The 2537 (63%) of patients received early enteral feeding (<48 h). The ICU and hospital mortality were 18.1% vs. 21.4% ($p = 0.01$) and 28.7% vs. 33.5% ($p = 0.001$), respectively, favoring the early feeding group, however in all adjusted analysis, the early feeding was again found to be independently associated with an increased risk of ventilator-associated pneumonias [47]. The overall beneficial effects of early enteral feeding in the more critically ill patients were explained as outweighing the detrimental effects of increased VAP rates, resulting in a significant survival advantage. Patients with lower disease severity may not carry this advantage however (the favorable effects of early feeding are offset by the increased mortality associated with developing a VAP in the less critically ill). Despite the increased VAP rate, the authors however concluded that the use of early enteral feeding in medical ICU patients offers an advantage in mortality, more clearly seen in the sickest patients. These studies hence would suggest that early enteral feeding is likely of most benefit to sicker medical ICU patients and the surgical ICU population.

Gastric Versus Post-pyloric Nutrition

In addition to the timing of initiation of enteral feeding, the site of nutrition delivery may have some bearing on VAP risk. Post-pyloric feeding has the theoretical advantage of reducing gastroesophageal reflux and hence aspiration pneumonia risk. A meta-analysis looking at 522 medical, neurosurgical, and trauma ICU patients, comparing gastric with post-pyloric feeding, found no reductions in the incidence of pneumonia in the post-pyloric group (OR 1.44, 95% CI 0.84–2.46, $p = 0.19$) [48]. Patients with a prior history of aspiration, high gastric residual volumes (>250 mL) and patients who had undergone gastric or major vascular surgery (potentially high-risk groups), however, were excluded from the trial. The European Society for Clinical Nutrition and Metabolism (ESPEN) guidelines hence could not recommend the use of the post-pyloric feeding as the preferred method [43]. A subsequent meta-analysis looked at 15 trials (11 of which were recruited from either a general or medical ICU). A significant reduction in VAP risk was noted in the patients who received post-pyloric nutrition (relative risk [RR] 0.63, 95% confidence interval [CI] 0.48–0.83, $p = 0.001$) but there was no association between tube position and the amount of aspiration [49]. The incongruity in these findings was attributed to the likely difficulty in defining aspiration versus micro-aspiration. The most recent and largest meta-analysis (41 studies conducted in ten countries and involving 3248 participants) did find that post-pyloric feeding was associated with a lower incidence of pulmonary aspiration, gastric reflux, and pneumonia ($p < 0.001$), less incidence of gastrointestinal complications including vomiting, nausea, diarrhea, abdominal distension, high gastric residual volume, and constipation ($p < 0.05$), and lastly a shorter length of mechanical ventilation, stay in ICU, and stay in hospital ($p < 0.001$), when compared with gastric feeding [50]. Hence, the routine use of post-pyloric feeding is likely beneficial for most ICU patients, and possibly more so for those who are at high risk of aspiration from gastric feeding [51, 52].

Stress Ulcer Prophylaxis

Gastrointestinal bleeding in critically ill patients is associated with significant morbidity and mortality [53]. Stress ulcer prophylaxis is therefore of major importance in the ICU on eligible patients. Gastric colonization and proliferation by potentially pathogenic organisms however increase with a higher gastric pH [54]. H_2-antagonists and antacids (used for stress ulcer prophylaxis in mechanically ventilated patients) may consequently increase such organism loads and theoretically increase the risk for ventilator-associated pneumonia [55]. An investigation of potentially increased VAP risk with various stress ulcer prophylactic agents has been conducted but with inconsistent results.

Sucralfate has been used as an alternative stress ulcer prophylactic agent. It protects the stomach lining by forming a protective barrier without affecting the gastric acid production and hence, may not increase the VAP risk. In a randomized controlled trial of 1200 mechanically ventilated patients, sucralfate was compared to an H_2 blocker as an alternate choice to prevent gastric ulceration, without increasing VAP rates [56]. There was no statistically significant difference in VAP rates between the ranitidine and the sucralfate group (19.1% vs. 16.2%, relative risk 1.18; 95% CI 0.92–1.51; $p = 0.19$). Sucralfate was however found to be associated with more gastrointestinal bleeding. It has been estimated that 3.8% of patients receiving sucralfate prophylaxis developed a clinically significant bleed versus 1.7% of the patients receiving ranitidine (relative risk, 0.44; 95% CI, 0.21–0.92; $p = 0.02$). Of note, however the source of bleeding could not be isolated in 19 of 33 patients hence not clearly indicating a gastric site of bleeding. Twenty randomized trials have been reviewed in several meta-analyses [55, 57–62]. Four of these meta-analyses also reported a significantly decreased incidence of ventilator-associated pneumonia with sucralfate therapy compared with H_2-antagonists [57–60] although three meta-analyses found trends in the reduction of rates of ventilator-associated pneumonia in patients given sucralfate but were statistically nonsignificant [55, 61, 62]. Three studies reported a statistically significant mortality decrease with sucralfate [55, 60, 61]. A later prospective cohort study of 747 patients by Borstain et al. found that sucralfate use was associated with a higher risk of early-onset VAP defined as pneumonia that occurred from day 3 to day 7 of MV (odds ratio 1.81, 95% CI 1.01–3.26) [63]. H_2 blockers and proton pump inhibitors were also both used in the trial but they were not associated with a statistically significant increase in VAPs. This discordant finding was potentially attributable to the formation of pharmacobezoars by sucralfate (bezoars composed of medications) which have been reported to cause such solid aggregates of indigestible materials which can contribute to intestinal obstruction and the potential promotion of bacterial overgrowth [64].

The data comparing stress ulcer prophylaxis with sucralfate and H_2-antagonists suggest an overall decrease in the incidence of ventilator-associated pneumonia with sucralfate. Stress ulcer prophylaxis with any agent however may increase the risk for ventilator-associated pneumonia [36]. Sucralfate may decrease risk when compared with H_2-antagonists but not when compared with placebo. Hence, in a patient that is at higher risk for the development of a stress ulcer, the benefits of sucralfate in limiting the development of a ventilator-associated pneumonia against the potential decrease in protection against gastrointestinal bleeding compared with H_2-antagonists must be weighed. Use of sucralfate in patients at low to moderate risk for gastrointestinal bleeding (those with no coagulopathy or need for prolonged mechanical ventilation) would be a reasonable approach [65].

Oral Antiseptics and Antibiotics

Oral antiseptics and antibiotics may decrease the bacterial load of aspirated oral and gastric secretions. Agents that have been investigated looking at a potential role for these agents in decreasing VAPs have been categorized as (1) oral antiseptic or antibiotic washes, (2) enteric antibiotics for oral decontamination, or (3) a combination of enteral and intravenous antibiotics for digestive decontamination. Aerosolized inhaled antibiotics have also been explored [66]. Povidone–iodine, iseganan (a topical antimicrobial peptide active against gram-positive bacteria, gram-negative bacteria, and yeasts used for the prevention of mucositis primarily in patients undergoing radiation treatment), and chlorhexidine are the major agents that have been assessed in randomized controlled trials in the topical group. Similarly, a combination of topical polymyxin, aminoglycoside, and amphotericin, and short courses of intravenous antimicrobial therapy have been investigated in the systemic antibiotic category.

Topical Oral Antiseptics

Topical chlorhexidine may be less prone to induced drug resistance due to the rapidity with which it acts [67]. Three trials found a decrease in VAPs with chlorhexidine [68–70] while eight did not show any benefit [71–78]. Houston et al. randomized 561 patients undergoing cardiac surgery to receive chlorhexidine gluconate oral rinse or a phenolic mixture [72]. The overall rate of VAPs was found not to be significantly lower in the chlorhexidine group (1.4% vs. 3.0%, $p = 0.21$) however in patients who were intubated for greater than 24 h a decrease in the VAP incidence was found (20% vs. 70%; $p = 0.02$). Deriso et al. also found that the VAP incidence was lower in patients undergoing cardiac surgery when randomized to chlorhexidine gluconate oral rinses (2.9% vs. 9.4%, $p < 0.05$) [71]. Similar findings were reported by Fourier et al. who randomized 60 to receive oral chlorhexidine or placebo in a multidisciplinary intensive care unit. The VAP incidence was again found to be lower in the treated group (odds ratio 0.27; 95% CI 0.07–0.96) [50]. Subgroup analysis of trials using chlorhexidine oral decontamination has suggested that such topical oral antiseptics may not be as effective in decreasing the gram-negative organisms [74]. Scannapieco et al. investigated the application of 0.12% chlorhexidine gluconate in 175 intubated trauma patients [78]. A quantitative measurement of oral respiratory pathogens revealed a reduction in *Staphylococcus aureus* but not of *Pseudomonas* or *Acinetobacter* in the dental plaque of the intervention group. Incidentally, no significant differences were found in the VAP rates in the treatment versus chlorhexidine groups (OR = 0.54, 95% CI = 0.23–1.25, $p = 0.15$).

Mechanical brushing of the teeth and mouth may be a more effective means of oral decontamination [79]. The amount of dental plaque increases with prolonged ICU admissions, with a strong correlation between bacterial colonization (in dental plaque) and development of nosocomial infections [80, 81] and a genetic homology between bacterial isolates from the dental plaque and lungs in patients diagnosed with a VAP [82]. There have also been concerns due to the potential increased risk of bacterial translocation with brushing [68, 79]. Mori et al. implemented brushing into an intensive oral hygiene protocol (2–3 times a day) which included (1) checking adequate cuff pressure before and after the cleaning, (2) suctioning the mouth before and after the intervention, (3) cleansing and rinsing the oral cavity with 300 mL of a weakly acidic using a toothbrush, and (4) cleaning the oral cavity using a swab soaked in povidone-iodine before and after brushing [83]. Intubated patients admitted to the medical surgical ICU prior to the implementation of the oral care protocol served as the historical controls. The incidence of VAPs, reported as episodes of pneumonia per 1000 ventilator days, was significantly lower with the implementation of oral care (3.9 vs. 10.4, $p > 0.001$). *P. aeruginosa* was the most frequently observed causative bacteria isolated both pre- and post-intervention, followed by MRSA and Candida. The number of potentially pathogenic bacteria examined however were significantly reduced after single oral care procedure.

Two meta-analyses of randomized controlled trials have found a potentially higher mortality rate with chlorhexidine [84, 85]. Klompas et al. found a non-significantly increased mortality in non-cardiac surgery patients (RR, 1.13, 95% CI, 0.99–1.29) [67]. Price et al. concluded that selective oropharyngeal decontamination was associated with a reduction in death but the use of oropharyngeal chlorhexidine was associated with an increase in mortality in adults in general intensive care units (odds ratio 1.25, 95% CI 1.05–1.50) [85]. There was no clear explanation for this effect except for the potential aspiration of chlorhexidine with subsequent worsening of the respiratory condition [84].

A subsequent Cochran review which included 35 RCTs (5374 participants) looked at four main comparisons: (1) chlorhexidine (mouth rinse or gel) versus placebo/usual care, (2) toothbrushing versus no toothbrushing, (3) powered versus manual toothbrushing, and (4) comparisons of oral care solutions [86]. Chlorhexidine compared to placebo or usual care was associated with a reduction in VAP (OR 0.60, 95% confidence intervals (CI) 0.47–0.77, $p < 0.001$). Fifteen patients (NNT 15 with a 95% CI of 10–34) would need to receive chlorhexidine oral decontamination to prevent one case of ventilator-associated pneumonia. This was however without any mortality benefit or decrease in duration of mechanical ventilation or ICU length of stay. The four RCTs did not report any benefit of toothbrushing (±CHX). Powered toothbrushing resulted in the same findings.

Although it still can be beneficial in specific settings, robust evidence to recommend its routine application of chlorhexidine for all mechanically ventilated patients is lacking. Given the possibility of harm, it should not be routinely recommended.

Enteral and Parenteral Antibiotics

Antibiotic prophylaxis can include any combination of oropharyngeal, intragastric, and intravenous antibiotics. Selective oropharyngeal decontamination (SOD) is the application of the topical antibiotic paste, usually containing tobramycin, polymyxin, colistin, and/or amphotericin B, to the oropharynx only, without enteral or empirical intravenous antibiotics. Selective digestive decontamination (SDD) consists of oropharyngeal and gastric application of non-absorbable antibiotics supplemented with a suspension (with the same antimicrobial agents) administered through the nasogastric tube along with a short course of an intravenous antibiotic, often cefotaxime or ciprofloxacin. Oropharyngeal antibiotics are applied as a paste, and gastric antibiotics are administered as a suspension through a nasogastric tube.

A meta-analysis looking at studies that implemented an SDD strategy found a statistically significant decrease in the incidence of bloodstream infections and mortality [87]. The 51 RCT trials included in the meta-analysis compared no treatment or placebo to oropharyngeal and/or intestinal administration of antibiotics as part of the SDD protocol, with or without a parenteral component. SDD significantly reduced overall bloodstream infections (OR of 0.73; 95% CI, 0.59–0.90; $p = 0.0036$). The subgroup analysis showed an even larger impact of SDD using parenteral and enteral antimicrobials on overall bloodstream infections (ORs of 0.63; 95% CI, 0.46–0.87; $p = 0.005$), bloodstream infections due to gram-negative bacteria 0.30 (95% CI, 0.16–0.56; $p < 0.001$), and overall mortality (0.74 (95% CI, 0.61–0.91; $p = 0.0034$)). Twenty patients need to be treated with SDD to prevent one gram-negative bloodstream infection and 22 patients to prevent one death.

De Smet et al. also looked at SDD in addition to SOD specifically as VAP preventative strategies in a trial which included 5939 patients [88]. In each of the 13 ICU, the three regimens (SDD, SOD, and standard care) were applied in random order over the course of 6 months. SOD included topical tobramycin, colistin, and amphotericin B to the oropharynx and stomach for 4 days and SDD composed of topical tobramycin, colistin, and amphotericin B to the oropharynx along with 4 days of intravenous cefotaxime. They did not find any difference in mortality rates for the whole group; however, the relative mortality was lower in the decontamination groups after adjusting for older age and for sicker patients. The 28-day adjusted odds of mortality for the SOD group was 0.86 (95% CI: 0.74–0.99) and 0.83 (95% CI: 0.72–0.97) for those assigned to SDD. There was no evidence of the emergence of antibiotic-resistant pathogens (fewer than 5% of isolates resistant to aminoglycosides, ciprofloxacin, or ceftazidime during the decontamination periods) or increased rates of detection of *C. difficile* toxin. A major criticism of this study however was the failure of treatment randomization which could affect the reliability of the results.

An additional seven meta-analyses of more than 40 randomized-controlled trials of SDD have also been published [89–95]. All seven meta-analyses reported a significant reduction in the risk for ventilator-associated pneumonia with the use of selective digestive tract decontamination. Four reported a significant reduction in mortality [89–91, 93]. Four separately analyzed trials used combined topical and systemic antibiotics and those that used topical antibiotics alone [89, 90, 93, 94]. While both approaches prevented ventilator-associated pneumonia, no mortality benefit occurred with topical prophylaxis alone [89, 90, 93, 94]. One of the meta-analyses showed an increased benefit in surgical compared with medical patients [89], while another showed no difference according to type of patient or severity of illness [90]. The reason for discordance among these meta-analyses likely resulted from differences in inclusion criteria, definitions of outcome measures, and analytic methodology. Studies of parenteral antibiotics alone have generally failed to show a benefit [96], although studies in patients with severe burns or coma have suggested a decreased incidence of VAPs [97, 98].

In a more recent study, Plantinga et al. performed a meta-analysis on six randomized trials using SDD with topical antibiotics [99]. About 57.8% of the subjects had a medical diagnosis, and 42.2% had a surgical reason for ICU admission. The effects of both SDD and SOD on hospital survival and ICU survival were not modified by the type of ICU admission but surgical patients appeared to have a greater decrease in ICU mortality and medical patients felt a greater impact on decreasing hospital mortality with SDD. SDD was associated with a 16% reduction in hospital mortality, and decontamination of the oropharynx and digestive tract with a combination of topical, oral, and parenteral antibiotics was associated with an 18% reduction in hospital mortality. Selective digestive decontamination was hence found to be more effective than selective oral decontamination alone (OR, 0.90; 95% CI, 0.82–0.97 for hospital death) performed in countries with low levels of antibiotic resistance.

Selective digestive tract decontamination seems to reduce the incidence of ventilator-associated pneumonia and when a combined topical and intravenous regimen is used, may reduce intensive care unit-related mortality [100]. A review of 32 studies of selective digestive tract decontamination however found that there may be an inverse relationship between methodological quality and benefit, suggesting that the findings of meta-analyses may be overly optimistic [101]. Although SDD overall has been found to be of benefit, it continues to carry serious concerns in regard to its long-term effects on affecting antibiotic resistance patterns and should not be currently recommended. Selective oral and digestive decontamination with antibiotics is therefore not recommended in settings with high baseline levels of antibiotic resistance.

Inhaled Antibiotics

Prophylactic inhaled antibiotics (such as gentamicin, polymyxins, tobramycin, and ceftazidime) administered via the respiratory tract have been investigated in several trials as a strategy to prevent VAPs and subsequently looked at collectively in a meta-analysis [66]. This review included eight trials of which five were RCTs and five were non-randomized trials. When just looking at the RCTs, VAPs were less likely in patients that received the prophylactic aerosolized antibiotic (odds ratio of 0.49; 95% CI: 0.32–0.76) although the trials did not report a mortality benefit. When the three non-randomized trials were included in the analysis; however, the VAP preventative benefit was no longer seen. Fewer patients were however colonized with *Pseudomonas aeruginosa* in the group that received the prophylaxis when looking at all eight trials (OR = 0.51, 95% CI = 0.30–0.86). Finally, although the emergence of resistant organisms was not seen (possibly due to the shorter duration of the inhaled antibiotic or the reduced use of systemic antibiotics), evidence from non-comparative studies support that this preventive strategy may lead to an increase in the emergence of resistant bacteria.

Probiotics

Similarly, probiotics (*Lactobacillus casei rhamnosus*; *Lactobacillus plantarum*; Synbiotic 2000FORTE; Ergyphilus; combination *Bifidobacterium longum* + *Lactobacillus bulgaricus* + *Streptococcus thermophilus*) have been investigated as a VAP preventative strategy. A Cochrane review of eight randomized controlled trials (1083 patients included) reported an association with lower VAP rates (odds ratio (OR) 0.70, 95% confidence interval (CI) 0.52–0.95) but no impact on duration of mechanical ventilation, ICU length of stay, mortality, or antibiotic utilization [102]. The overall quality of the evidence however was low. A subsequent trial found lower VAP rates in the 235 patients randomized to the probiotic group (containing *Bacillus subtilis* and *Enterococcus faecalis*) 0.5 g three times daily through a nasogastric feeding tube for no longer than 14 days. The incidence of microbiologically confirmed VAP in the probiotics group was lower when compared to the control patients (36.4 vs. 50.4%, $p = 0.031$). No differences were again found in the incidence of clinically suspected VAP, duration of mechanical ventilation, length of hospital stay, mortality, or antimicrobial consumption [103]. A recent meta-analysis including 18 RCTs involving 4893 patients showed that probiotics reduced the incidence of VAPs (RR 0.68, 95% CI 0.55–0.84) but also concluded that due to the low quality of pooled evidence, and an observed loss of benefit when the analyses were restricted to the higher quality investigations (double-blinded or adequately randomized studies), sufficient evidence for the use of could not be provided to conclude that probiotics are of benefit for the prevention of VAP in ICU patients [104].

Avoidance of Sedation and Paralytic Agents

Sedation holidays (when appropriate) have been implemented in the ICU on mechanically ventilated patients to minimize additional ventilator days (secondary to excessive and residual sedation). This is now standard practice in the ICU to minimize delays in weaning and liberation from mechanical ventilation. Spontaneous-awakening trials have been shown to decrease the time to liberation by approximately 2 days ($p < 0.01$) and reduced ICU stay by 3.5 days ($p = 0.02$) [105].

Cook et al. conducted a study of 1014 mechanically ventilated patients in over 16 ICUs. About 17.5% developed a VAP on day 9.0 ± 5.9 after admission to the intensive care unit (median, 7 days; interquartile range, 5–10 days) with an increase in cumulative risk over time [106]. The daily hazard rate for developing a VAP however decreased after day 5 (3.3% at day 5, 2.3% at day 10, and 1.3% at day 15). Witnessed aspiration (risk ratio, 3.25; CI, 1.62–6.50) and exposure to paralytic agents (risk ratio, 1.57; CI, 1.03–2.39) were identified as independent predictors for the development of a VAP. There is substantial evidence that daily sedative interruptions decrease duration of mechanical ventilation, length of hospitalization, and mortality [107–109]. Early sedative administration between the first day and the fourth day of invasive mechanical ventilation was independently found to increase the risk for VAPs. In subsequent multivariate analysis, the administration of sedatives prior to intubation was also significantly associated with an increased number of VAPs (RR, 15.69; 95% CI, 1.62–152.06) [110]. Minimizing sedatives and avoiding paralytics are important strategies for the prevention of VAPs supported by a high level of evidence.

Endotracheal Tubes with Subglottic Secretion Aspiration Ports

The pooled secretions above the inflated endotracheal cuff can become colonized by potentially pathogenic organisms [111, 112]. Aspiration of this contaminated fluid into the lower respiratory tract is thought to contribute to the development of ventilator-associated pneumonias [113, 114]. Endotracheal tubes engineered with a dorsal lumen above the endotracheal cuff (which can remove such pooled subglottic secretions) have been investigated in several randomized trials to decrease this risk but with conflicting results [115–122]. Three of these trials demonstrated a reduction in VAP rates, with no change in mechanical ventilation days, ICU length of stay, hospital length of stay, or mortality, while two studies did not show any advantage. Mahul et al. used an intermittent (hourly) subglottic secretion drainage (SDD) in patients intubated for more than 3 days and found a reduction (no-SSD: 29.1%,

SSD: 13%) and a delay to diagnosis of a VAP (no-SSD: 8.3 ± 5 days, SSD: 16.2 ± 11 days) [115]. The intervention group was however also paired with either sucralfate or antacids. The group that received sucralfate was not associated with a significantly lower incidence of pneumonia (antacids: 23.6%, sucralfate: 17.8%), but was associated with lower colonization rate in subglottic and gastric aspirates. Valles et al. used a continuous suction protocol in a general ICU population and found a decrease in the overall incidence of VAPs in the intervention group (19.9 episodes/1000 ventilator days vs. 39.6 episodes/1000 ventilator days; RR, 1.98; 95% CI, 1.03–3.82) [100]. Bouza et al. did not find an overall reduction in VAPs. When analyzing patients that were intubated for greater than 48 h; however, (patients in both groups were enrolled at the time of intubation with many being extubated earlier than 48 h) he did demonstrate a reduction in the incidence of VAPs, ICU length of stay, and duration of mechanical ventilation [116]. A decrease in antibiotic prescription was noted in the intervention group with potential savings to offset the cost of the modified tube. Kollef et al. did not see any differences in regard to the primary outcome with the patients being enrolled consecutively at the time of intubation [117]. A delay in VAP onset was found however when compared to controls (5.6 ± 2.3 days compared to 2.9 ± 1.2 days $p = 0.006$; $p = 0.006$).

A meta-analysis by Dezfulian et al. reviewed 896 patients from five studies that were randomized to either a subglottic secretion drainage or a standard endotracheal tube care. A reduction in the incidence of VAPs by nearly half was found (risk ratio [RR] = 0.51; 95% confidence interval [CI] = 0.37–0.71), but by primarily reducing early-onset pneumonia (pneumonia occurring within 5–7 days after intubation) [123]. When only looking at the four studies which recruited patients expected to require 72 h of mechanical ventilation, secretion drainage also shortened the duration of mechanical ventilation by 2 days (95% CI: 1.7–2.3 days), the length of stay in the intensive care unit by 3 days (95% CI: 2.1–3.9 days), and delayed the onset of pneumonia by 6.8 days (95% CI: 5.5–8.1 days). Limiting the trials to patients ventilated for longer periods does increase their power but limits their generalizability to routine ICU care due to the poor predictability of length of intubation. Carroff et al. in another meta-analysis looking at 3369 patients found that subglottic secretion drainage was associated with lower ventilator-associated pneumonia rates (risk ratio, 0.58; 95% CI, 0.51–0.67; $I^2 = 0\%$) but could not demonstrate a decrease in the duration of mechanical ventilation, length of stay, ventilator-associated events, mortality, or antibiotic usage [124]. They reasoned that this may have been a consequence of the analysis being underpowered (particularly for mortality). The lower attributable mortality of early-onset pneumonia compared to that of late-onset pneumonia may have also negated any potential mortality benefit. A more recent meta-analysis by Pozuelo-Carrascosa et al. [125] looking at 29 studies (9 systematic reviews with meta-analysis and 20 RCTs) found a reduced VAP incidence (risk ratio (RR) 0.56, 95% CI 0.48–0.63; $I^2 = 0\%$, $p = 0.841$) in addition to a reduction in mortality (RR 0.88, 95% CI 0.80–0.97; $I^2 = 0\%$, $p = 0.888$). No decreases in the duration of mechanical ventilation, ICU, or hospital length of stay were however seen.

Patients undergoing prolonged mechanical ventilation seem to benefit more from subglottic secretion drainage (SSD), however other than a higher economic cost, these modified tubes are likely underutilized due to the absence of factors allowing accurate prediction of prolonged mechanical ventilation. Up to a third of patients are liberated from mechanical ventilation sooner than 72 h when longer respiratory support was predicted, hence making it difficult to identify patients who are most likely to benefit from this VAP prevention strategy [118, 119]. In addition, consistent decreases in mortality, ICU, and hospital length of stay have not yet been demonstrated. In summary, there may be a small subset of patients ventilated for intermediate lengths of time who would benefit from endotracheal tubes equipped with subglottic secretion aspiration ports but prospectively identifying these patients is impractical and hence cannot currently be recommended for general use.

Silver-Coated Endotracheal Tubes

Silver has broad-spectrum antimicrobial activity in vitro [108] and can reduce bacterial adhesion to devices [109, 110] and block biofilm formation on devices in animal models [111]. Silver-coated tubes have been developed with silver ions micro dispersed in a proprietary polymer, on the inner and outer lumen, to provide a potential antimicrobial effect. The polymer itself may also block bacterial adhesion to the endotracheal tube [112–115]. Silver has been used extensively in the burn population and is generally considered safe and non-toxic [116, 117].

The North American Silver-Coated Endotracheal Tube (NASCENT) looked at silver-coated endotracheal tubes in a prospective randomized, single-blind, multicenter trial [118]. About 2003 participants anticipated to require mechanical ventilation for more than 24 h were enrolled from 54 centers. Fewer VAPs were diagnosed in the intervention group (4.8%; 95% confidence interval [CI], 3.4–6.6%) than in the control group (7.5%; 95% CI, 5.7–9.7%). Silver-coated endotracheal tubes were also found to result in a later VAP diagnosis ($p = 0.005$). The authors concluded a relative risk reduction of 34% ($p = 0.03$) with a number needed to treat to prevent 1 VAP approximating 37 patients intubated for more than 24 h (95% CI: 19–369); however, when further analysis was performed to exclude organisms not typically considered pulmonary pathogens on a bronchoalveolar lavage culture (yeast, enterococcus, coagulase-negative Staphylococcus, and normal flora), the benefits of using the silver-coated tube were no longer found to be significant ($p = 0.08$) [119]. A NASCENT cohort (93 patients) was subsequently reanalyzed, in a retrospective review of those subjects diagnosed with a VAP and intubated for greater than 24 h, looking at the effect on mortality when using the modified tube [120]. Only VAPs involving multidrug-resistant bacteria as methicillin-resistant *Staphylococcus aureus* (MRSA), *Pseudomonas aeruginosa*, *Acinetobacter baumannii*, *Stenotrophomonas maltophilia*, and *Burkholderia cepacia* were included in this analysis. The silver-coated ETT was reported to be associated with reduced mortality (5/37 [14%] vs. 20/56 [36%], $p = 0.03$). The mortality rate was approximately 60% lower for patients in the silver group than for those in the control group (14% vs. 36%; $p = 0.03$). Unexpectedly, patients without a VAP had a 17% higher mortality in the silver group that in the control group (31% vs. 26%, $p = 0.03$). This finding could not be explained by any of the analysis conducted in the study. A Cochrane review which included three eligible RCT trials (including the NASCET trial) with a total of 2081 participants could not draw conclusions about hospital mortality, device-related complications, duration of intubation, and length of hospital and intensive care unit stay [121]. Silver-coated tubes hence cannot be included as a VAP prevention measure.

Ventilator Weaning and Extubation Protocols

The presence of an endotracheal tube increases the probability of developing nosocomial pneumonia with the risk being proportional to the length of time a patient is on mechanical ventilation [106, 126, 127]. Ventilator weaning strategies incorporating daily screening of respiratory function, a trial of spontaneous breathing, and notification of the physician of successful results have been markedly successful in decreasing patients' ventilator and ICU days (median duration of mechanical ventilation reduced to 4.5 days from 6 days in the control group ($p = 0.003$) without an increased risk of reintubation) [128]. A randomized, controlled trial involving 128 adult patients introduced daily interruptions of sedative infusion medication on intubated patients in a medical intensive care unit until they were awake. These sedation holidays with subsequent resumption of infusion titrated to patient wakefulness shortened the median duration of mechanical ventilation to 4.9 days compared with 7.3 days in the control group ($p = 0.004$) without increased complications. The median intensive care length of stay was also reduced from 9.9 to 6.4 days ($p = 0.02$) [105]. Girard et al. found that the combination of daily assessment of readiness to wean and daily sedative interruption together versus daily assessment of readiness to wean alone reduced the median duration of mechanical ventilation by 3.1 days, intensive care length of stay by 3.8 days, and hospital length of stay by 4.1 days [129].

Re-intubations have been associated with an increased risk of VAPs likely due to the risk of aspiration of pathogens from the oropharynx by patients with subglottic dysfunction after several days of endotracheal intubation [130–132]. Tracking unplanned extubations and implementing measures to decrease these events (0.8–2.2 per 100 endotracheal tube-days) should be part of routine review in an ICU [133–135]. The combined protocols did not however result in excessive re-intubations, and selected patients may also be supported by the use of noninvasive mechanical ventilation both as an initial measure and in select cases to allow early liberation from the mechanical ventilator to further decrease ventilator days [28]. Implementation of daily assessments of readiness to be taken off mechanical ventilation and ventilator liberation protocols hence holds a high level of evidence in the prevention of VAPs.

Early Tracheostomy

Early tracheostomy is a common practice when a prolonged intubation is anticipated. Early tracheostomy has been demonstrated to decrease the risk of developing a VAP. The timing of the intervention however has been defined differently in many studies. Rumbak et al. defined early tracheostomy as earlier than 48 h versus after 14 days among 120 patients in a medical ICU likely to need ventilation for more than 14 days [136]. The ventilator and weaning practices in both groups were the same with all the tracheostomies placed percutaneously under bronchoscopic guidance. The early tracheostomy group showed significantly less mortality (31.7% vs. 61.7%), fewer pneumonias (5% vs. 25%), and a lower rate of accidental extubations (0% vs. 10%). The cumulative frequency of pneumonia in the early tracheostomy group was 80% lower than the delayed group ($p < 0.001$), and the mortality was 50% lower in the early tracheotomy compared with the delayed group ($p < 0.005$). The intervention group also had a shorter ICU stay (4.8 ± 1.4 vs. 16.2 ± 3.8 days) and a shorter duration of mechanical ventilation (7.6 ± 2.0 vs. 17.4 ± 5.3 days). This may have been a function of less sedation in the early tracheostomy group and ability to change the inner cannula of the tracheostomy, hence preventing the buildup of biofilm.

Most other studies comparing early with either late tracheostomy or prolonged intubation have found no differences in VAP rates [137–146]. Blot et al. showed that mortality, duration of mechanical ventilation, duration of ICU stay, and incidence of infections did not differ between patients randomized to undergo a tracheostomy within 4 days when compared to patients who remained intubated with an endotracheal tube for at least 14 days [144]. An RCT study looked at early tracheotomy (after 6–8 days) and late tracheotomy (after 13–15 days). Ventilator-associated pneumonias were observed in 30 patients in the early tracheotomy group (14%; 95% confidence interval [CI], 10–19%) and in 44 patients in the late tracheotomy group (21%; 95% CI, 15–26%) ($p = 0.07$) with a hazard ratio of developing ventilator-associated pneumonia of 0.66 (95% CI, 0.42–1.04) demonstrating also no statistical benefit of early tracheostomy [105]. A meta-analysis looking at nine studies and 2040 patients (early tracheostomy defined as a tracheostomy ≤10 days of intubation) demonstrated a reduction in the use of sedation but did not demonstrate that the early tracheostomy resulted in a reduced risk of a VAP (RR = 0.84; 95% CI = 0.66–1.08; $p = 0.17$). Benefits in mortality [relative risk = 0.88; 95% CI = 0.76–1.00; $p = 0.06$], duration of MV (weighted mean difference (WMD) = −4.46 days; 95% CI = −12.61 to 3.69 days; $p = 0.28$), and length of ICU stay (WMD = −7.57 days; 95% CI = −15.42 to 0.29 days; $p = 0.06$) were not seen [146].

Several subsequent studies were included in a more recent meta-analysis comparing VAP incidence in early (<7 days) vs. late tracheostomy [147]. This meta-analysis included a total 17 RCTs and 3145 patients. Early tracheotomy was associated with a decrease in the incidence of VAPs (OR, 0.59 [95% CI, 0.35–0.99] days) and more ventilator-free days (mean difference [MD], 1.74 [95% CI,

0.48–3.00]). Early tracheotomy also resulted in fewer ICU days (MD, −6.25 [95% CI, −11.22 to −1.28] days) but without any difference in mortality. Hence, early tracheostomy may have some clinical benefit in preventing VAPS in severely ill patients likely to need prolonged ventilation but there is currently insufficient data to determine the impact on duration of mechanical ventilation, length of stay, or mortality.

Ventilator Circuit Management Strategies

Avoiding Routine Changes of Ventilator Circuits

Methods of ventilator circuit management may affect rates of ventilator-associated pneumonia. Preventing or eliminating the bacterial colonization of respiratory tubing could decrease rates of ventilator-associated pneumonias [148]. Colonization of the tubing with potentially pathogenic organisms has been found to mostly originate from the patient [149]. Craven et al. demonstrated that changing the ventilator circuit frequently (every 24 h vs. every 48 h) increased the risk of pneumonia (odds ratio [OR] 2.5, 95% confidence interval [CI] 1.3–4.8) [150]. Dreyfuss et al. also looked at replacing the ventilator circuitry at 48 h versus no change until after 48 h and found no difference in the VAP rates between the groups (11 of 35 and 8 of 28 in Groups 1 and 2, respectively; $p = 0.8$) [151]. Colonization by gram-positive and gram-negative bacteria in the tubing did not differ between the groups. Hence, not changing ventilator circuits appears not to increase the rate of nosocomial pneumonias while not wasting resources (both economic and personnel time) that such circuit changes would require [152]. Additional studies have also shown that there is no benefit in decreasing VAP incidence with frequent circuit exchanges [153–158]. Kotilainen et al. specifically looked at a delayed periodic change of the ventilator circuit (every 72 h vs. weekly changes). There was no difference in VAPs (9.1% vs. 6.2% $p = 0.44$).

Periodic changing of ventilator circuits may have an even lower impact on VAPs when humidified moisture exchangers (HMEs) due to the minimal fluid condensation in the respiratory circuit with its use [159]. There were no differences in VAP incidence when comparing circuit changes at 48 h versus no routine changes when only using HMEs (23.0% vs. 22.9%, $p = 0.98$), concluding that routine circuit exchanges when using a HME is of even less benefit. Changing the ventilator circuit when needed (visibly soiled or malfunctioning tubing) rather than on a fixed schedule hence has a high level of evidence in having no impact on VAP rates or patient outcomes with the economic benefit of decreasing costs.

Heat and Moisture Exchangers or Heated Humidifiers

The use of mechanical ventilation requires conditioning of the ventilator delivered breaths to prevent drying of the mucus and endobronchial periciliary surface by moisture evaporation. Due to the bypassing of inherent mechanisms which contribute to the addition of moisture to the inspired air, resulting from the placement of an artificial airway, mucous clearance is hampered and drying can damage the airway. Heated humidifiers (HH) can prevent this by adding back some moisture by passing over a heated water reservoir. This can however result in the pooling of excess condensation in the tubing of the ventilator circuit. Heat and moisture exchangers (HMEs) are an alternate way to condition the air by capturing heat and moisture from the patient on exhalation. The main difference between the two would be that HH delivers more moisture (44 mg of water vapor per liter of gas) when compared to an HME (26–32 mg of water vapor per liter of gas). Mucociliary dysfunction has been found to only occur after 24–48 h with an absolute humidity level of less than 32 mg water vapor per liter [160]. A randomized study however found the morphological integrity of the respiratory epithelium of 41 patients receiving mechanical ventilation for more than 5 days was compromised less when using a HH at 32 mg H20/L with a relative humidity of 100% versus just using an HME [161].

HMEs were however found to have a statistical benefit in a prospective randomized trial looking at 280 trauma patients who underwent routine circuit changes every 7 days [162]. Kirton et al. randomized patients to either an HME (changed every 24 h) or to a conventional heated wire humidifier. The HME nosocomial VAP rate was lower (6%) compared to 16% in the HH group ($p < 0.05$) with an additional reduction in total ICU days in the HME group. A large meta-analysis pooling the results from nine trials [160–168] including this study revealed a reduction in the relative risk of developing a VAP in the HME group (0.7; 95% CI: 0.50–0.94), with a larger effect on patients ventilated for at least 7 days (five RCTs, relative risk 0.57) [169]. The Kirton et al. study was however the only positive study in the meta-analysis. Two non-randomized studies not included in the review did reveal results in favor of HH [170, 171] but two subsequent randomized trials found no significant differences in VAP rates when comparing HHs and HMEs [172, 173]. The majority of the studies found no significant differences between the two systems [160–173], with several suggesting a likely lower incidence of VAP when using the HH [170–175]. The use of HME in patients who are expected to need mechanical ventilation for 24–48 h can be recommended, whereas HH may be a better choice in patients expected to be intubated for a longer time.

Suctioning Systems: Closed Versus Open Tracheal Suctioning System

The suction of respiratory secretions is necessary in patients with an artificial airway to remove respiratory secretions. This can be done with an open tracheal suctioning system (OTSS) or a closed tracheal suctioning system (CTSS). OTSS uses single-use, disposable suctioning catheters, and CTSS uses reusable suctioning catheters enveloped in a protective plastic and equipped with a suction valve, hence avoiding direct contact of the aspiration catheter. The closed system is not routinely changed unless there is soiling or physical damage (e.g., compromise of protective envelope) and does not require the patient to be disconnected from the respiratory circuit to suction. Only one study has reported a lower incidence of VAP using CTSS [176]. The prospective randomized study reported a non-adjusted lower incidence rate of VAP in circuits equipped with CTSS (7.32 vs. 15.89 per 1000 patient-days, $p = 0.07$). Subsequent meta-analyses by Vonberg et al. [177] and Jongerden et al. [178], however, did not find any benefits of using the closed suctioning system. Two additional randomized studies also found no significant differences in either total VAP incidence or exogenous (bacteria introduced from outside of the patient) VAP incidence [179, 180].

Monitoring Endotracheal Tube Cuff Pressure

The inflatable cuff close to the distal end of the endotracheal tube helps to keep the tube in position in the trachea and also prevents the escape of delivered volumes around the tube. The cuff may also protect against colonized secretions leaking down into the lower respiratory tract. Too much pressure in the cuff may conversely result in tracheal damage however. An intracuff pressure less than 30 cmH_2O has been found to prevent tracheal injury [181, 182]. Rello et al. assessed the risk of pneumonia in patients intubated less than 8 days and demonstrated a trend toward an increased risk of pneumonia (relative risk 2.57, 95% CI = 0.78–8.03) in patients intubated with an intracuff pressure maintained below 20 cmH_2O. In that same cohort, the risk was more significant if the patient was not on antibiotics (relative risk 4.23, 95% CI = 1.12–15.92) [183]. A single-center prospective trial compared frequent cuff pressure assessments using a manometric syringe every 8 h, with a targeted pressure of 24–30 cmH_2O versus infrequent cuff pressure monitoring [184]. There was no advantage to more frequent versus less frequent cuff pressure monitoring. The occurrence of VAPs was similar for both groups (3.6% vs. 5.8%, $p = 0\ 0.37$). The evidence is hence supportive of maintaining an optimal cuff pressure without the need for frequent monitoring.

VAP Prevention Bundles

The bundling of proven infection preventative care processes has been associated with significant and sustained reductions in health care associated conditions, including central line-associated bloodstream infections [185]. Similarly, VAP prevention bundles theoretically should have a greater impact on decreasing VAPs than each intervention individually. Many institutions have devised their own bundle protocols [186–190]; however, there is no consensus on what would constitute an optimal VAP prevention bundle [191, 192].

Blamoun et al. implemented a ventilator bundle (VB) in their medical ICU and compared VAP rates before and after introducing the protocol [187]. The bundle included (1) use of contact isolation when indicated, (2) routine MRSA screening, (3) hand hygiene, (4) oral hygiene for intubated patients, (5) respiratory therapist-driven ventilator liberation protocols including sedation holidays, spontaneous breathing trials (SBT) with notification to the intensivist of readiness to extubate, (6) early tracheostomy (<12 days) if failing the spontaneous breathing trials, and (7) head of bed elevation to 30–45°. The modified aspect of the VB in this study was to include a group of respiratory therapist-driven protocols to focus on minimizing the number of days of intubation. A statistically significant reduction in ventilator-associated pneumonia (VAP), from a median of 14.1 cases/103 ventilator days (interquartile range [IQR] 5 12.1–20.6) to 0 cases/103 ventilator days (IQR 5 0–1.1) was noted ($p = 0.0006$). Hawe et al. looked at how to implement a VAP prevention bundle—initially introduced as a laminated protocol posted by the ventilator in every patient room followed by actively engaging with the team with a method of process improvement [188]. Semi-recumbent patient positioning (30–45° angle), oral care with chlorhexidine, the use of subglottic suction/drainage endotracheal tubes, daily sedation holidays, daily assessments for ventilator weaning, and endotracheal tubing management (including the use of an HME) were implemented in the bundle. VAPs did not decrease until the bundle was actively implemented in the second phase with daily audits of adherence. VAPs dropped from 49 episodes (19.2/1000 ventilator days) when passively implemented to 10 VAPs (7.5/1000 ventilator days) during the active implementation period. There was also a trend toward a lower unit mortality during the active implementation period ($p = 0.06$).

Another VAP prevention protocol was investigated as part of a "Pneumonia Zero" initiative in 181 participating ICUs conducted during a national Spanish multimodal intervention trial implementing a comprehensive evidence-based ventilator-associated pneumonia prevention bundle [193]. The bundle included seven mandatory interventions: (1) education in optimal airway handling, (2) strict hand hygiene with alcohol before airway management, (3) maintenance of cuff pressure, (4) oral hygiene with chlorhexidine, (5) semi-recumbent positioning when able, (6) ventilator day reduction protocols, and (7) the avoidance of elective changes of ventilator circuits, humidifiers, and endotracheal tubes. Additional measures such as selective decontamination of the digestive tract or selective oropharyngeal decontamination, continuous aspiration of subglottic secretions, and short course (2–3 doses) of systemic antibiotics after intubation of patients with decreased consciousness at the time of intubation were encouraged but were only maintained as optional components of the mandatory bundle. The bundle resulted in a decrease in VAPs from 2.4% to 1.9% ($p < 0.0001$). Participating ICUs that continued the use of the implemented bundle for a longer period of time (19–21 months) found further decreases in the VAP incidence to 1.2% ($p < 0.0001$).

Speck et al. identified potential interventions to be included in a VAP bundle with a review of guidelines and literature, but also implemented a 2-step modified Delphi method (structured communication technique and decision-making tool) to gain consensus on the final list of interventions to be included [194]. After collaborating with an interdisciplinary group of clinical experts, the VAP prevention bundle focused on five bedside care processes, which were evidence-based and manageable interventions and which were selected by a large and diverse group of clinical experts that kept the bundle's implementation in mind hence providing a structured approach for developing a new VAP prevention bundle. Obtaining clinician input on which interventions to include increases the likelihood that providers will adhere to the bundle.

References

1. Kollef MH. Epidemiology and risk factors for nosocomial pneumonia. Emphasis on prevention. Clin Chest Med. 1999;20:653–70.
2. Chastre J, Fagon JY. Ventilator-associated pneumonia. Am J Respir Crit Care Med. 2002;165:867–903.
3. Cook DJ, Kollef MH. Risk factors for ICU-acquired pneumonia. JAMA. 1998;279:1605–6.
4. Langer M, Cigada M, Mandelli M, Mosconi P, Tognoni G. Early onset pneumonia: a multicenter study in intensive care units. Intensive Care Med. 1987;13:342–6.
5. Strausbaugh L. Nosocomial respiratory infections. In: Mandell GL, Bennett JE, Dolin R, editors. Principles and practice of infectious diseases. Philadelphia, PA: Churchill Livingstone; 2000. p. 3020–7.
6. American Thoracic Society. Hospital-acquired pneumonia in adults: diagnosis, assessment of severity, initial antimicrobial therapy, and preventive strategies. A consensus statement, American Thoracic Society, November 1995. Am J Respir Crit Care Med. 1996;153:1711–25.
7. Park DR. The microbiology of ventilator-associated pneumonia. Respir Care. 2005;50(6):742–65.
8. Rello J, Ausina V, Ricart M, Castella J, Prats G. Impact of previous antimicrobial therapy on the etiology and outcome of ventilator associated pneumonia. Chest. 1993;104(4):1230–5.
9. Yu VL, Singh N. Excessive antimicrobial usage causes measurable harm to patients with suspected ventilator-associated pneumonia. Intensive Care Med. 2004;30(5):735–8.
10. Dennesen PJ, van der Ven AJ, Kessels AG, Ramsay G, Bonten MJ. Resolution of infectious parameters after antimicrobial therapy in patients with ventilator-associated pneumonia. Am J Respir Crit Care Med. 2001;163(6):1371–5.
11. Rello J, Ricart M, Ausina V, Net A, Prats G. Pneumonia due to Haemophilus influenzae among mechanically ventilated patients. Incidence, outcome, and risk factors. Chest. 1992;102(5):1562–5.
12. Shah PM. Staphylococcus aureus in lower respiratory infections: clinical relevance of antimicrobial resistance. Semin Respir Infect. 2001;16(3):196–202.
13. Stevens DL. Community-acquired Staphylococcus aureus infections: increasing virulence and emerging methicillin resistance in the new millennium. Curr Opin Infect Dis. 2003;16(3):189–91.
14. Montero A, Corbella X, Ariza J. Clinical relevance of Acinetobacter baumannii ventilator-associated pneumonia. Crit Care Med. 2003;31(10):2557–9.
15. Baraibar J, Correa H, Mariscal D, Gallego M, Valles J, Rello J. Risk factors for infection by Acinetobacter baumannii in intubated patients with nosocomial pneumonia. Chest. 1997;112(4):1050–4.
16. Dellit TH, Chan JD, Nathens AB, Skerrett SJ, Hooton TM. Development of ventilator-associated pneumonia guidelines based on local microbiology and resistance patterns. Proceedings of the 42nd Annual Meeting of the Infectious Diseases Society of America, 2004 Sept 30–Oct 3, Boston, Massachusetts. A216.

17. Rello J, Ausina V, Ricart M, Puzo C, Quintana E, Net A, Prats G. Risk factors for infection by Pseudomonas aeruginosa in patients with ventilator-associated pneumonia. Intensive Care Med. 1994;20(3):193–8.
18. Rello J, Rue M, Jubert P, Muses G, Sonora R, Valles J, Niederman MS. Survival in patients with nosocomial pneumonia: impact of the severity of illness and the etiologic agent. Crit Care Med. 1997;25(11):1862–7.
19. Kollef MH, Silver P, Murphy DM, et al. The effect of late-onset ventilator-associated pneumonia in determining patient mortality. Chest. 1995;108:1655–62.
20. Rochwerg B, Brochard L, Elliott MW, Hess D, Hill NS, Nava S, Paolo Navalesi (Members of the Steering Committee), Antonelli M, Brozek J, Conti G, Ferrer M, Guntupalli K, Jaber S, Keenan S, Mancebo J, Mehta S, Suhail Raoof (Members of the Task Force). Official ERS/ATS clinical practice guidelines: noninvasive ventilation for acute respiratory failure. Eur Respir J. 2017;50:1602426.
21. Hilbert G, et al. Noninvasive ventilation in immunosuppressed patients with pulmonary infiltrates, fever, and acute respiratory failure. N Engl J Med. 2001;344:481–7.
22. Pingleton SK, Fagon JY, Leeper KV Jr. Patient selection for clinical investigation of ventilator-associated pneumonia: criteria for evaluating diagnostic techniques. Chest. 1992;102:553S–6S.
23. Rochwerg B, Granton D, Wang DX, et al. High flow nasal cannula compared with conventional oxygen therapy for acute hypoxemic respiratory failure: a systematic review and meta-analysis. Intensive Care Med. 2019;45:563–72.
24. Granton D, Chaudhuri D, Wang D, et al. High-flow nasal cannula compared with conventional oxygen therapy or noninvasive ventilation immediately post extubation: a systematic review and meta-analysis. Crit Care Med. 2020;48:e1129–36.
25. Chaudhuri D, Granton D, Wang DX, et al. High-flow nasal cannula in the immediate postoperative period: a systematic review and meta-analysis. Chest. 2020;158:1934–46.
26. Yasuda H, Okano H, Mayumi T, et al. Post-extubation oxygenation strategies in acute respiratory failure: a systematic review and network meta-analysis. Crit Care (London). 2021;25:135.
27. Frat JP, Thille AW, Mercat A, et al. High-flow oxygen through nasal cannula in acute hypoxemic respiratory failure. N Engl J Med. 2015;372:2185–96.
28. Conti G, Antonelli M, Navalesi P, et al. Noninvasive vs. conventional mechanical ventilation in patients with chronic obstructive pulmonary disease after failure of medical treatment in the ward: a randomized trial. Intensive Care Med. 2002;28:1701–7.
29. Jurjevic M, Matic I, Sakic-Zdravcevic K, et al. Mechanical ventilation in chronic obstructive pulmonary disease patients, noninvasive vs. invasive method (randomized prospective study). Coll Antropol. 2009;33:791–7.
30. Ferrer M, Esquinas A, Arancibia F, et al. Noninvasive ventilation during persistent weaning failure: a randomized controlled trial. Am J Respir Crit Care Med. 2003;168:70–6.
31. Nava S, Ambrosino N, Clini E, et al. Noninvasive mechanical ventilation in the weaning of patients with respiratory failure due to chronic obstructive pulmonary disease. A randomized, controlled trial. Ann Intern Med. 1998;128:721–8.
32. Brochard L, Mancebo J, Wysocki M, Lofaso F, Conti G, Rauss A, et al. Noninvasive ventilation for acute exacerbations of chronic obstructive pulmonary disease. N Engl J Med. 1995;333:817–22.
33. Burns KE, Adhikari NK, Meade MO. A meta-analysis of noninvasive weaning to facilitate liberation from mechanical ventilation. Can J Anaesth. 2006;53:305–15.
34. Keyt H, Faverio P, Restrepo MI. Prevention of ventilator-associated pneumonia in the intensive care unit: a review of the clinically relevant recent advancements. Indian J Med Res. 2014;139(6):814–21.
35. Gunasekera P, Gratrix A. Ventilator-associated pneumonia. BJA Educ. 2016;16(6):198–202.

36. Kollef MH. Ventilator-associated pneumonia. A multivariate analysis. JAMA. 1993;270(16):1965–70.
37. Torres A, Serra-Batlles J, Ros E, et al. Pulmonary aspiration of gastric contents in patients receiving mechanical ventilation: the effect of body position. Ann Intern Med. 1992;116(7):540–3.
38. Drakulovic MB, Torres A, Bauer TT, Nicolas JM, Nogue S, Ferrer M. Supine body position as a risk factor for nosocomial pneumonia in mechanically ventilated patients: a randomised trial. Lancet. 1999;354(9193):1851–8.
39. van Nieuwenhoven CA, Vandenbroucke-Grauls C, van Tiel FH, Joore HC, van Schijndel RJ, van der Tweel I, Ramsay G, Bonten MJ. Feasibility and effects of the semirecumbent position to prevent ventilator-associated pneumonia: a randomized study. Crit Care Med. 2006;34(2):396–402.
40. Bercault N, Wolf M, Runge I, Fleury J-C, Boulain T. Intra hospital transport of critically ill ventilated patients: a risk factor for ventilator-associated pneumonia—a matched cohort study. Crit Care Med. 2005;33:2471–8.
41. Pingleton SK. Enteral nutrition as a risk factor for nosocomial pneumonia. Eur J Clin Microbiol Infect Dis. 1989;8:51–5.
42. Winterbauer RH, Durning RB, Barron E, et al. Aspirated nasogastric feeding solution detected by glucose strips. Ann Intern Med. 1981;95:67–8.
43. Cataldi-Belcher EL, Seltzer MH, Slocum BA, et al. Complications occurring during enteral nutrition support: a prospective study. JPEN. 1983;7:546–52.
44. Reignier R, Mercier E, Le Gouge A, et al. Effect of not monitoring residual gastric volume on risk of ventilator-associated pneumonia in adults receiving mechanical ventilation and early enteral feeding: a randomized controlled trial. JAMA. 2013;309(3):249.
45. Marik PE, Zaloga GP. Early enteral nutrition in acutely ill patients: a systematic review. Crit Care Med. 2001;29:2264–70.
46. Ibrahim EH, Mehringer L, Prentice D, et al. Early versus late enteral feeding of mechanically ventilated patients: results of a clinical trial. JPEN J Parenter Enteral Nutr. 2002;26:174–81.
47. Artinian V, Krayem H, DiGiovine B. Effects of early enteral feeding on the outcome of critically ill mechanically ventilated medical patients. Chest. 2006;129:960–7.
48. Marik PE, Zaloga GP. Gastric versus post-pyloric feeding: a systematic review. Crit Care. 2003;7:R46–51.
49. Jiyong J, Tiancha H, Huiquin W, Jingfen J. Effect of gastric versus post-pyloric feeding on the incidence of pneumonia in critically ill patients: observations from traditional and Bayesian random-effects meta-analysis. Clin Nutr. 2013;32:8–15.
50. Liu Y, Wang Y, Zhang B, Wang J, Xiao Q. Gastric-tube versus post-pyloric feeding in critical patients: a systematic review and meta-analysis of pulmonary aspiration- and nutrition-related outcomes. Eur J Clin Nutr. 2021;75:1337–48.
51. Silk DB, Gow NM. Postoperative starvation after gastrointestinal surgery. Early feeding is beneficial. BMJ. 2001;323:761–2.
52. Lewis SJ, Egger M, Sylvester PA, Thomas S. Early enteral feeding versus 'nil by mouth' after gastrointestinal surgery: systematic review and meta-analysis of controlled trials. BMJ. 2001;323:773–6.
53. Cook DJ, Fuller HD, Guyatt GH, Marshall JC, Leasa D, Hall R, et al. Risk factors for gastrointestinal bleeding in critically ill patients. Canadian Critical Care Trials Group. N Engl J Med. 1994;330:377–81.
54. Donowitz LG, Page MC, Mileur BL, Guenthner SH. Alteration of normal gastric flora in critical care patients receiving antacid and cimetidine therapy. Infect Control. 1986;7:23–6.
55. Cook DJ, Reeve BK, Guyatt GH, Heyland DK, Griffith LE, Buckingham L, et al. Stress ulcer prophylaxis in critically ill patients. Resolving discordant meta-analyses. JAMA. 1996;275:308–14.

56. Cook D, Guyatt G, Marshall J, et al. A comparison of sucralfate and ranitidine for the prevention of upper gastrointestinal bleeding in patients requiring mechanical ventilation. Canadian Critical Care Trials Group. N Engl J Med. 1998;338:791–7.
57. Messori A, Trippoli S, Vaiani M, Gorini M, Corrado A. Bleeding and pneumonia in intensive care patients given ranitidine and sucralfate for prevention of stress ulcer: meta-analysis of randomised controlled trials. BMJ. 2000;321:1103–6.
58. Tryba M, Cook DJ. Gastric alkalinization, pneumonia, and systemic infections: the controversy. Scand J Gastroenterol Suppl. 1995;210:53–9.
59. Cook DJ. Stress ulcer prophylaxis: gastrointestinal bleeding and nosocomial pneumonia. Best evidence synthesis. Scand J Gastroenterol Suppl. 1995;210:48–52.
60. Tryba M. Sucralfate versus antacids or H2-antagonists for stress ulcer prophylaxis: a meta-analysis on efficacy and pneumonia rate. Crit Care Med. 1991;19:942–9.
61. Tryba M. Prophylaxis of stress ulcer bleeding. A meta-analysis. J Clin Gastroenterol. 1991;13(Suppl 2):S44–55.
62. Cook DJ, Laine LA, Guyatt GH, Raffin TA. Nosocomial pneumonia and the role of gastric pH. A meta-analysis. Chest. 1991;100:7–13.
63. Bornstain C, Azoulay E, De Lassence A, et al. Sedation, sucralfate, and antibiotic use are potential means for protection against early-onset ventilator-associated pneumonia. Clin Infect Dis. 2004;38:1401–8.
64. Stack PE, Thomas E. Pharmacobezoar: an evolving new entity. Dig Dis. 1995;13:356–64.
65. Saint S, Matthay MA. Risk reduction in the intensive care unit. Am J Med. 1998;105:515–23.
66. Falagas ME, Siempos II, Bliziotis IA, Michalopoulos A. Administration of antibiotics via the respiratory tract for the prevention of ICU-acquired pneumonia: a meta-analysis of comparative trials. Crit Care (London, England). 2006;10(4):R123.
67. Klompas M, Speck K, Howell MD, et al. Reappraisal of routine oral care with chlorhexidine gluconate for patients receiving mechanical ventilation: systematic review and meta-analysis. JAMA Intern Med. 2014;174:751–61.
68. Fourrier F, Cau-Pottier E, Boutigny H, Roussel-Delvallez M, Jourdain M, Chopin C. Effects of dental plaque antiseptic decontamination on bacterial colonization and nosocomial infections in critically ill patients. Intensive Care Med. 2000;26(9):1239–47.
69. Genuit T, Bochicchio G, Napolitano LM, Mccarter RJ, Roghman MC. Prophylactic chlorhexidine oral rinse decreases ventilator associated pneumonia in surgical ICU patients. Surg Infect. 2001;2(1):5–18.
70. Segers P, Speekenbrink RG, Ubbink DT, Van Ogtrop ML, De Mol BA. Prevention of nosocomial infection in cardiac surgery by decontamination of the nasopharynx and oropharynx with chlorhexidine gluconate: a randomized controlled trial. JAMA. 2006;296(20):2460–6.
71. Deriso AJ II, Ladowski JS, Dillon TA, Justice JW, Peterson AC. Chlorhexidine gluconate 0.12% oral rinse reduces the incidence of total nosocomial respiratory infection and nonprophylactic systemic antibiotic use in patients undergoing heart surgery. Chest. 1996;109(6):1556–61.
72. Houston S, Hougland P, Anderson JJ, Larocco M, Kennedy V, Gentry LO. Effectiveness of 0.12% chlorhexidine gluconate oral rinse in reducing prevalence of nosocomial pneumonia in patients undergoing heart surgery. Am J Crit Care. 2002;11(6):567–70.
73. Fourrier F, Dubois D, Pronnier P, et al. Effect of gingival and dental plaque antiseptic decontamination on nosocomial infections acquired in the intensive care unit: a double-blind placebo-controlled multicenter study. Crit Care Med. 2005;33(8):1728–35.
74. Koeman M, Van Der Ven AJ, Hak E, et al. Oral decontamination with chlorhexidine reduces the incidence of ventilator-associated pneumonia. Am J Respir Crit Care Med. 2006;173(12):1348–55.
75. Tantipong H, Morkchareonpong C, Jaiyindee S, Thamlikitkul V. Randomized controlled trial and meta-analysis of oral decontamination with 2% chlorhexidine solution for the prevention of ventilator associated pneumonia. Infect Control Hosp Epidemiol. 2008;29(2):131–6.

76. Bellissimo-Rodrigues F, Bellissimo-Rodrigues WT, Viana JM, et al. Effectiveness of oral rinse with chlorhexidine in preventing nosocomial respiratory tract infections among intensive care unit patients. Infect Control Hosp Epidemiol. 2009;30(10):952–8.
77. Panchabhai TS, Dangayach NS, Krishnan A, Kothari VM, Karnad DR. Oropharyngeal cleansing with 0.2% chlorhexidine for prevention of nosocomial pneumonia in critically ill patients: an open-label randomized trial with 0.01% potassium permanganate as control. Chest. 2009;135(5):1150–6.
78. Scannapieco FA, Yu J, Raghavendran K, et al. A randomized trial of chlorhexidine gluconate on oral bacterial pathogens in mechanically ventilated patients. Crit Care (London, England). 2009;13(4):R117.
79. Caton JG, Blieden TM, Lowenguth RA, Frantz BJ, Wagener CJ, Doblin JM, Stein SH, Proskin HM. Comparison between mechanical cleaning and an antimicrobial rinse for the treatment and prevention of interdental gingivitis. J Clin Periodontol. 1993;20:172–8.
80. Nardi G, Di Silvestre AD, De Monte A, Massarutti D, Proietti A, Grazia Troncon M, Lesa L, Zussino M. Reduction in gram-positive pneumonia and antibiotic consumption following the use of a SDD protocol including nasal and oral mupirocin. Eur J Emerg Med. 2001;8:203–14.
81. Scannapieco FA, Rethman MP. The relationship between periodontal diseases and respiratory diseases. Dent Today. 2003;22:79–83.
82. Heo SM, Haase EM, Lesse AJ, Gill SR, Scannapieco FA. Genetic relationships between respiratory pathogens isolated from dental plaque and bronchoalveolar lavage fluid from patients in the intensive care unit undergoing mechanical ventilation. Clin Infect Dis. 2008;47(12):1562–70.
83. Mori H, Hirasawa H, Oda S, Shiga H, Matsuda K, Nakamura M. Oral care reduces incidence of ventilator associated pneumonia in ICU populations. Intensive Care Med. 2006;32:230–6.
84. Price R, MacLennan G, Glen J. Selective digestive or oropharyngeal decontamination and topical oropharyngeal chlorhexidine for prevention of death in general intensive care: systematic review and network meta-analysis. BMJ. 2014;348:g2197.
85. Zhao T, Wu X, Zhang Q, Li C, Worthington HV, Hua F. Oral hygiene care for critically ill patients to prevent ventilator-associated pneumonia. Cochrane Database Syst Rev. 2020;12(12):CD008367.
86. Klompas M. Oropharyngeal decontamination with antiseptics to prevent ventilator-associated pneumonia: rethinking the benefits of chlorhexidine. Semin Respir Crit Care Med. 2017;38:381–90.
87. Silvestri L, Van Saene HK, Milanese M, Gregori D, Gullo A. Selective decontamination of the digestive tract reduces bacterial bloodstream infection and mortality in critically ill patients. Systematic review of randomized, controlled trials. J Hosp Infect. 2007;65(3):187–203.
88. De Smet AM, Kluytmans JA, Cooper BS, et al. Decontamination of the digestive tract and oropharynx in ICU patients. N Engl J Med. 2009;360(1):20–31.
89. Nathens AB, Marshall JC. Selective decontamination of the digestive tract in surgical patients: a systematic review of the evidence. Arch Surg. 1999;134:170–6.
90. D'Amico R, Pifferi S, Leonetti C, Torri V, Tinazzi A, Liberati A. Effectiveness of antibiotic prophylaxis in critically ill adult patients: systematic review of randomized controlled trials. BMJ. 1998;316:1275–85.
91. Hurley JC. Prophylaxis with enteral antibiotics in ventilated patients: selective decontamination or selective cross-infection? Antimicrob Agents Chemother. 1995;39:941–7.
92. Kollef MH. The role of selective digestive tract decontamination on mortality and respiratory tract infections. A meta-analysis. Chest. 1994;105:1101–8.
93. Heyland DK, Cook DJ, Jaeschke R, Griffith L, Lee HN, Guyatt GH. Selective decontamination of the digestive tract. An overview. Chest. 1994;105:1221–9.
94. Meta-analysis of randomized controlled trials of selective decontamination of the digestive tract. Selective Decontamination of the Digestive Tract Trialists' Collaborative Group. BMJ. 1993;307:525–32.

95. Vandenbroucke-Grauls CM, Vandenbroucke JP. Effect of selective decontamination of the digestive tract on respiratory tract infections and mortality in the intensive care unit. Lancet. 1991;338:859–62.
96. Lode H, Höffken G, Kemmerich B, Schaberg T. Systemic and endotracheal antibiotic prophylaxis of nosocomial pneumonia in ICU. Intensive Care Med. 1992;18(Suppl 1):S24–7.
97. Kimura A, Mochizuki T, Nishizawa K, Mashiko K, Yamamoto Y, Otsuka T. Trimethoprim-sulfamethoxazole for the prevention of methicillin-resistant Staphylococcus aureus pneumonia in severely burned patients. J Trauma. 1998;45:383–7.
98. Sirvent JM, Torres A, El-Ebiary M, Castro P, de Batlle J, Bonet A. Protective effect of intravenously administered cefuroxime against nosocomial pneumonia in patients with structural coma. Am J Respir Crit Care Med. 1997;155:1729–34.
99. Plantinga NL, de Smet AMGA, Oostdijk EAN, de Jonge E, Camus C, Krueger WA, Bergmans D, Reitsma JB, Bonten MJM. Selective digestive and oropharyngeal decontamination in medical and surgical ICU patients: individual patient data meta-analysis. Clin Microbiol Infect. 2018;24:505–13.
100. Pittet D, Eggimann P, Rubinovitch B. Prevention of ventilator-associated pneumonia by oral decontamination: just another SDD study? Am J Respir Crit Care Med. 2001;164:338–9.
101. Van Nieuwenhoven CA, Buskens E, Van Tiel FH, Bonten MJ. Relationship between methodological trial quality and the effects of selective digestive decontamination on pneumonia and mortality in critically ill patients. JAMA. 2001;286(3):335–40.
102. Bo L, Li J, Tao T, et al. Probiotics for preventing ventilator-associated pneumonia. Cochrane Database Syst Rev. 2014;(10):CD009066.
103. Zeng J, Wang CT, Zhang FS, et al. Effect of probiotics on the incidence of ventilator-associated pneumonia in critically ill patients: a randomized controlled multicenter trial. Intensive Care Med. 2016;42:1018–28.
104. Cheema HA, Shahid A, Ayyan M, Mustafa B, Zahid A, Fatima M, Ehsan M, Athar F, Duric N, Szakmany T. Probiotics for the prevention of ventilator-associated pneumonia: an updated systematic review and meta-analysis of randomised controlled trials. Nutrients. 2022;14:1600.
105. Kress JP, Pohlman AS, O'Connor MF, Hall JB. Daily interruption of sedative infusions in critically ill patients undergoing mechanical ventilation. N Engl J Med. 2000;342:1471–7.
106. Cook DJ, Walter SD, Cook RJ, et al. Incidence of and risk factors for ventilator-associated pneumonia in critically ill patients. Ann Intern Med. 1998;129:433–40.
107. Girard TD, Kress JP, Fuchs BD, Thomason JW, Schweickert WD, Pun BT, et al. Efficacy and safety of a paired sedation and ventilator weaning protocol for mechanically ventilated patients in intensive care (awakening and breathing controlled trial): a randomized controlled trial. Lancet. 2008;371:126–34.
108. Kollef MH, Levy NT, Ahrens TS, Schaiff R, Prentice D, Sherman G. The use of continuous IV sedation is associated with prolongation of mechanical ventilation. Chest. 1998;114:541–8.
109. Schweickert WD, Gehlbach BK, Pohlman AS, Hall JB, Kress JP. Daily interruption of sedative infusions and complications of critical illness in mechanically ventilated patients. Crit Care Med. 2004;32:1272–6.
110. Liu J, Zhang S, Chen J, Mao Y, Shao X, Li Y, Cao J, Zheng W, Zhang B, Zong Z. Risk factors for ventilator-associated events: a prospective cohort study. Am J Infect Control. 2019;47:744–9.
111. Johanson WG, Pierce AK, Sanford JP. Changing pharyngeal bacterial flora of hospitalized patients. Emergence of gram-negative bacilli. N Engl J Med. 1969;281(21):1137–40.
112. Johanson WG Jr, Pierce AK, Sanford JP, Thomas GD. Nosocomial respiratory infections with gram-negative bacilli. The significance of colonization of the respiratory tract. Ann Intern Med. 1972;77(5):701–6.
113. Craven DE, Steger KA. Nosocomial pneumonia in mechanically ventilated adult patients: epidemiology and prevention in 1996. Semin Respir Infect. 1996;11:32–53.

114. Johanson WG, Dever LL. Nosocomial pneumonia. Intensive Care Med. 2003;29(1):23–9.
115. Mahul P, Auboyer C, Jospe R, et al. Prevention of nosocomial pneumonia in intubated patients: respective role of mechanical subglottic secretions drainage and stress ulcer prophylaxis. Intensive Care Med. 1992;18(1):20–5.
116. Bouza E, Perez MJ, Munoz P, Rincon C, Barrio JM, Hortal J. Continuous aspiration of subglottic secretions in the prevention of ventilator-associated pneumonia in the postoperative period of major heart surgery. Chest. 2008;134(5):938–46.
117. Kollef MH, Skubas NJ, Sundt TM. A randomized clinical trial of continuous aspiration of subglottic secretions in cardiac surgery patients. Chest. 1999;116(5):1339–46.
118. Valles J, Artigas A, Rello J, et al. Continuous aspiration of subglottic secretions in preventing ventilator-associated pneumonia. Ann Intern Med. 1995;122(3):179–86.
119. Smulders K, Van Der Hoeven H, Weers-Pothoff I, Vandenbroucke-Grauls C. A randomized clinical trial of intermittent subglottic secretion drainage in patients receiving mechanical ventilation. Chest. 2002;121(3):858–62.
120. Lorente L, Lecuona M, Jimenez A, Mora ML, Sierra A. Influence of an endotracheal tube with polyurethane cuff and subglottic secretion drainage on pneumonia. Am J Respir Crit Care Med. 2007;176(11):1079–83.
121. Yang CS, Qiu HB, Zhu YP, et al. Effect of continuous aspiration of subglottic secretions on the prevention of ventilator-associated pneumonia in mechanically ventilated patients: a prospective, randomized, controlled clinical trial. Zhonghua Nei Ke Za Zhi. 2008;47(8):625–9.
122. Zheng RQ, Lin H, Shao J, et al. A clinical study of subglottic secretion drainage for prevention of ventilation associated pneumonia. Zhongguo Wei Zhong Bing Ji Jiu Yi Xue. 2008;20(6):338–40.
123. Dezfulian C, Shojania K, Collard HR, et al. Subglottic secretion drainage for preventing ventilator-associated pneumonia: a meta-analysis. Am J Med. 2005;118(1):11–8.
124. Caroff DA, Li L, Muscedere J, Klompas M. Subglottic secretion drainage and objective outcomes. Crit Care Med. 2016;44(4):830–40.
125. Pozuelo-Carrascosa DP, Herráiz-Adillo Á, Alvarez-Bueno C, et al. Subglottic secretion drainage for preventing ventilator-associated pneumonia: an overview of systematic reviews and an updated meta-analysis. Eur Respir Rev. 2020;29:190107.
126. Torres A, Aznar R, Gatell JM, et al. Incidence, risk, and prognosis factors of nosocomial pneumonia in mechanically ventilated patients. Am Rev Respir Dis. 1990;142:523–8.
127. Myny D, Depuydt P, Colardyn F, Blot S. Ventilator associated pneumonia in a tertiary care ICU: analysis of risk factors for acquisition and mortality. Acta Clin Belg. 2005;60:114–21.
128. Ely EW, Baker AM, Dunagan DP, et al. Effect on the duration of mechanical ventilation of identifying patients capable of breathing spontaneously. N Engl J Med. 1996;335(25):1864–9.
129. Girard TD, Kress JP, Fuchs BD, et al. Efficacy and safety of a paired sedation and ventilator weaning protocol for mechanically ventilated patients in intensive care (awakening and breathing controlled trial): a randomized controlled trial. Lancet. 2008;371(9607):126–34.
130. Torres A, Gatell JM, Aznar E, El-Ebiary M, Puig de la Bellacasa J, González J. Reintubation increases the risk of nosocomial pneumonia in patients needing mechanical ventilation. Am J Respir Crit Care Med. 1995;152:137–41.
131. Leal-Noval SR, Márquez-Vacaro JA, García-Curiel A, et al. Nosocomial pneumonia in patients undergoing heart surgery. Crit Care Med. 2000;28:935–40.
132. Kollef MH, von Harz B, Prentice D, et al. Patient transport from intensive care increases the risk of developing ventilator-associated pneumonia. Chest. 1997;112:765–73.
133. Lorente L, Huidobro MS, Martín MM, Jiménez A, Mora ML. Accidental catheter removal in critically ill patients: a prospective and observational study. Crit Care. 2004;8:229–33.
134. Chiang AA, Lee KC, Lee JC, Wei CH. Effectiveness of a continuous quality improvement program aiming to reduce unplanned extubation: a prospective study. Intensive Care Med. 1996;22:1269–71.

135. Carrión M, Ayuso D, Marcos M, et al. Accidental removal of endotracheal and nasogastric tubes and intravascular catheters. Crit Care Med. 2000;28:63–6.
136. Rumbak MJ, Newton M, Truncale T, Schwartz SW, Adams JW, Hazard PB. A prospective, randomized, study comparing early percutaneous dilational tracheotomy to prolonged translaryngeal intubation (delayed tracheotomy) in critically ill medical patients. Crit Care Med. 2004;32:1689–94.
137. Bouderka MA, Fakhir B, Bouaggad A, Hmamouchi B, Hamoudi D, Harti A. Early tracheostomy versus prolonged endotracheal intubation in severe head injury. J Trauma. 2004;57:251–4.
138. Rodríguez JL, Steinberg SM, Luchetti FA, Gibbons KJ, Taheri PA, Flint LM. Early tracheostomy for primary airway management in the surgical critical care setting. Surgery. 1990;108:655–9.
139. Saffle JR, Morris SE, Edelman L. Early tracheostomy does not improve outcome in burn patients. J Burn Care Rehabil. 2002;23:431–8.
140. Brook AD, Sherman G, Malen J, Kollef MH. Early versus late tracheostomy in patients who require prolonged mechanical ventilation. Am J Crit Care. 2000;9:352–9.
141. Niederman MS, Ferranti RD, Zeigler A, Merrill WW, Reynolds HY. Respiratory infection complicating longterm tracheostomy. The implication of persistent gramnegative tracheobronchial colonization. Chest. 1984;85:39–44.
142. El-Naggar M, Sadagopan S, Levine H, Kantor H, Collins VJ. Factors influencing choice between tracheostomy and prolonged translaryngeal intubation in acute respiratory failure: a prospective study. Anesth Analg. 1976;55:195–201.
143. Sugerman HJ, Wolfe L, Pasquale MD, et al. Multicenter, randomized, prospective trial of early tracheostomy. J Trauma. 1997;43:741–7.
144. Blot F, Similowski T, Trouillet JL, et al. Early tracheotomy versus prolonged endotracheal intubation in unselected severely ill ICU patients. Intensive Care Med. 2008;34(10):1779–87.
145. Terragni PP, Antonelli M, Fumagalli R, Faggiano C, Berardino M, Pallavicini FB, Miletto A, Mangione S, Sinardi AU, Pastorelli M, Vivaldi N, Pasetto A, Della Rocca G, Urbino R, Filippini C, Pagano E, Evangelista A, Ciccone G, Mascia L, Ranieri VM. Early vs late tracheotomy for prevention of pneumonia in mechanically ventilated adult ICU patients. A randomized controlled trial. JAMA. 2010;303(15):1483–9. https://doi.org/10.1001/jama.2010.447.
146. Meng L, Wang C, Li J, Zhang J. Early vs late tracheostomy in critically ill patients: a systematic review and meta-analysis. Clin Respir J. 2016;10:684–92.
147. Chorath K, Hoang A, Rajasekaran K, Moreira A. Association of early vs late tracheostomy placement with pneumonia and ventilator days in critically ill patients: a meta-analysis. JAMA Otolaryngol Head Neck Surg. 2021;147(5):450–9.
148. Craven DE, Kunches LM, Kilinsky V, Lichtenberg DA, Make BJ, McCabe WR. Risk factors for pneumonia and fatality in patients receiving continuous mechanical ventilation. Am Rev Respir Dis. 1986;133(5):792–6.
149. Craven DE, Goularte TA, Make BJ. Contaminated condensate in mechanical ventilator circuits: a risk factor for nosocomial pneumonia? Am Rev Respir Dis. 1984;129(4):625–8.
150. Craven DE, Connolly MG Jr, Lichtenberg DA, Primeau PJ, McCabe WR. Contamination of mechanical ventilators with tubing changes every 24 or 48 hours. N Engl J Med. 1982;306(25):1505–9.
151. Dreyfuss D, Djedaini K, Weber P, Brun P, Lanore JJ, Rahmani J, et al. Prospective study of nosocomial pneumonia and of patient and circuit colonization during mechanical ventilation with circuit changes every 48 hours versus no change. Am Rev Respir Dis. 1991;143(4 Pt 1):738–43.
152. Tablan OC, Anderson LJ, Arden NH, Breiman RF, Butler JC, McNeil MM, the Hospital Infection Control Practice Advisory Committee, Centers for Disease Control and Prevention. Guideline for prevention of nosocomial pneumonia. Am J Infect Control. 1994;22(4):247–92.

153. Fink JB, Krause SA, Barrett L, Schaaff D, Alex CG. Extending ventilator circuit change interval beyond 2 days reduces the likelihood of ventilator-associated pneumonia. Chest. 1998;113:405–11.
154. Han JN, Liu YP, Ma S, et al. Effects of decreasing the frequency of ventilator circuit changes to every 7 days on the rate of ventilator-associated pneumonia in a Beijing hospital. Respir Care. 2001;46:891–6.
155. Gastmeier P, Wendt C, Ruden H. Breathing circuit exchange in intensive care. Once daily once weekly? Anaesthesist. 1997;46:943–8.
156. Long MN, Wickstrom G, Grimes A, Benton CF, Belcher B, Stamm AM. Prospective, randomized study of ventilator associated pneumonia in patients with one versus three ventilator circuit changes per week. Infect Control Hosp Epidemiol. 1996;17:14–9.
157. Hess D, Burns E, Romagnoli D, Kacmarek RM. Weekly ventilator circuit changes. A strategy to reduce costs without affecting pneumonia rates. Anesthesiology. 1995;82:903–11.
158. Kotilainen HR, Keroac MA. Cost analysis and clinical impact of weekly ventilator circuit changes in patients in intensive care unit. Am J Infect Control. 1997;25:117–20.
159. Lorente L, Lecuona M, Galván R, Ramos MJ, Mora ML, Sierra A. Periodically changing ventilator circuits is not necessary to prevent ventilator-associated pneumonia when a heat and moisture exchanger it is used. Infect Control Hosp Epidemiol. 2004;25:1077–82.
160. Williams R, Rankin N, Smith T, Galler D, Seakins P. Relationship between the humidity and temperature of inspired gas and the function of the airway mucosa. Crit Care Med. 1996;24:1920–9.
161. Hurni JM, Feihl F, Lazor R, Leuenberger P, Perret C. Safety of combined heat and moisture exchanger filters in long-term mechanical ventilation. Chest. 1997;111:686–91.
162. Kirton OC, DeHaven B, Morgan J, Morejon O, Civetta J. A prospective, randomized comparison of an in-line heat moisture exchange filter and heated wire humidifiers: rates of ventilator-associated early-onset (community-acquired) or late-onset (hospital-acquired) pneumonia and incidence of endotracheal tube occlusion. Chest. 1997;112:1055–9.
163. Martin C, Perrin G, Gevaudan MJ, Saux P, Gouin F. Heat and moisture exchangers and vaporizing humidifiers in the intensive care unit. Chest. 1990;97:144–9.
164. Roustan JP, Kienlen J, Aubas S, Du Cailar J. Comparison of hydrophobic heat and moisture exchangers with heated humidifier during prolonged mechanical ventilation. Intensive Care Med. 1992;18:97–100.
165. Dreyfuss D, Djedaïni K, Gros I, et al. Mechanical ventilation with heated humidifiers or heat and moisture exchangers: effects on patient colonization and incidence of nosocomial pneumonia. Am J Respir Crit Care Med. 1995;151:986–92.
166. Branson R, Davis K, Campbell RS, Johnson DJ, Porembka DT. Humidification in the intensive care unit. Prospective study of a new protocol utilizing heated humidification and a hygroscopic condenser humidifier. Chest. 1993;104:1800–5.
167. Kollef MH, Shapiro SD, Boyd V, et al. A randomized clinical trial comparing an extended-use hygroscopic condenser humidifier with heated-water humidification in mechanically ventilated patients. Chest. 1998;113:759–67.
168. Memish ZA, Oni GA, Djazmati W, Cunningham G, Mah MW. A randomized trial to compare the effects of a heat and moisture exchanger with a heated humidifying system on the occurrence rate of ventilator-associated pneumonia. Am J Infect Control. 2001;29:301–5.
169. Kola A, Eckmanns T, Gastmeier P. Efficacy of heat and moisture exchangers in preventing ventilator-associated pneumonia: meta-analysis of randomized controlled trials. Intensive Care Med. 2005;31:5–11.
170. Cohen IL, Weinberg PF, Alan I, Rowinsky GS. Endotracheal tube occlusion associated with the use of heat and moisture exchangers in the intensive care unit. Crit Care Med. 1988;16:277–9.

171. Blin F, Fraïsse F, Chauveau P, et al. Incidence of nosocomial pneumonias among 1788 ventilated patients in 6 ICU according to the type of humidification used. Intensive Care Med. 1996;22(Suppl 1):S324.
172. Lacherade JC, Auburtin M, Cerf C, et al. Impact of humidification systems on ventilator-associated pneumonia: a randomized multicenter trial. Am J Respir Crit Care Med. 2005;172:1276–82.
173. Boots RJ, George N, Faoagali JL, Druery J, Dean K, Heller RF. Double-heater-wire circuits and heat- and moisture exchangers and the risk of ventilator-associated pneumonia. Crit Care Med. 2006;34:687–93.
174. Misset B, Escudier B, Rivara D, Leclercq B, Nitenberg G. Heat and moisture exchanger vs heated humidifier during long-term mechanical ventilation. A prospective randomized study. Chest. 1991;100:160–3.
175. Lorente L, Lecuona M, Jiménez A, Mora ML, Sierra A. Ventilator-associated pneumonia using a heated humidifier or a heat and moisture exchanger-randomized controlled trial [ISRCTN88724583]. Crit Care. 2006;10:R116.
176. Combes P, Fauvage B, Oleyer C. Nosocomial pneumonia in mechanically ventilated patients, a prospective randomised evaluation of the Stericath closed suctioning system. Intensive Care Med. 2000;26:878–82.
177. Vonberg R-P, Eckmanns T, Welte T, Gastmeier P. Impact of the suctioning system (open vs. closed) on the incidence of ventilation-associated pneumonia: meta-analysis of randomized controlled trials. Intensive Care Med. 2006;32:1329–35.
178. Jongerden IP, Rovers MM, Grypdonck MH, Bonten MJ. Open and closed endotracheal suction systems in mechanically ventilated intensive care patients: a meta-analysis. Crit Care Med. 2007;35(1):260–70.
179. Lorente L, Lecuona M, García C, Mora ML, Sierra A. Ventilator-associated pneumonia using a closed versus an open tracheal suction system. Crit Care Med. 2005;33:115–9.
180. Lorente L, Lecuona M, Jiménez A, Mora ML, Sierra A. Tracheal suction by closed system without daily change versus open system. Intensive Care Med. 2006;32:538–44.
181. Lewis FR Jr, Schiobohm RM, Thomas AN. Prevention of complications from prolonged tracheal intubation. Am J Surg. 1978;135:452–7.
182. Wain JC. Postintubation tracheal stenosis. Chest Surg Clin N Am. 2003;13:231–46.
183. Rello J, Sonora R, Jubert P, Artigas A, Rue M, Valles J. Pneumonia in intubated patients: role of respiratory airway care. Am J Respir Crit Care Med. 1996;154:111–5.
184. Letvin A, Kremer P, Silver PC, Samih N, Reed-Watts P, Kollef MH. Frequent versus infrequent monitoring of endotracheal tube cuff pressures. Respir Care. 2018;63:495–501.
185. Pronovost PJ, Berenholtz SM, Needham DM. Translating evidence into practice: a model for large scale knowledge translation. BMJ. 2008;337:a1714. https://doi.org/10.1136/bmj.a1714.
186. Cocanour CS, Peninger M, Domonoske BD, et al. Decreasing ventilator associated pneumonia in a trauma ICU. J Trauma. 2006;61(1):122–129; discussion 129–30.
187. Blamoun J, Alfakir M, Rella ME, et al. Efficacy of an expanded ventilator bundle for the reduction of ventilator-associated pneumonia in the medical intensive care unit. Am J Infect Control. 2009;37(2):172–5.
188. Hawe CS, Ellis KS, Cairns CJ, Longmate A. Reduction of ventilator associated pneumonia: active versus passive guideline implementation. Intensive Care Med. 2009;35(7):1180–6.
189. Rello J, Lode H, Cornaglia G, Masterton R. A European care bundle for prevention of ventilator-associated pneumonia. Intensive Care Med. 2010;36(5):773–80.
190. Berenholtz S, Pham J, Thompson D, Needham D, Lubomski L, Hyzy R, Welsh R, Cosgrove S, Sexton B, Colantuoni E, Watson S, Goeschel C, Pronovost P. Collaborative cohort study of an intervention to reduce ventilator-associated pneumonia in the intensive care unit. Infect Control Hosp Epidemiol. 2011;32(4):305–14.

191. Wip C, Napolitano L. Bundles to prevent ventilator-associated pneumonia: how valuable are they? Curr Opin Infect Dis. 2009;22(2):159–66.
192. Zilberberg MD, Shorr AF, Kollef MH. Implementing quality improvements in the intensive care unit: ventilator bundle as an example. Crit Care Med. 2009;37(1):305–9.
193. Álvarez-Lerma F, et al. Prevention of ventilator-associated pneumonia: the multimodal approach of the Spanish ICU "pneumonia zero" program. Crit Care Med. 2018;46:181–8.
194. Speck K, Rawat N, Weiner NC, Tujuba HG, Farley D, Berenholtz S. A systematic approach for developing a ventilator-associated pneumonia prevention bundle. Am J Infect Control. 2016;44(6):652–6.

Chapter 6
Infection Prevention Challenges in the Medical Intensive Care Unit (MICU)

Brandy McKelvy, Jennifer Cortes, and Anabelle Keene

Introduction

In this chapter, we will discuss a variety of issues that occur in patients requiring hospital stays in the medical intensive care unit (MICU) for a long period of time. Patients who are admitted to the MICU frequently have protracted disease states. We will examine some of the challenges encountered while taking care of patients who are at risk for prolonged hospital stays and at risk for many secondary and hospital-acquired infections. Preventing secondary infections in patients on chronic mechanical ventilation and in those who require frequent readmissions is one of the most important ways to decrease ICU length of stay. We will examine the troubles which emerged while taking care of complicated medical conditions such as COVID-19 with immunosuppression both of which put patients at risk for prolonged ICU stays and nefarious infections.

This chapter will explore some of the challenges associated with avoidance of infection in critically ill patients with prolonged mechanical ventilation and those with tracheostomy. We will describe the difficulties that occur with prolonged intubation and mechanical ventilation requiring tracheostomy and the options to reduce ventilator-associated pneumonia (VAP) in patients with respiratory failure with tracheostomy. We will confer the need, risks, and benefits of tracheostomy placed in

B. McKelvy (✉)
McGovern Medical School, Houston, TX, USA
e-mail: Brandy.J.McKelvy@uth.tmc.edu

J. Cortes
Department of Pharmacy, Memorial Herman Hospital-TMC, Houston, TX, USA
e-mail: Jennifer.Cortes@memorialhermann.org

A. Keene
Memorial Herman Hospital-TMC, Houston, TX, USA
e-mail: Anabelle.Keene@memorialhermann.org

M. Ellsworth, L. Ostrosky-Zeichner (eds.), *Infection Prevention in the Intensive Care Setting*, https://doi.org/10.1007/978-3-031-67062-6_6

patients with prolonged mechanical ventilation regardless of the underlying lung pathology including those on ECMO.

We will identify emerging infections witnessed in the immunocompromised COIVD-19 patients and describe some ideas to screen for and mediate the risk of secondary infections. We will discuss the evolution of prolonged mechanical ventilation in COVID-19 patients over the last 2 years with the increased risk of opportunistic infections.

COVID-19 patients frequently require extracorporeal membrane oxygenation (ECMO) support. These patients require extended ECMO runs, previously the average time was 2 weeks, but now has extended to 3–6 months, or sometimes longer. Patients require mechanical ventilator for the majority of time on ECMO and eventually need a tracheostomy. Despite the growing number of patients on ECMO since the beginning or the pandemic, there are currently no adequate guideline recommendations on how to prevent infections in the ECMO population.

Unique challenges found in the MICU include stress ulcer prophylaxis because MICU patients have more comorbidities that increase their risk for gastrointestinal bleeding. We will review the use of proton pump inhibitors (PPIs) in the ICU and how they convey a risk of infection.

Mechanical Ventilation and the MICU

Patients admitted to the MICU are more likely to have diseases that will need prolonged intubation and mechanical ventilation. These are patients with conditions such as hypoxic respiratory failure due to Adult-Respiratory Distress Syndrome (ARDS). ARDS can occur due to viral illness including COVID-19, other viruses (influenza A, etc), or disease states such as pancreatitis, bacterial and aspiration pneumonias, sepsis, and sometimes trauma and burns. Many patients with ARDS will require mechanical ventilation greater than 2 weeks and likely need placement of tracheostomy. Patients with other types of chronic lung diseases like chronic obstructive pulmonary disease (COPD), interstitial lung disease (ILD), or cystic fibrosis may require long-term ventilation necessitating a tracheostomy. Another group of patients admitted to the MICU who require prolonged mechanical ventilation are those with neuromuscular disorders, severe deconditioning with critical care myopathy/neuropathy and those with spinal cord injuries with paraplegia or tetraplegia.

MICU in the Time of COVID-19

Since the pandemic began, patients with COIVD-19 and ARDS have been requiring extended stays on mechanical ventilation. The nationwide average time on the ventilator has at least doubled. Bain et al., reported the median duration of mechanical ventilation within patients with COVID-19 to be 13.5 days compared with their pre-pandemic data: viral ARDS = 7.5 days, bacterial ARDS = 8.0 days, and culture negative ARDS = 7.0 days [1]. ICUs across the country have seen increased length of stay due to COVID-19 infections. In patients who have ARDS and also require ECMO, we are seeing even longer days on mechanical ventilation up to 6 months or more. The current average length of stay at our intuition for patients on ECMO and mechanical ventilation is 58.22 days with a median time of 44 days. The longest duration of mechanical ventilation and ECMO is 174 days [unpublished data Memorial Hermann-TMC]. The risk of secondary infections of the lung, catheter-related infections or urinary tract infections has also increased with extended ICU legnths of stay.

COVID-19 and Secondary Infections

Hyper-inflammation and cytokine storm syndrome (CSS) are among the major causes of acute respiratory distress syndrome (ARDS), multi-organ failure, and death due to severe acute respiratory syndrome SARS-Cov-2 [2]. Immunosuppression is being used to mitigate hyper-inflammation and cytokine storm syndrome (CSS) in COVID-19 patients [3]. Immunosuppressive therapies which have been investigated include corticosteroids (dexamethasone, hydrocortisone, methylprednisolone), JAKs inhibitors (ruxolitinib, baricitinib, tofacitinib), IL-6 blockers (tocilizumab), IL-1 blockers (anakinra, canakinumab), TNF-α blockers (infliximab), and GM-CSF blockers (Mavrilimumab) [3]. In the pre-COVID-19 era, each of these drugs was known to be a risk factor for opportunistic infections. Immunosuppressive therapy is used for a number of autoimmune diseases to alter their immune status; however, this is an important risk factor for opportunistic infections [4]. As such, appropriate precautions are normally taken to screen patients for latent or undiagnosed infections prior to administration of treatments. Additionally, these drugs are delivered in a stable outpatient setting. Infusing a medication in patients who would not have previously qualified for therapies makes them extremely immunocompromised while in a very dangerous environment.

In recent studies of patients with COVID-19 infection, immunosuppressive therapy has shown promising results for control of the cytokine storm syndrome (CSS) in severe cases [2]. Meanwhile, several opportunistic infections have been reported in COVID-19 patients including: *Aspergillus* spp., *Candida* spp., *Cryptococcus neoformans*, *Pneumocystis jirovecii*, mucormycosis, *Cytomegalovirus* (CMV), *Herpes simplex virus* (HSV), *Strongyloides stercoralis*, *Mycobacterium tuberculosis*, and *Toxoplasma gondii* [2]. We have witnessed most of the above secondary infections, and additionally, histoplasmosis, at our institution. The targeted immunotherapies are not routinely used in the in-patient setting, and the standard of care requires patients be screened for many infections before the medication is given which was frequently ignored in the emergent setting.

Due to a combination of the virus and drug-induced immunosuppression, critically ill patients with COVID-19 have an even higher risk of developing a secondary infection. These secondary infections can aggravate the severity of illness and increase the risk of death [5]. A recent multicenter study described a cumulative incidence of VAP of 50% in patients with COIVD-19 admitted to the ICU [6]. In the study by De Bruyn et al., almost two-thirds of patients included suffered with a secondary pneumonia (64.9%) [5]. Treatment with corticosteroids was associated with a higher likelihood of acquiring a secondary bacterial infection ($p = 0.0004$) [5]. Pathogens found in this study were grouped as gram-negative bacilli (82%), gram-positive cocci (66%), and gram-negative cocci (24%), with another 19.7% having aspergillosis [5]. This rate is three times higher than the incidence of secondary pneumonia in critically-ill patients not infected with COVID-19 (13.5–23%) reported by Melsen et al. [7]. A large multicenter study, performed in 36 European ICUs, identified gram-negative bacilli, mainly *Pseudomonas aeruginosa*, *Enterobacter* species, and *Escherichia coli* as the most common bacteria involved in secondary pneumonia in COVID-19 patients [6].

Attempting infection prevention in this patient population has become exceedingly challenging. Prolonged use of central lines, dialysis lines, and urinary catheters put each of these patients at risk for nosocomial infection. The use of high dose steroids and immune-modulators can lead to increase in VAP, catheter-related infections (CLABSI), urinary infections (CAUTI), and infections not normally seen in the MICU such as endemic fungal infections in ventilated patients, reactivation of latent viral infections, and tuberculosis. Increased amounts of candida infections and increased numbers of resistant gram-negative bacteria have also occurred. Avoidance of line-associated infections in patients who stay in a high-risk environment for a protracted length of time has been difficult.

Decreasing Opportunistic Infections in MICU Patients

Identification of the pathogens responsible for the development of secondary infections in critically ill COVID-19 patients generates new possibilities including individually tailored empiric antibiotic therapy in patients with early signs of a secondary infection [5]. Identification of risk factors associated with secondary bacterial infections may lead to development of new prevention strategies [5]. Currently, we are able to identify risks and have isolated many pathogens but do not have a perfect prevention schema. Strategies for early identification of opportunist pathogens in patients with COIVD-19 and immunosuppression may give opportunity for directed therapy and an associated decrease in mortality. Screening for aspergillus and candida should be considered in the group of patients with prolonged intubation and mechanical ventilation, especially after high dose steroids or immunosuppression.

The primary challenge surrounding diagnosis and treatment of COVID-19-associated opportunistic infections (CAOIs) is earlier recognition [2]. Early diagnosis and treatment are paramount to managing aspergillosis among COVID-19 patients. Serologic tests with β-D-glucan (BDG) and galactomannan antigen are recommended for diagnosis of candidiasis. Early diagnosis and treatment of COVID-19-associated candidiasis (CAC) are important for management of the disease; however, multidrug resistant species are a major obstacle to CAC management [2]. Future consideration may be given to prophylactic strategies for COVID-19 patients especially for those who received immunosuppressive therapy or who have underlying diseases, and patients admitted to the ICU who receive invasive mechanical ventilation.

As it currently stands, the risk of secondary infections associated with the administration of steroids is outweighed by the positive treatment effect on the virus itself. Much more needs to be learned and much to be discovered in the ways of screening, identification, treatment, and prevention of secondary infections. Protocolized screening of patients with the recommended labs outlined by the FDA drug label prior to administration of the immune-modulators and matching what is standard of care in the outpatient setting is one way to identify which patients are at risk for getting secondary infections and which microbes to target.

Ventilator-Associated Pneumonia (VAP)

Ventilator-associated pneumonia is the most common nosocomial infection in the ICU with an incidence ranging from 8% to 28% depending on the various studies and patient populations. VAP carries a high mortality rate; overall, attributable mortality ranges from 0 to 50% [8]. Patients who developed VAP have increased length of stay in the hospital by 7–9 days with an excess cost of up to $40,000.

VAP is difficult to define but there is agreement that it occurs after 48 hours of mechanical ventilation. The criteria can be subjective, and there is no one universal definition. There are different methods available to diagnose VAP. Available for use are the Centers for Disease Control and Prevention (CDC)/National Healthcare safety network (NHSN) approach, the clinical pulmonary infection score (CPIS), and the Johnson Criteria. Each employs different combinations of radiographic, clinical, microbiologic, physiologic, and laboratory parameters. Additionally, there is a spectrum of disease severity which can occur including: colonization of the tube, tracheostomy site infection, ventilator-associated tracheitis (VAT), and full-blown pneumonia (VAP). Not every institution obtains cultures of a patient's secretions and if the sample only comes from the airway and not the actual alveoli, it may not represent true pneumonia. There are inconsistencies in how the samples are obtained. Overall, it becomes difficult to define a secondary bacterial pneumonia while in the ICU.

Patients may differ in how they react physiologically to a new ventilator-associated infection. This ranges from changes in oxygen requirements, hypoxemia, increases in PEEP (positive-end-expiratory pressure) requirement, fever, elevated white blood cell count, change in secretions, new infiltrates on chest X-ray, to hemodynamic variations and sepsis or septic shock. However, in the immunocompromised patients who have received high-dose steroids and immune-modulators while in the ICU and are acutely ill, new infections can have a lot more consequence and require attention and intervention.

Ventilator-Associated Pneumonia Pathogens

The typical pathogens in patients in the MICU consist of mostly gram-negative rods. These bugs can colonize the plastic used in tracheal devices making it difficult to confirm an active infection in the alveoli from colonization of the airway, or just biofilm buildup.

For patients who have aspiration pneumonia, the pathogens are normally from the upper airway flora and deemed as such on cultures, so aspiration pneumonia tends to be a clinical diagnosis using radiographic findings along with oxygenation changes, fever, elevated white blood cell count, and possible cultures from the lower respiratory tract [9]. If a patient is colonized in the upper airway identified with MRSA PCR from the nares, then these bacteria can also cause pneumonia. Alternatively, MRSA is a well-known hospital pathogen which patients can become infected with after being hospitalized or while on mechanical ventilator. Frequently, VAP will consist of bugs that come from gastrointestinal flora such as *Escherichia coli*, enterococcus, *Pseudomonas*, and others. Micro-aspiration of oropharyngeal secretions contaminated with endogenous flora around the endotracheal tube cuff is the major route for microbial invasion [8].

The longer a patient stays in the hospital and on a ventilator, the risk of multidrug resistant (MDR) pathogens increases. These include gut organisms *Pseudomonas aeruginosa*, *Acinetobacter baumannii*, Enterobacteriaceae (*Klebsiella pneumoniae*, *Escherichia coli*, *Citrobacter freundii*, *Enterobacter* spp.), the health care-associated organism [*Staphylococcus aureus* (MRSA)], and the opportunistic bacteria *Stenotrophomonas maltophilia*. These are the types of infections we frequently see in patients on prolonged mechanical ventilation including those in the MICU at Memorial Hermann Hospital-TMC.

Hematogenous spread from infected intravascular catheters, ascending urinary tract infections, ascending cholangitis, wound or joint infections, or other distal sources or translocation of gastrointestinal tract lumen flora can occur, making it difficult to identify the primary source of infection. Further details on VAP are covered in other chapters in the book, but we will cover items relevant to prolong mechanical ventilation and tracheostomy infection prevention in this chapter to avoid too much overlap.

Prolonged Mechanical Ventilation (PMV) and Tracheostomy

Prolonged mechanical ventilation is defined as >2 weeks of mechanical ventilation. Frequently, after 2 weeks with an endotracheal tube for ventilation, patients will undergo a procedure to produce a tracheostomy tube (trach). A trach is a more permanent and comfortable way to ventilate patients for a longer period of time. Of all hospitalized patients requiring mechanical ventilation, approximately 10% will receive a tracheostomy [10] but this number is on the rise especially since the pandemic started. The longer a patient is on a ventilator, there is an increased chance for a secondary infection to develop, typically the rate reported is 0.05/events/patient ventilator day. Patients who remain intubated with a standard endotracheal tube are at increased risk of compilations such as tracheal stenosis, tracheal-esophageal fistula, and breakdown of skin around the face and mouth.

Patients are classically defined as chronically mechanically ventilated once they require ventilation for greater than 30 days. These types of patients mostly commonly require tracheostomy (which is reversible) to maintain long-term ventilation (if/when safe to perform). There are similar concerns with infections in both endotracheal tube (ETT) and tracheostomy patient populations; however, those with a trach are at risk for tracheitis, colonization of the tube, and not necessarily ventilator-associated pneumonia. We will make notations as to when these situations differ in this chapter.

Intubation with an ETT increases the risk of infection. The presence of the tube bypasses the normal host defenses including cough, adduction of the vocal cords, and the mucociliary clearance of the airway. This leads to a direct pathway for oral pathogens to enter the lungs, especially if the ETT cuff is not adequately inflated. The presence of a foreign body made of plastic also allows for formation of a biofilm of bacteria that can colonize the airway and, at times, lead to infection. The prevalence of long-term care facility (LTCF) residents with tracheostomy devices lies at 1.4%, although most of them do not require mechanical ventilation [11]. Not being attached to a ventilator circuit decreases the associated risk of infections. The infections most frequently associated with tracheostomy devices are either tracheobronchitis or pneumonia [12].

Benefits and Risk of Tracheostomy

There are many advantages to tracheostomy but it does not always significantly decrease the risk of infection [13]. The available studies show inconsistent results regarding decrease in VAP. This is likely due to the various methodologies applied in the studies over the years. Regardless, with a trach in place, this allows the vocal cords to close, reducing the amount of oropharyngeal secretions aspirated and lessens the bacterial biofilm formation inside of the tracheostomy cannula [14]. This, in theory, along with better access to pulmonary toilet, improved oral hygiene and more rapid weaning from the ventilator should decrease the risk of VAP [15]. The case–control study by Nseir et al., demonstrated a tracheostomy is independently associated with a decreased risk for VAP [15]. This study was completed in 2007, and further studies have not reliably shown a decrease in VAP in patients with tracheostomy. Because of their rigid design, shorter length, and removable inner cannula (to allow for evacuation of secretions), airflow resistance and associated work of breathing should be less with tracheostomies relative to endotracheal tubes [16–18].

Financial expenditures to support the care of tracheostomy patients are among the highest of any diagnostic or procedural group (DRG) [19]. Tracheostomy enables transfer of patients requiring prolonged ventilator support to less resource-intensive settings (such as LTACHs or step-down units) effectively increasing the capacity of ICUs to provide care for more acutely ill individuals [20]. Tracheostomy allows clinicians to be more aggressive in weaning attempts [21]. This differs from an endotracheal tube that would have to be replaced if a patient fails extubation, which then requires re-sedation and puts the patient at risk of the procedure and for aspiration during the reintubation. The presence of a tracheostomy promotes oral hygiene and pulmonary toilet, enhances patient comfort, provides airway security, and allows eventual oral nutrition and speech [16, 22]. Tracheostomy allows for easier communication, lip reading, and subsequent vocalization. Emergent intubation and/or multiple intubations increase the risk of VAP, prolonged MV via an endotracheal tube increases the rate of VAP, and repeated extubation and reintubation increase the risk of VAP, all reasons tracheostomy can be of value.

Delayed tracheostomy is also associated with higher incidence of long-term airway stenosis [23].

There are some disadvantages to tracheostomy. One risk is that of dislodgement, especially in the prone position. Prone positioning has previously been shown to decrease mortality in ARDS patients. During the COVID-19 pandemic, proning was increasingly utilized. Thus, one should be cautious about too early of placement of a trach if the patient is still in severe ARDS and might need to be placed in a prone position. Tracheostomy is normally placed during the recovery phase, but when a patient still requires mechanical ventilation. Conversely, because of the prolonged duration of ECMO cannulation in the COVID-19 patients, early tracheostomy has routinely been performed, recognizing with the use of ECMO, an ARDS patient would circumvent the need for proning. Typically, the risk of bleeding associated with trach placement is minimal. However, since the pandemic we have seen a much higher number of patients with tracheal bleeding, because those on ECMO require continuous infusion of anti-coagulation and thus have a much higher risk of bleeding once a trach is in place.

Tracheostomy and Tracheostomy in COVID-19 Patients

The timeline for patients on mechanical ventilation to undergo tracheostomy varies depending on the ICU location and the clinical diagnosis. Patients with trauma or neurologic injury may receive a trach as early as day 3 in the surgical-trauma or neurosurgical intensive care units. Patients who require tracheostomy in the cardiovascular ICU have to wait 14 days to prevent risk of mediastinitis in those who have had sternotomies for valve replacement, aortic repair, or bypass surgeries. Patients who have upper airway obstruction such as angioedema or otolaryngology (ENT) patients with tumors require tracheostomy but are usually only on the ventilator for the first 24 h and will rapidly get to trach collar, not requiring mechanical ventilation. For patients in a MICU, one typically starts considering tracheostomy in patients not expected to be extubated by day 10–14. In MICU patients with acute respiratory failure, and no additional comorbidities, earlier tracheostomy may lead to an unnecessary procedure. In the TracMan trial, only 45.5% patients randomized to the late tracheostomy group ultimately underwent the procedure [24]. Several studies show if you wait up to 2 weeks, approximately 50% of patients will be successfully extubated and not require trach. Historical data suggests the majority of patients in this time frame would be liberated from mechanical ventilation without need for tracheostomy [25].

In the last 2 years with COVID-19, the number of tracheostomies performed in the MICU has increased nearly 500% [unpublished data Memorial Hermann-TMC]. The length of stay in the ICU and length of stay on the ventilator have increased substantially. In the review by Saad et al., in patients with COVID-19 ARDS, the ICU length of stay (LOS) was 41 days (33.0–54.0), the time on mechanical ventilation was 35.0 days (27.0–46.0), and the time on mechanical ventilation after transfer to LTAC was an additional 11.0 days (5.8–26.0) [26]. The time, effort, and resource usage for these patients are extraordinary. In a 2-month review by the Head and Neck Surgery group in New York, there was no significant benefit or harm to patients or providers when performing tracheostomy on COVID-19 ARDS patients. They reported the median time to discontinuation of mechanical ventilation from intubation was 26.5 days for the early tracheostomy group and 31 days for the late tracheostomy group, with mean time on vent 33.49 days (8–101) [27]. The median length of stay in the hospital was 40 days for the early trach group and 49 days for the late trach group with mean LOS 51.29 (21–92) days [27]. Overall, in the last 2 years, there have been many more tracheostomies performed nationwide and much longer stays in the ICU and on the ventilator.

Prevention of Tracheostomy-Associated Infections

To minimize the risk of infection, a respiratory program should be introduced to reduce the potential of aspiration, minimize atelectasis, and provide cleaning for respiratory therapy equipment [28]. Education and training in the handling and clean care of tracheostomy devices are key to infection control. In addition, sedation should be minimized and good oral care provided [11]. Appropriate hand hygiene and gloving should be performed during manipulation of the tracheostomy device [11]. Long-term care facility (LTCF) providers must to be educated and trained in the handling and clean care of tracheostomy devices. An individualized treatment protocol addressing adequate removal of airway secretions and providing satisfactory airway humidity should be implemented for residents with chronic tracheostomy devices [29]. Weaning and decannulation will have the greatest impact on reducing the risk of infection [11]. Accordingly, the recommendations from the IDSA and other national guidelines regarding prevention of VAP should be applied to patients on a ventilator whether it is via a standard endotracheal tube or a tracheostomy tube.

Prevention of VAP and Tracheostomy-Associated Infections

IDSA Guidelines Recommended Multiple Ways to Help Prevent VAP

Hand Washing

As is discussed in other chapters in this book, hand washing is the number one way to prevent infection of any type in any of the ICUs. Doctors are reported to be the worst at hand hygiene compliance. Staff education and high compliance with hand washing and alcohol-based hand rubbing must be enforced. Good hand hygiene before and after contact with patients, respiratory devices, or objectis contaminated with respiratory secretions must be performed. After contact with a patient, a health care worker's hands can become transiently colonized with pathogenic and antibiotic-resistant bacteria which can be then transferred to other patients. Hand soaps containing an antiseptic agent such as chlorhexidine, or alcohol-based hand rubs have been shown to effectively reduce bacterial counts on hands when used properly.

Using Gloves While Handling Respiratory Secretions

This is clearly an extension of hand hygiene and should always be done. We will not belabor that point other than to mention appropriate use of gloves by healthcare providers is also critical to preventing spread of disease in the ICU. Transmission from health care providers is known to contribute to VAP. There are reported outbreaks of pathogens that are linked to certain nurses and/or respiratory therapists. The water supply in a patient's room such as sinks or faucets can serve as a reservoir for bacteria. Aseptic techniques should be used when changing a tracheostomy tube. In addition to gloves, sterile fluid should be used when removing secretions from respiratory suction catheters or ETTs for cleaning purposes.

Staff Education

Adequate education of health care workers regarding healthcare-associated pneumonia, infection prevention, and prevention methods is critical to implementing any protocols to reduce infections including VAP. All health care staff (RTs, RNs, and MDs) should understand, they are potential carriers and spreaders of pathogens. MRSA is the most common gram-positive bacteria found to colonize health care workers.

ICU Staffing Levels: Limited Staff/Staffing Rations/New Staff

In a multicenter, retrospective cohort study among 2606 patients admitted to an ICU after abdominal aortic surgery, patients cared for in ICUs that reported nurse-to-patient ratio of 1:3 or greater on either day or night shifts were at greater risk of respiratory complications including postoperative pneumonia [30]. During COVID-19 pandemic, there were significant problems with reduced staffing.

This can lead to lapses in infection control practices when nurses are overworked, overextended and are taking care of increased numbers of patients. Studies show a substantial proportion of VAP could be avoided if nurse staffing could be maintained at a higher level. This relationship was independent of patient, age comorbidity, level of surgical urgency, ICU size, and hospital procedure volume [30]. Another study demonstrated that lower nurse-to-patient ratio was associated with increased risk for late onset ventilator-associated pneumonia [31]. The optimal level of nursing staffing and experience to minimize the risk of infection are not completely determined and may vary among the types of ICUs.

Oral Hygiene

Keeping the teeth and mouth clean, preventing the buildup of dental plaque on teeth, and decreasing secretions in the mouth may help reduce the risk of developing VAP. Oral hygiene care (OHC) with either chlorhexidine mouthwash or gel reduces the odds of developing VAP by 30–40% in critically ill adults depending on the study. However, there is no evidence OHC affects mortality, duration of mechanical ventilation, or duration of ICU stay [32]. There is no consensus data as to how often, what quantity, or which technique should be used to apply the chlorhexidine. Each institution creates their own protocol. There is minimal systemic absorption of chlorhexidine, and there are low adverse effects including unpleasant taste, dysgeusia, mild oral mucosa irritation, and staining of teeth. The conflicting data pose a challenge to hospitals, but the benefit-to-risk ratio favors its usage. The most commonly studied regimen is 0.12% (10–15 mL) at least twice daily [32].

Avoiding Unnecessary Intubation

Non-invasive positive pressure ventilation (NIPPV) use increased significantly during COVID-19 pandemic. Previously, there were certain patient populations in which use of NIPPV was studied and evidence-based. These conditions include mild to moderate COPD exacerbations, acute cardiogenic pulmonary edema, and patients with pneumonia who are immune-compromised. This data was originally reported in the 2009 study by Nava and Hill [33]. NIPPV can prevent unnecessary endotracheal intubation which can decrease the chance of VAP. Subsequent meta-analysis in 2015 on the use of NIPPV suggests that the survival benefit may be lost when NIPPV is applied late as a rescue therapy [34]. In the original randomized control trial by Antonelli et al., patients ventilated noninvasively had a significantly lower rate of both pneumonia (3% vs. 25%) and sinusitis (0 vs. 6%) [35]. Since the pandemic, NIPPV has increasingly been used to avoid intubation in COVID-19 ARDS patients. The results have been mixed, and the data is not clear at this time if NIPPV is the preferred method of ventilation in this patient population.

Minimalizing Sedation and Paralytic Agents

Sedating agents and paralytic use reduce the ability for patients to cough. Sedation holidays to assess preparedness for weaning and eventual extubation greatly reduce the risk for VAP by reducing the time on vent. There is extensive data indicating the need to limit the use of sedation and paralytics to hasten liberation from the ventilator. Continuous sedation is more common in the acute phase of illness and lessens as the patient's physiologic parameters improve. The shortest duration of mechanical ventilation conveys the least risk of VAP. The insertion of tracheostomy normally allows for more rapid sedation weaning with a controlled and more easily replaceable airway. Sedation should be minimized, if possible, in the tracheostomy patients.

Avoiding Naso-Tracheal Intubation and Naso-Grastic Tubes

Nasogastric intubation bypasses the normal mucosal defenses of the upper and lower respiratory tract and leaves the patients at risk for healthcare-associated sinusitis and pneumonia [36]. Naso-tracheal intubation can lead to sinusitis as early as 3 days due to blocking of the sinus ostia. Naso-tracheal intubation is rarely used and only in patients who cannot otherwise be orally intubated such as cases with masses, jaw trauma, or presence of hardware. However, nasogastric tubes are frequently used for feedings in the MICU. Oral-gastric tubes are preferred but have to be removed when the ETT is removed, they are uncomfortable and can cause gagging in awake patients. In patients with tracheostomies, temporary feeding tubes will be needed, if patient is liberated from mechanical ventilation, they can undergo a swallowing trial. Many of the long-term trach patients and trach patients on ventilation will not be able to swallow and will require percutaneous gastrostomy tubes (PEGs) which are also potentially reversible.

Adequate Endotracheal Tube Cuff Pressure

The ETT cuff pressure (P_{cuff}) should be maintained at 20–30 cm H_2O to prevent leakage of contaminated oropharyngeal secretions and gastric contents around the cuff and into the lower respiratory tract. It is recommended checking the cuff pressure be part of the routine ventilator checks the respiratory therapists perform on a daily basis to minimize seepage into the lower respiratory tract. Once patients have tracheostomies, the cuff will need to be inflated while the patient is still requiring a mechanical ventilator. Once the patient is off MV, the cuff will be deflated to allow the patient to vocalize, another reason the sedation should be minimized. Over inflation of the ETT cuff carries the risk of tracheal ischemia and tracho-esophageal fistula formation (>30 cm H_2O).

Aspiration of Subglottic Secretions

Subglottic suctioning of oropharyngeal secretions using a specially designed endotracheal tube has been shown to reduce the incidence of ventilator-associated pneumonia [37]. Theoretically, aspiration of subglottic secretions with a specialized tube should lessen the burden of aspirated organisms. However, there is significant increase in the price of these specialized tubes over standard tubes, and the cost effectiveness of this strategy needs further investigation. Additionally, the smaller inner luminal diameter increases airway resistance. Furthermore, if patients are intubated at outside hospitals, in ER, or by those who do not stock the tubes, this would require a tube exchange which can put the patient at additional risk. Thus, there are significant limitations, and their use has not been universally adopted. There is evidence subglottic secretion suctioning via a regular ETT decreases incidence of VAP, duration of mechanical ventilation and delays VAP onset [37]. However, there is no evidence that subglottic secretion suctioning reduces mortality, duration of mechanical ventilation or length of stay [37]. Subglottic suctioning and oral suctioning should also occur before the balloon on the ETT is deflated for depth adjustment or removal.

Use of Silver-Coated Endotracheal Tubes

Silver-coated ETTs slowly release silver cations. These silver ions appear to have a strong antimicrobial effect, and silver has been used for many centuries to treat and prevent infections. The use of silver-coated endotracheal tubes has been shown to reduce the incidence of VAP and mortality [38, 39]. However, the cost of these tubes has been prohibitive for their widespread usage.

Enteral Nutrition Versus Parenteral Nutrition

Enteral feeding is an area which remains controversial. Most authors recommend enteral feeding over parenteral feeding. The evidence to support this is easy to find; enteral nutrition reduces the risk of infections related to central venous catheters. Enteral nutrition prevents villous atrophy of the intestinal mucosa that can lead to increased bacterial translocation. Based on what is known about the risk of over distention of the stomach and the risk of vomiting and aspiration, physicians shy away from the practice of gastric feeding compared to post pyloric feeding. But there is no consistent evidence to support this idea. The debate regarding early vs. late enteral feeding and the controversy over post-pyloric feeding continue. One older study demonstrated delaying feeding by 5 days decreased the risk of VAP; however, this falls within the average time on vent for most patients. The practice of delayed feeding in ventilated patients may decrease VAP but leads to caloric deficiency in a vulnerable patient population with many comorbidities, so this practice is not recommended. Post-pyloric feeding is endorsed when placement of the tube is feasible per the Cochrane systematic review [40]. Delays in placement of post-pyloric tubes can lead to decreased caloric intake in patients while the tube is being appropriately positioned. Multiple studies have examined post-pyloric versus gastric feedings with regard to incidence of aspiration and development of VAP. These studies were small and inconclusive. In a meta-analysis, post-pyloric feedings reduced the incidence of VAP and increased the nutrition delivered [41]. However, no single trial demonstrated post-pyloric tube feedings prevented VAP.

Restricted Transfusion

Many critical care guidelines recommend restrictive transfusion practices for multiple reasons. Blood transfusions have been shown to have important effects on immunologic function, increasing the risk of infection. The pathway to ventilator-associated pneumonia prevention is less clear, however. One study of trauma patients found a decreased risk of VAP with hemoglobin (Hgb) limited to 7 g/dL. In the Croce, et al. trial, the number of patients diagnosed with VAP was 2.2% in those who received no blood transfusion and 19.4% in patients who received blood transfusion after the first 48 hours of resuscitation [42]. Another study looked at the association between transfusions and ventilator-associated events (VAE). Because of the spectrum of diagnoses (VAE, infection-related ventilator-associated complication, possible VAP, or probable VAP), a simple change in the amount of oxygen or PEEP required on the ventilator can suggest a VAP. However, with transfusions, other physiologic changes can occur including pulmonary edema, volume overload, atelectasis, or transfusion-related lung injury (TRALI) affecting oxygenation other than just pneumonia. Wang, et al., concluded that compared to patients without transfusion, the risk of VAE was significantly higher in patients with red blood cell (RBC) transfusions greater than 3 units (HR 1.73; 95% CI 1.25–2.40; $p = 0.001$) [43]. Thus, restricted transfusions can decrease the number of times a patient might be under surveillance for a ventilator event, but it is harder to say it actually averts VAP.

Limiting transfusion to only those with Hgb <7 g/dL in the MICU patient population has already been shown to decrease mortality and ICU complications. The Shorr et al., group observed an increased risk of late onset (>5 days on vent) VAP with Odds Ratio 2.16, 95% CI 1.27–3.66 and demonstrated a positive dose–response relationship (with more transfusions patients were at higher risk for VAP) [44]. The TRICC trial by Hebert and colleagues found no significant differences in overall mortality in a mixed ICU patient population but organ failure was reduced in the restrictive transfusion group [45]. It is also known that leukocyte-depleted red blood cell transfusions can help reduce VAP in selected patient populations. Patients who stay in the ICU for a prolonged period of time and especially patients with trach and on ECMO require many units of RBC transfusions owing to the fact they are on blood thinners to maintain the ECMO circuit which then increases the risk of secondary VAP. Patients in the MICU who receive continuous renal replacement therapy (CRRT) are also at risk for multiple blood transfusions since they routinely lose blood if the filter clots.

Selective Oropharyngeal Decontamination and Selective Digestive Decontamination

Selective oropharyngeal decontamination (SOD) and selective digestive decontamination (SDD) have been studied for many years. This involves the use of topical oral antibiotics for SOD and oral and intestinal antibiotics, often with a systemic antibiotics added during the first few days of the regimen for SDD, with the goal being the elimination of potential pathogens from the oropharynx and/or gastrointestinal (GI) tract. With the eradication of endogenous bacterial sources, infection may be avoided. SOD and SDD are effective in reducing the incidence of VAP in the ICU. SDD with systemic antimicrobial therapy also reduces mortality. Importantly, the main concern associated with the use of SOD or SDD remains the development and spread of antimicrobial resistance. Overall, the currently available evidence does not support the use of SOD or SDD as a preventive strategy on a large scale, particularly in settings with endemic cross-transmission of multi-drug resistant (MDR) micro-organisms, especially in an ICU like MICU where there are many pathogens in patients with prolonged ventilator stays. This is not in practice at many institutions including our own.

Keeping Head of the Bed >30°

This is a low cost, easy intervention but one that is frequently overlooked. Patients are laid flat for bathing, turning, or during transport and forgotten to be sat back up. In some ICUs, patients can only be upright for a limited amount of time due to intracranial pressure issues, surgical restrictions, and femoral location of life-support lines including heart catheterization devices, intra-aortic blood pumps (IABP), or ECMO cannulas. Since the COVID-19 pandemic, with a large rise in the use of ECMO circuits in patients with ARDS in the MICU, there have been more limitations in keeping patients upright. That practice which bled over into newer staff, coupled with lack of education as to why the ECMO patients are a special situation, has resulted in a lot of head of bed elevation at <30°. A review by the Cochrane library in 2015 showed reduced risk of clinically suspected VAP with semi-recumbent position (30°–60°) compared to supine position (0–10%). This consisted of a review of eight trials with 759 participants, and the rate for VAP was 14.3% vs. 40.2% [46].

Only Changing Ventilator Circuits When Soiled or at 7 Days

Contamination of mechanical ventilators tubing, ventilator circuits, and moisture exchangers can also be a source of infection. “Breaking” of the circuit prematurely can contribute to infection. Ventilator breathing circuit components should not be changed more frequently than every 48 hours. Circuit change intervals of 7 and 30 days have lower risk for VAP than 2-day intervals, yielding substantial reductions in morbidity as well as labor and supply costs [47].

Use of Heated Moisture Exchangers

Condensate should be periodically drained from mechanical ventilator tubing while avoiding flow of condensate toward the patient. Use of heat and moisture exchangers (HMEs) instead of heated humidifiers can decrease the amount of condensate in the mechanical ventilator tube thereby decreasing the fluid which can get into the ETT and thus decrease the risk of VAP. For patients who are maintained on ventilators for a prolonged period of time, it is suggested that this interchange be made. This exchange can also decrease the effective dead space on the vent circuit which can be of value in severe ARDS patients, such as those with COVID-19, but cannot be used in patients with excess secretions or risk for airway obstruction, which can lead to increased work of breathing.

Cleaning of Respiratory Equipment

Contaminated respiratory equipment has been implicated as the source of outbreaks of nosocomial pneumonia. Devices that generate aerosols such as nebulizer reservoirs, devices used for humification, and multidose medications nebulizers have all been associated with outbreaks caused by hydrophilic bacteria [36]. Bronchoscopes have also been a source of health care-associated pneumonia in the ICU and usually are a result of an incomplete or compromised disinfection between procedures. The more recent use of disposable bronchoscopes (Ambu scope®) has helped attenuate this risk. Incomplete cleaning of ventilators or high-flow oxygen delivery devices can also put the patient at risk [36]. Sterile water should be used to fill bubbling humidifiers and nebulizers rather than tap water [36]. Devices used on multiple patients (portable respirators, oxygen sensors, Ambu bags, etc.) if not disposable, should undergo sterilization or high-level disinfection each time between patient use.

Suctioning devices themselves can be contaminated with health care-associated bacteria quite quickly. Sole et al., found that most suctioning equipment including the Yankauer® suction devices and suction tubing are colonized with a potential pathogen within 24 hour of use [48]. There is no available standard storage device used for the oral suction cannulas, and they frequently fall onto the floor, touch the bed or left on the ventilator uncovered. Newer devices which have their own protection sheath and catheters which are disposable or used for only 24 hours are available at some institutions.

Additional Methods Not Covered in This Chapter

Isolation to prevent cross contamination with MDR pathogens
Surveillance of ventilated patient to determine trends and detect outbreaks of VAP
Surveillance cultures of high-risk patients
Rotational antibiotics schema

Use of Bundles to prevent VAP

Each of the individual interventions can reduce the risk of VAP whether it may be patients with ETTs or patients with trachs. Combining some elements can reduce risk even further. The use of bundles has been shown to significantly reduce ventilator-associated pneumonia. Bundles typically consist of elevation of head of bed, oral care every 4 h, peptic ulcer disease prophylaxis (discussed later), deep vein thrombosis prophylaxis, and daily sedation vacation/assessment to extubate. Insurance of bundle compliance is critically important to maintain prevention.

The Use of Extracorporeal Membrane Oxygenation in MICU and Antimicrobial Prophylaxis

Extracorporeal membrane oxygenation (ECMO) provides gas exchange with or without cardiovascular hemodynamic support with the use of an oxygenator, a device that uses a semipermeable membrane to separate the blood compartment from the gas compartment. There are two types of ECMO, veno-arterial (VA) and veno-venous (VV). In both modalities, deoxygenated blood is removed from the body through a large drainage cannula placed in a central vessel and is pumped through an oxygenator where blood is oxygenated and carbon dioxide is removed. Blood is returned to the patient via a large reinfusion cannula into a central vessel. VA ECMO is primarily used for circulatory and respiratory support; therefore, blood is removed from a central vein and returned via an artery. VV ECMO is solely for respiratory support; the blood is removed and returned from a central vein while the patient's heart continues to circulate the oxygenated blood [49, 50]. VV ECMO is becoming an increasingly common therapy in intensive care units across the world. Numerous randomized clinical trials, cohort studies, and case series have reported the use of VV ECMO in acute respiratory distress syndrome (ARDS) largely caused by an infection, as a bridge to lung transplantation, for acute chronic obstructive pulmonary disease exacerbation, for status asthmaticus, in massive pulmonary embolism, and for acutely decompensated pulmonary hypertension [50].

The benefits of ECMO must be weighed against the risk of complications. Complications can occur as a result of the device, mechanically, or because of indirect effects on the organs [50]. The ELSO registry reports an overall prevalence of culture proven infection in 11.1% of patients but a meta-analysis reported significant infections to be 30.4% [51]. The rate of acquiring an infection per 1000 days of ECMO is 30.6 for adults [52]. Acquiring a hospital infection is associated with increased morbidity and mortality [53]. The prevalence has been reported to be up to 45% with the most common being bloodstream, surgical site, urinary tract and respiratory tract infections [54]. The timing in the development of infections has not been fully elucidated. Early infections are most likely be related to insertion of cannulas as opposed to late infections which would be a result of maintenance; however, the overall prevalence of infection was reported to be highest in adult patients who were maintained on ECMO for greater than 14 days (51.6%) compared to those requiring ECMO for ≤7 days (12.8%) [53].

In patients receiving ECMO for respiratory failure, the most common organisms identified in the respiratory tract were yeast, *Staphylococcus aureus*, and *Pseudomonas* spp. The most common bacteria isolated in the bloodstream were coagulase-negative staphylococci (15.9%), *Candida* (12.7%), *Enterococcus* spp., and *Staphylococcus aureus* [55]. These organisms were identified in culture but the prevalence may not be reflective of a true active infection. Patients can be colonized with these organisms or could have already been infected prior to the initiation of ECMO.

Patients receiving ECMO are at risk for developing ICU-related nosocomial infections such as ventilator-associated pneumonia (VAP), catheter-related bloodstream infections (CRBSI), and catheter-associated urinary tract infections (CAUTI). A single center observational study of mostly VV ECMO reported nosocomial infection rates of 55%. VAPs were found to be the most common along with a high prevalence of multidrug resistant organisms. In patients who developed a nosocomial infection, there was greater overall mortality, duration of mechanical ventilation, duration of ECMO, and intensive care unit (ICU) length of stay [56]. In addition to the development of nosocomial infections as seen in other critically-ill patients, it is hypothesized ECMO patients have additional physiologic factors that may increase their susceptibility to develop infections. When initially placed on ECMO, exposure of a patient's blood to the extracorporeal membrane activates a variety of coagulation and inflammatory cascades. Pro-inflammatory levels rise along with activation of the intrinsic and extrinsic coagulation pathways, complement system, and the contact system that results in leukocyte activation [57]. Many other factors have also been identified for increasing risk of infections during ECMO runs. Older patients, patients with autoimmune comorbidities likely secondary to chronic immunosuppression, a higher Sequential Organ Failure Assessment (SOFA) score prior to cannulation, VA ECMO compared to VV ECMO, and longer duration of ECMO runs (greater than 20 days) have all be shown to increase risk of infection [58].

Despite the risk for infections, the ELSO general guidelines for all ECLS cases recommend using appropriate antibiotics for a documented infection but there is no standard policy regarding the use of prophylactic antibiotics solely for the indication of ECMO [59]. Previously, the ELSO Infectious Disease Task Force also did not recommend routine use of prophylactic antibiotics beyond 48 h after cannulation except for patients at high risk such as a prolonged open chest or in immunocompromised hosts. The task force recommended prevention of nosocomial infections using the following strategies: reduce unnecessary breaking of lines, use sterile practices and needleless hubs for all connection and access sites, use chlorhexidine for disinfection, isolate patients with contaminated wounds, serious or multidrug resistant infections, frequent hand washing, use VAP prevention bundles, oral and gastrointestinal decontamination as deemed appropriate, early enteral nutrition or a dedicated venous access line for parenteral nutrition, avoidance and removal of all unnecessary central lines, and avoide use of long-term intravenous access during ECMO course [58].

The current guideline recommendations from the task force are likely secondary to lack of high-quality randomized-controlled trials evaluating the benefit and harm of antibiotic prophylaxis. A review of nine studies was conducted to evaluate the evidence for antibiotic prophylaxis in preventing a nosocomial infection. None of the studies reviewed found a correlation or reduced risk of infection related to prophylaxis [52]. A more recent retrospective cohort study evaluated the efficacy of antibiotics in ECMO patients. The authors identified over 9000 patients and propensity-matched patients to a prophylaxis versus control group. They found a significant reduction for in-hospital mortality (56.4% vs. 59.8%) and development of nosocomial pneumonia (12.9% vs. 15.3%) versus the control group [60]. Although the authors classified the patients into a prophylaxis group, it was difficult to discern if patients actually received prophylactic or empiric antibiotics as some patients did not receive antibiotics for up to 48 h after initiation of ECMO [61]. Further prospective randomized trials need to be completed to get a better understanding of the role of antibiotic prophylaxis.

Without high-quality evidence and lacking supporting guidelines despite the continued concern for increased risk of infections, it is expected that practices regarding antibiotic prophylaxis in ECMO patients would vary among institutions. In 2011, a multi-institutional survey of practice patterns of ELSO centers confirmed the heterogeneity. A 37-question web-based survey was developed and distributed to ECMO centers in order to gain a better understanding of prescribing and surveillance practice patterns. Sixty-eight percent of the centers that responded administer prophylactic antibiotics, of which 65% are part of a standardized protocol. Antibacterial prophylaxis is administered at 42% of the centers, and 3% only administered to a specific patient population. The majority of centers use at least two antibacterial agents for prophylaxis. Among centers that use prophylaxis as part of a protocol, the most common single agent was a first-generation cephalosporin. Of centers that prescribe prophylaxis based on physician preference, vancomycin was the most common single agent antibiotic. For centers that use combination antibiotics as part of their protocol or per physician choice, there was a lot of variation with vancomycin, third-generation cephalosporins, penicillin-derived combinations, and aminoglycosides being the most common. The antibacterial prophylaxis was prescribed for the duration of ECMO cannulation at the majority of the centers, with others reporting prophylaxis pre-cannulation and for a limited amount of time. Only 2% of centers administer routine antifungal medications and 13% in selective cases. Surveillance cultures were reported at 64 centers with 100% obtaining blood cultures and approximately 50% urine and sputum. The frequency of surveillance cultures varied from every 24 hour down to once a week or only on admission [54]. A more recent survey aimed to identify common practices to prevent bloodstream infections specifically from ELSO centers. A quarter of the respondents reported an infection prevention bundle or checklist is used during cannulation, and less than half reported a maintenance bundle is normally used. Approximately 50% of the responders reported routine antimicrobial prophylaxis with ampicillin + aminoglycoside or a cephalosporin being the most common. Routine surveillance cultures were reported in 34.2% of the responses [62]. It is clear from both surveys there is not a clear practice or consensus in terms of use of antibiotics, choice of antibiotics, or duration of antibiotics.

Routine and prolonged use of antimicrobial prophylaxis raises some concerns with published evidence regarding the fear of antimicrobial-associated injury. Antimicrobials can cause harm via multiple mechanisms: selection of disease resistant bacteria leading to a multidrug resistant infection, anaphylaxis or idiosyncratic drug reactions, disruption of the microbiome, and mitochondrial dysfunction resulting in cellular dysfunction [63]. Unnecessary or excessively broad-spectrum antibiotics can also increase a patient's risk of developing a secondary infection or predispose them to sepsis [63]. The use of non-clinically indicated antibiotics in hospitalized patients can be associated with an adverse drug event (ADE). For every 10 days of excess antibiotic therapy, there is a 3% increased risk of an ADEs including *C. difficile* infection, and gastrointestinal, renal, or hematologic abnormalities [64]. More importantly, reduced exposure to antibiotics in critically-ill patients has been associated with a reduced risk-adjusted mortality [63].

The limited current evidence does not support routine use of antimicrobial prophylaxis in patients receiving ECMO support but unfortunately, acquiring an infection can lead to prolonged hospitalization, increased complications and mortality. ECMO centers should establish a multidisciplinary team to develop a protocol for preventing infections using bundles and a standard antimicrobial prophylaxis regimen that balances the antimicrobial harm alongside prevention of nosocomial infections. Considering the striking increase in use of ECMO devices since the beginning of the pandemic in COVID-19 patients, there is an urgent need to establish protocols for antibiotic and antifungal prophylaxis.

The Use of Proton Pump Inhibitors for Stress Ulcer Prophylaxis (SUP) in the MICU

Primary prevention of stress-related mucosal bleeding from the upper gastrointestinal tract is known as stress ulcer prophylaxis (SUP) [65]. Stress ulcers are ulcerations of the upper gastrointestinal tract (esophagus, stomach, and duodenum) that occur after hospitalization [66]. Approximately 4% of critically ill patients will develop stress ulcers during their hospitalization [67]. It is common practice to start SUP on most all patients admitted to the ICU. Currently, around two-thirds of patients without risk factors receive treatment, two-thirds continue to get treatment upon transfer from the ICU, and one-third are discharged home on therapy without a new indication [68].

Because of their disease states, patients in the MICU are at highest risk to develop stress ulcers during their hospital stay. In a meta-analysis by Bardou et al., the patients at risk for stress ulcers were those on mechanical ventilation >48 h and patients with coagulopathy [68]. The study by Cook et al., from 1994 revealed patients with respiratory failure requiring mechanical ventilation for >48 h had an Odds Ratio of 15.6 (p value <0.001) of developing stress ulcers [69]. Additionally, the same study by Cook et al., and the study by Laine et al., in 2008 showed patients with coagulopathy (platelet count <50,000 platelets/m^3, INR >1.5 or partial thromboplastin time more than two times control value) had an Odds Ratio 4.3 (p value <0.001) for development of GI bleeding from stress ulcers [69, 70]. The rest of the meta-analysis by Bardou et al., identified additional risk factors with Odds Ratios between 1 and 2 to be: maximum creatinine, acute kidney injury, acute respiratory failure, age associations, acute hepatic injury, chronic hepatic injury, and male sex [68]. The majority of patients with these conditions will be hospitalized in the MICU making it a unique opportunity to assess and appropriately prescribe SUPs for the right indications.

PPIs work by blocking the gastric H^+/K^+ ATPase enzyme, which inhibits gastric acid secretion [71]. PPI therapy is highly effective for the treatment of a variety of gastrointestinal disorders including gastroesophageal reflux disease (GERD), peptic ulcer disease (PUD), *Helicobacter pylori* (*H. pylori*) infections, and other hypersecretory conditions. PPIs are now one of the most frequently prescribed drug classes in the world, as they combine a high level of efficacy with low toxicity [72].

Many stress ulcer prophylaxis recommendations are based on older literature. Current studies have shown that stress ulcer prophylaxis should be limited to patients considered to be at high risk for clinically significant bleeding [65]. Critically-ill patient populations which have shown benefit from stress ulcer prophylaxis include patients with: mechanical ventilation *without* enteral nutrition, chronic liver disease (defined as one or more of the following: portal hypertension,

Table 6.1 Criteria for stress ulcer prophylaxis in the Medical ICU

Mechanical ventilation *without* enteral nutrition
Chronic liver disease: 1 or more of:
• Portal hypertension
• Cirrhosis
• History of variceal bleeding
• History of hepatic encephalopathy
Concerning coagulopathy: 1 or more of:
• Platelets <50,000/m^3
• INR above 1.5
• PT above 20 s
Two or more moderate risk factors:
• Shock (1 or more of: continuous infusion of vasopressors or inotropes, systolic blood pressure (SBP) < 90 mmHg, mean arterial blood pressure < 70 mmHg, or plasma lactate level 4 mmol/L or above)
• Sepsis
• Acute kidney injury
• Mechanical ventilation *with* enteral nutrition

cirrhosis, history of variceal bleeding, history of hepatic encephalopathy), significant coagulopathy (one or more of the following: platelets <50,000/m^3, INR > 1.5, PT > 20 s), and two or more moderate risk factors for stress ulcers including shock, sepsis, AKI, and/or mechanical ventilation *with* enteral nutrition [66] (Table 6.1).

PPIs have been used in most critically-ill patients for SUP during the last three decades and have been recommended by Surviving Sepsis Campaign guidelines [73] since they were first published in 2004. Orders for SUP have been built into ICU admission and ventilator initiation order sets to make sure they are not forgotten, consequently, this has contributed to their overuse in the ICU. The medications used in SUP are typically proton pump inhibitors (PPIs) or histamine H_2-receptor antagonists (H_2-blockers), though PPIs are the drug class used predominantly. The PPIs most commonly used in the MICU include pantoprazole, omeprazole, and lansoprazole.

Over the last decade, there have been numerous studies and publications regarding PPI use and the increased risk of hospital-acquired infections. PPIs are prescribed in the ICU to prevent stress-related mucosal bleeding from the upper gastrointestinal tract. However, research has found PPI use in critically-ill patients to be associated with an increased risk of both hospital-acquired pneumonia (HAP) [74] and *Clostridium difficile* infection (CDI) [75]. Additional research has linked the reduction of gastric acid from PPI use with the increased risk of hospital-acquired pneumonia (HAP) [76] and *Clostridium difficile* infections (CDI) [77]. The increased risk of infection is thought to be due to a higher bacterial load in the stomach secondary to the higher pH from the inhibition of gastric acid production. Gastric acid is an important barrier to colonization and infections by invading pathogens [76]. The gastric lumen normally maintains a pH of less than 2. PPIs raise the intra-gastric pH to over 4 for 10.5–16.8 hours depending on the particular PPI and milligram dose administered [76]. Raising the gastric pH levels can lead to bacterial overgrowth. However, an elevated intra-gastric pH of over 4 is recommended to treat *GERD*, PUD, and *H. pylori* infections [76]. PPIs can lead to delayed gastric emptying, increased gastric contents, and increased pressure on the lower esophageal sphincter [76]. The increase pressure against the lower esophageal sphincter which may then increase the risk of subsequent aspiration of both the gastric contents and the bacteria, causing increased risk of HAP [76]. The increased risk of CDI in PPI use is suspected to be caused from the inhibited gastric acid production leading to the proliferation of spores and their ability to convert to a vegetative form of *C. difficile* [75].

One method which can be employed in the MICU to prevent infections is reducing proton pump inhibitor (PPI) use in critically-ill patients. PPI use should be restricted to patients with acknowledged risk factors. Daily reassessment for the need of continued SUP and specifically PPI use in the ICU should be undertaken, and this can help attenuate some of the healthcare-associated infections. The MICU at our institution has decreased PPI usage by educating providers and registered nurses about the increased risks of infections and the appropriate criteria for critically-ill patients who benefit from stress ulcer prophylaxis, listed in Table 6.1.

Conclusion

Taking care of patients in the medical intensive care unit comes with a host of challenges. Ensuring these patients the safest and least dangerous stay in the ICU is difficult. Each day a patient is in the ICU poses a threat. Patients with prolonged mechanical ventilation no matter what the original cause of respiratory failure can achieve benefit from tracheostomy placement but are still at risk for infection. The same precautions must be taken for trach patients as the endotracheal tube patient to reduce the risk for ventilator-related infections. Similar protocols should be applied in both groups.

COVID-19 patients have risk of developing VAP but they are further immunocompromised with high-dose steroids and immunomodulators making them very susceptible to additional secondary and opportunistic infections. Diligent watch is required since there, as of yet, no standardized tools for infection prevention in this patient population. Future opportunities remain to identify ways of screening and early detention for patients in jeopardy.

Another group of patients in the MICU are those on ECMO. Patients on ECMO with COVID-19 ARDS are at very high risk for healthcare-associated infections due to their many devices and long lengths of stay. Unfortunately, there are no guidelines to address antimicrobial prophylaxis for these patients either. Many ECMO centers routinely provide antibiotic prophylaxis for ECMO patients but this varies among the institutions.

Lastly, PPIs and SUP are used extensively in most ICUs. This routine practice is coming under scrutiny because of their overuse without indication, the cost associated with over prescribing, and the risk of VAP and *C. difficile* in some patient populations. They should be reserved for high-risk patients when the risk of bleeding outweighs the risk of VAP from pH-modifying agents.

References

1. Bain W, Yang H, Shah FA, et al. COVID-19 versus non-COVID 19 acute respiratory distress syndrome. Ann Am Thorac Soc. 2021;18(7):1202–10.
2. Abdoli A, Falahi S, Kenarkoohi A. COVID-19 associated opportunistic infections: a snapshot on the current reports. Clin Exp Med. 2021;23:1–20.
3. Alijotas-Reig J, Esteve-Valverde E, Belizna C, Selva-O'Callaghn A, Perdos-Gea J, Quintana A, et al. Immunomodulatory therapy for the management of severe COVID-19. Beyond the anti-viral therapy: a comprehensive review. Autoimmune Rev. 2020;19(7):102569.
4. Fishman JA. Opportunistic infections—coming to the limits of immunosuppression? Cold Spring Harb Perspect Med. 2013;3(10):a015669.
5. De Bruyn A, Verellen S, Bruckers L, Geebelen L, Callebaut I, De Pauw I, Stessel B, Dubois J. Secondary infection in COIVD-19 critically ill patients: a retrospective single-center evaluation. BMC Infect Dis. 2022;22:207–13.
6. Rouze A, Martin-Loeches I, Povoa P, Makris D, Artigas A, Bouchereau M, et al. Relationship between SARS-CoV-2 infection and the incidence of ventilator associated lower respiratory tract infections: a European mufti-center cohort study. Intensive Care Med. 2021;47(2):188–98.
7. Melsen WG, Rovers MM, Groenwold RH, Bergmans DC, Camus C, Bauer TT, et al. Attributable mortality of ventilator-associated pneumonia: a meta-analysis of individual patient data from randomized prevention studies. Lancet Infect Dis. 2013;13(8):665–71.
8. Landelle C, Pittet D. Guide to infection control the healthcare setting: mechanical ventilation from the International Society for Infection Diseases. Chapter update; 2018.
9. Grasselli G, Cattaneo E, Florio G. Secondary infections in critically ill patients with COVID-19. Crit Care. 2021;25(1):317.
10. Stelfox HT, Crimi C, Berra L, et al. Determinants of tracheostomy decannulation: an international survey. Crit Care. 2008;2(1):R26.
11. Crnich CJ, Drinka P. Medical device-associated infections in the long-term care setting. Infect Dis Clin N Am. 2012;26(1):143–64.
12. Ahmed QA, Niederman MS. Respiratory infections in the chronically critically ill patient. Ventilator-associated pneumonia and tracheobronchitis. Clin Chest Med. 2001;22(1):71–85.
13. Terragni PP, Antoneli M, Fumagalli R, et al. Early vs late tracheostomy for prevention of pneumonia in mechanically ventilated adult ICU patients: a randomized controlled trial. JAMA. 2010;303:1483–9.
14. Lin W-C, Chen C-W, Wang J-D, Tsai L-M. Is tracheostomy a better choice than translaryngeal intubation for critical ill patients requiring mechanical ventilation for more than 14 days? A comparison of short-term outcomes. BMC Anesthesiol. 2015;15:181–8.
15. Nseir S, Di Pompeo C, Jozefowicz E, Cavestri B, Brisson H, Nyunga M, Soubrier S, Durocher A. Relationship between tracheotomy and ventilator associated pneumonia, a case-control study. Eur Respir J. 2007;30:314–20.
16. Heffner JE, Hess D. Tracheostomy management in the chronically ventilated patient. Clin Chest Med. 2001;22:55–69.
17. Heffner JE. Timing of tracheostomy in mechanically ventilated patients. Am Rev Respir Dis. 1993;147:768–71.
18. Shah C, Kollef MH. Endotracheal tube intraluminal volume loss among mechanically ventilated patients. Crit Care Med. 2004;32:120–5.
19. HCUP. Fact book 7: procedures in US hospitals. 2003.
20. Freeman BD, Morris PE. Tracheostomy practice in adults with acute respiratory failure. Crit Care Med. 2012;40(10):2890–6.
21. Freeman BD. Indications for and management of tracheostomy. In: Fink M, editor. Textbook of critical care. 6th ed. Philadelphia, PA: Elsevier; 2011. p. 369–72.
22. Plummer AL, Gracey DR. ACCP consensus conference on artificial airways in patients receiving mechanical ventilation. Chest. 1989;96:178–80.

23. Piazza C, Filauro M, Dikkers FG, et al. Long-term intubation and high rate of tracheostomy in COIVD-19 patients might determine and unprecedented increase of airway stenosis: a call to action from the European Laryngological Society. Eur Arch Otorhinolaryngol. 2021;278(1):1–7.
24. Young D, Harrison D, Cuthbertson BH, Rowan K. Effect of early vs late tracheostomy placement on survival in patient receiving mechanical ventilation: the TracMan randomized trial. JAMA. 2013;309(20):2121–9.
25. Freeman BD, Borecki IB, Coopersmith CM, et al. Relationship between tracheostomy timing and duration of mechanical ventilation in critically ill patients. Crit Care Med. 2005;33:2513–20.
26. Saad M, Laghi FA Jr, Brofman J, Undevia NS, Shaikh H. Long-term acute care hospital outcomes of mechanically ventilated patients with coronavirus disease 2019. Crit Care Med. 2022;50(2):256–62.
27. Kwak PE, Connors JR, Benedict PA, et al. Early outcomes from early tracheostomy for patients with COIVD-19. JAMA Otolaryngol Head Neck Surg. 2021;147(3):239–44.
28. Smith PW, Bennett G, Bradley S, et al. SSHEA/APIC Guideline: infection prevention and control in the long-term care facility. Am J Infect Control. 2008;36(7):504–35.
29. Wright SE, Vandahm K. Long-term care of the tracheostomy patient. Clin Chest Med. 2003;24(3):473–87.
30. Dang D, Johantgen ME, Pronovost PJ, et al. Postoperative complications: does intensive care unit staff nursing make a difference? Heart Lung. 2002;31:219–28.
31. Hugonnet S, Uckay I, Pittet D. Staffing level: a determinant of late-onset ventilator associate pneumonia. Crit Care. 2007;11(4):R80.
32. Hua F, Xie H, Worthington HV, Furness S, Zhang Q, Li C. Oral hygiene care for critically ill patients to prevent ventilator associate pneumonia. Cochrane Database Syst Rev. 2016;(10):CD008367.
33. Nava S, Hill N. Non-invasive ventilation in acute respiratory failure. Lancet. 2009;374:250–9.
34. Cabrini L, Landoni G, Oriani A, Plumari VP, Nobile L, Greco M, Pain L, Beretta L, Zangrillo A. Noninvasive ventilation and survival in acute care settings: a comprehensive systematic review and meta-analysis of randomized controlled trials. Crit Care Med. 2015;43(4):880–8.
35. Antonelli M, Conti G, Rocco M, et al. A comparison of noninvasive positive-pressure ventilation and conventional mechanical ventilation in patient with acute respiratory failure. N Engl J Med. 1998;339:429–35.
36. Honda H, Warren DK, Kollef MH. Chapter 4: Infection prevention and surveillance in the intensive care unit. In: Principles of critical care. 4th ed. McGraw Hill; 2015.
37. Smulders K, van der Hans H, Weers-Pothoff I, et al. A randomized clinical trial of intermittent subglottic secretion drainage in patients receiving mechanical ventilation. Chest. 2002;121:858–62.
38. Kollef MM, Afresa B, Anzueto A, et al. Silver coated endotracheal tubes and the incidence of ventilator-associated pneumonia: the NASCEN randomized trial. JAMA. 2008;300(7):805–13.
39. Afresa B, Shorr AF, Anzueto AR, et al. Association between a silver-coasted endotracheal tube and reduced mortality in patients with ventilator associated pneumonia. Chest. 2010;137(5):1015–21.
40. Alkhawaja S, Martin C, Butler RJ, Gwadry-Sridhar F. Post-pyloric gastric tube feeding for preventing pneumonia and improving nutritional outcomes in critically ill adults. Cochrane Database Syst Rev. 2015;2015(8):CD008875.
41. Heyland DK, Dover R, Dhaliwal R, Greenwood J. Optimizing the benefits and minimizing the risks of enteral nutrition in the critically ill: role of small bowel feeding. JPEN J Parenter Enteral Nutr. 2002;26:S51–7.
42. Croce M, Tolley EA, Claridge JA, Fabian TC. Transfusions result in pulmonary morbidity and death after a moderate degree of injury. J Trauma Injury Infect Crit Care. 2005;59:19–24.
43. Wang W, He W, Zhue S, et al. Association between blood transfusion and ventilator-associated events: a nested case-control study. Infect Control Hosp Epidemiol. 2022;43:597–602.

44. Shorr AF, Dug M-S, Kelly KM, Kollef MH, the CRIT Study Group. Red blood cell transfusion and ventilator-assocaited pneumonia: a potential link? Crit Care Med. 2004;32(3):666–74.
45. Hebert PC, Wells G, Blajchman MA, et al. A multicenter, randomized, controlled clinical trial of transfusion requirements in critical care (TRICC). N Engl J Med. 1999;340:409–17.
46. Wang L, Li X, Yang Z, Tang X, Yuan Q, Deng L, Sun X. Semi-recumbent position versus supine position for the prevention of ventilator-associate pneumonia in adults requiring mechanical ventilation. Cochrane Database Syst Rev. 2016;(1):CD009946.
47. Fink JB, Krause SA, Barret L, Schaff D, Alex CG. Extending ventilator circuit change interval beyond 2 days reduces the likelihood of ventilator associated pneumonia. Chest. 1998;113(2):405–11.
48. Sole ML, Poalillo FE, Byers JF, Ludy JE. Bacterial growth in secretions and on suction equipment or orally intubated patients: a pilot study. Am J Crit Care. 2002;11:141–9.
49. Abrams D, Combes A, Brodie D. Extracorporeal membrane oxygenation in cardiopulmonary disease in adults. J Am Coll Cardiol. 2014;63:2769–78. https://doi.org/10.1016/j.jacc.2014.03.046.
50. Brodie D, Slutsky AS, Combes A. Extracorporeal life support for adults with respiratory failure and related indications: a review. JAMA. 2019;322:557–68. https://doi.org/10.1001/jama.2019.9302.
51. Cheng R, Hachamovitch R, Kittleson M, et al. Complications of extracorporeal membrane oxygenation for treatment of cardiogenic shock and cardiac arrest: a meta-analysis of 1,866 adult patients. Ann Thorac Surg. 2014;97:610–6. https://doi.org/10.1016/j.athoracsur.2013.09.008.
52. O'Horo JC, Cawcutt KA, De Moraes G, et al. The evidence base for prophylactic antibiotics in patients receiving extracorporeal membrane oxygenation. ASAIO J. 2016;2:6–10. https://doi.org/10.1097/MAT.0000000000000287.
53. Bizzarro MJ, Conrad SA, Kaufman DA, Rycus P. Extracorporeal Life Support Organization Task Force on Infections, Extracorporeal Membrane Oxygenation: infections acquired during extracorporeal membrane oxygenation in neonates, children, and adults. Pediatr Crit Care Med. 2011;12:277–81. https://doi.org/10.1097/PCC.0b013e3181e28894.
54. Kao LS, Fleming GM, Escamilla R, et al. Antimicrobial prophylaxis and infection surveillance in extracorporeal membrane oxygenation patients: a multi-institutional survey of practice patterns. ASAIO J. 2011;57:231–8. https://doi.org/10.1097/MAT.0b013e31820d19ab.
55. Abrams D, Grasselli G, Schmidt M, et al. ECLS-associated infections in adults: what we know and what we don't know yet. Intensive Care Med. 2020;6:182–91. https://doi.org/10.1007/s00134-019-05847-z.
56. Grasselli G, Scaravilli V, Di Bella S, et al. Nosocomial infections during extracorporeal membrane oxygenation: incidence, etiology, and impact on patients' outcome. Crit Care Med. 2017;5:1726–33. https://doi.org/10.1097/CCM.0000000000002652.
57. Millar JE, Fanning JP, McDonald CI, McAuley DF, Fraser JF. The inflammatory response to extracorporeal membrane oxygenation (ECMO): a review of the pathophysiology. Crit Care Med. 2016;20:387. https://doi.org/10.1186/s13054-016-1570-4.
58. Biffi S, Di Bella S, Scaravilli V, et al. Infections during extracorporeal membrane oxygenation: epidemiology, risk factors, pathogenesis, and prevention. Int J Antimicrob Agents. 2017;50:9–16. https://doi.org/10.1016/j.ijantimicag.2017.02.025.
59. https://www.elso.org/Portals/0/ELSO%20Guidelines%20General%20All%20ECLS%20Version%201_4.pdf.
60. Kondo Y, Ohbe Aso S, et al. Efficacy of prophylactic antibiotics during extracorporeal membrane oxygenation a nationwide cohort study. Ann Am Thorac Soc. 2021;18:1861–7. https://doi.org/10.1513/AnnalsATS.202008-974OC.
61. Montrucchio G, Zagagnoni M, Brazzi L. Antimicrobial prophylaxis in extracorporeal membrane oxygenation: is the debate still open? Ann Am Thorac Soc. 2022;9:870–1. https://doi.org/10.1513/AnnalsATS.202111-1290LE.
62. Glater-Welt LB, Schneider JB, Zinger MM, et al. Nosocomial bloodstream infections in patients receiving extracorporeal life support: variability in prevention practices: a survey of

the extracorporeal life support organization members. J Intensive Care Med. 2016;31:654–9. https://doi.org/10.1177/0885066615571540.
63. Arulkumaran N, Routledge M, Schlebusch S, et al. Antimicrobial-associated harm in critical care: a narrative review. Intensive Care Med. 2020;46:225–35. https://doi.org/10.1007/s00134-020-05929-3.
64. Tamma PD, Avdic E, Li DX, et al. Association of adverse events with antibiotic use in hospitalized patients. JAMA Intern Med. 2017;177:1308–15. https://doi.org/10.1001/jamainternmed.2017.1938.
65. Barletta JF, Bruno JJ, Buckley MS, Cook DJ. Stress ulcer prophylaxis. Crit Care Med. 2016;44(7):1395–405. https://doi.org/10.1097/ccm.0000000000001872.
66. Cook D, Guyatt G. Prophylaxis against upper gastrointestinal bleeding in hospitalized patients. N Engl J Med. 2018;378(26):2506–16. https://doi.org/10.1056/nejmra1605507.
67. Ye Z, Reintam Blaser A, Lytvyn L, Wang Y, Guyatt GH, Mikita JS, Roberts J, Agoritsas T, Bertschy S, Boroli F, Camsooksai J, Du B, Heen AF, Lu J, Mella JM, Vandvik PO, Wise R, Zheng Y, Liu L, Siemieniuk RAC. Gastrointestinal bleeding prophylaxis for critically ill patients: a clinical practice guideline. BMJ. 2020;368:l6722. https://doi.org/10.1136/bmj.l6722.
68. Bardou M, Quenot J-P, Barkun A. Stress-related mucosal disease in the critically ill patient. Nat Rev Gastroenterol Hepatol. 2015;12:98–107.
69. Cook DJ, et al. Risk factors for gastrointestinal bleeding in critical ill patients. Canadian Critical Care Trials Group. N Engl J Med. 1994;330:377–81.
70. Laine L, et al. Lower gastrointestinal events in a double-blind trial of the cyclo-oxygenase-2 selective inhibitor etoricoxib and the traditional non-steroidal anti-inflammatory drug diclofenac. Gastroenterology. 2008;135:1517–25.
71. Shin JM, Sachs G. Pharmacology of proton pump inhibitors. Curr Gastroenterol Rep. 2008;10(6):528–34. https://doi.org/10.1007/s11894-008-0098-4.
72. Forgacs I, Loganayagam A. Overprescribing proton pump inhibitors. BMJ. 2008;336(7634):2–3. https://doi.org/10.1136/bmj.39406.449456.be.
73. Dellinger RP, Carlet JM, Masur H, Gerlach H, Calandra T, Cohen J, Gea-Banacloche J, Keh D, Marshall JC, Parker MM, Ramsay G, Zimmerman JL, Vincent JL, Levy MM. Surviving Sepsis Campaign guidelines for management of severe sepsis and septic shock. Crit Care Med. 2004;32(3):858–73. https://doi.org/10.1097/01.ccm.0000117317.18092.e4.
74. Moayyedi P, Leontiadis GI. The risks of PPI therapy. Nat Rev Gastroenterol Hepatol. 2012;9(3):132–9. https://doi.org/10.1038/nrgastro.2011.272.
75. Trifan A, Stanciu C, Girleanu I, Stoica OC, Singeap AM, Maxim R, Chiriac SA, Ciobica A, Boiculese L. Proton pump inhibitors therapy and risk of Clostridium difficile infection: systematic review and meta-analysis. World J Gastroenterol. 2017;23(35):6500–15. https://doi.org/10.3748/wjg.v23.i35.6500.
76. Fohl AL. Proton pump inhibitor-associated pneumonia: not a breath of fresh air after all? World J Gastrointest Pharmacol Ther. 2011;2(3):17. https://doi.org/10.4292/wjgpt.v2.i3.17.
77. Dial S. Risk of Clostridium difficile diarrhea among hospital inpatients prescribed proton pump inhibitors: cohort and case-control studies. Can Med Assoc J. 2004;171(1):33–8. https://doi.org/10.1503/cmaj.1040876.

Chapter 7
Infection Prevention in the Surgical ICU

Chelsea Guy-Frank, Ryan Rihani, and Lillian S. Kao

Introduction

Hospital-associated infections (HAIs) are a significant problem in intensive care unit (ICU) patients, with studies reporting HAI rates of up to almost 50% [1]. Furthermore, surgical and trauma ICU patient populations incur additional risks for infection related to their surgical procedures or injury. Although the type and prevalence of HAIs may vary based on the surgical population, there are general principles for infection prevention that can be applied across subgroups.

C. Guy-Frank
Center for Surgical Trials and Evidence-Based Practice, McGovern Medical School, University of Texas Health Science Center at Houston, Houston, TX, USA

R. Rihani
Center for Surgical Trials and Evidence-Based Practice, McGovern Medical School, University of Texas Health Science Center at Houston, Houston, TX, USA

Department of Anesthesiology, Critical Care and Pain Medicine, McGovern Medical School, University of Texas Health Science Center at Houston, Houston, USA

L. S. Kao (✉)
Center for Surgical Trials and Evidence-Based Practice, McGovern Medical School, University of Texas Health Science Center at Houston, Houston, TX, USA

Department of Surgery, McGovern Medical School, University of Texas Health Science Center at Houston, Houston, USA
e-mail: Lillian.S.Kao@uth.tmc.edu

M. Ellsworth, L. Ostrosky-Zeichner (eds.), *Infection Prevention in the Intensive Care Setting*, https://doi.org/10.1007/978-3-031-67062-6_7

Overview of Prevention Strategies

Several general important strategies for infection prevention include general hygiene and bathing, oral hygiene, glycemic control, nutritional optimization, antimicrobial prophylaxis, mobilization, respiratory training, and MRSA screening and decolonization.

General Hygiene and Bathing

Maintenance of clean, hydrated, dry, and non-irritated skin can help reduce the risk of surgical site infections (SSIs), wound infections, and pressure injuries. This starts in the preoperative phase and should be maintained in the surgical ICU. However, the choice of cleansing agent for routine ICU use is controversial; in particular, the effectiveness of chlorhexidine (CHG) washes or washcloths has been debated. Meta-analyses of preoperative bathing have failed to demonstrate a significant benefit in SSI reduction with CHG versus unmedicated soap [2, 3]. Similarly, a Cochrane review did not find sufficient evidence in critically ill patients for CHG bathing over non-CHG bathing strategies (soap and water or non-CHG cloths) for prevention of HAIs [4]. Other meta-analyses suggest that daily CHG bathing reduces HAIs in adult ICU patients, but that CHG bathing does not occur routinely and that the effectiveness is greatest among high-risk patients [5]. In addition to questions about effectiveness, there are concerns about increased CHG resistance with widespread daily use due to CHG reducing only gram-positive but not gram-negative bacteremia [6]. Thus, use of routine CHG bathing may depend on underlying baseline risk for the given surgical ICU population.

Oral Hygiene and Care

Oral disease is common and associated with non-communicable diseases like cancer and diabetes, a reduced quality of life, and even lower survival [7]. It is also associated with postoperative infectious complications, most notably pneumonia [8–10]. Proposed pathways that link oral disease to infectious complications include increased pathogenic bacterial load and inflammation leading to higher risk with aspiration, pathogenic colonization of the stomach and direct seeding, and transient bacteremia with hematogenous spread of infection [11, 12].

Oral hygiene is a component of many perioperative and ICU care bundles. However, studies report conflicting results with regard to reduction in HAIs and other outcomes such as mortality and length of stay (LOS). A Cochrane review found that CHG mouth rinse/gel as part of an oral hygiene protocol likely reduces the incidence of ventilator associated pneumonia (VAP) but has no effect on mortality or ICU LOS compared to placebo or usual care [13]. Additionally, toothbrushing (± antiseptics) may reduce VAP compared to oral hygiene protocols without toothbrushing (± antiseptics), as mechanical debridement may be better at disrupting biofilms compared to rinses. Comparatively, other studies found oral CHG use to be independently associated with an increased risk of oral mucositis and death, specifically in mechanically ventilated non-cardiac surgery and across all ICU patients [6, 14, 15]. The use of CHG may affect nitric oxide homeostasis, which may be associated with increased risk of ICU-acquired sepsis and mortality [6]. A recent multicenter stepped wedge cluster randomized trial reported that de-adoption of CHG mouthwash from oral care did not have any impact on mortality and may have improved oral health [16]. Despite the conflicting data specifically on CHG-based oral care, oral hygiene overall is important for general health and reduction of HAIs. Protocols should focus more on mechanical oral cleansing rather than rely on CHG-based oral rinses or gels.

Glycemic Control

General

Acute stress hyperglycemia in the perioperative period, in both diabetics and non-diabetics, increases the risk of postoperative infectious complications [3, 17]. In the 2000s, intensive glucose control (blood glucose 80–120 mg/dL) was recommended compared to conventional treatment (insulin if glucose >215 mg/dL and maintenance of glucose 180–200 mg/dL) in surgical ICU patients to reduce mortality based on a randomized trial of 1548 cardiac surgery patients [18]. However, intensive glucose control had variable effectiveness in subsequent trials and was associated with increased rates of hypoglycemia. Based on the NICE-SUGAR trial, a multicenter medical/surgical ICU study comparing intensive (blood glucose 81–108 mg/dL) versus conventional glucose control (144–180 mg/dL), intensive glucose control was abandoned based on increased 90-day mortality in the intensive glucose control group [19]. Although subgroup analysis suggested that trauma patients and those receiving corticosteroids may still benefit from intensive glucose control, a more conservative recommended range was adopted by many critical care societies.

Over the past decade, there have since been several systematic reviews/meta-analyses with mixed results and recommendations of blood glucose targets and the safety of intensive glycemic control. A meta-analysis by Yao et al. examining medical, surgical, and mixed ICUs found reduced rate of all-cause mortality, infection rate, acquired sepsis, and ICU LOS, although more hypoglycemia risk, with intensive glucose control compared to conventional glucose control [20]. Wang et al. examined surgery patients only and found lower total postoperative infections and short-term (30-day) mortality; de Vries et al. found lower SSI risk but no effect on mortality, with both showing higher risk of hypoglycemia with intensive glucose control compared to conventional glucose control [21, 22]. The discordance across outcomes may be explained by the patient populations included, the feeding parameters (enteral and/or parenteral), variation in monitoring, and variation in target blood glucose levels. Currently, exact cut-offs of blood glucose recommendations vary, and ultimately, glycemic control protocols must balance the benefits of tighter glucose control with the risks of hypoglycemia.

Burn

With the stress response seen in burn patients, there are increases in catecholamine, glucagon, and glucocorticoid production, leading to enhanced glycogenolysis and protein breakdown, with subsequent hyperglycemia [23]. Recent evidence has demonstrated that hyperglycemia in severely burned patients is especially detrimental, associated with increased infections and sepsis, a higher incidence of pneumonia, catabolism, hypermetabolism, and post-burn mortality [24, 25]. Pham and colleagues showed in a retrospective study in 2005 that intensive insulin therapy to maintain normoglycemia in severely burned children can be safely and effectively implemented in the burn unit and seems to lower infection rates and improve survival [26]. A study published in 2008 evaluating American Burn Association verified burn centers demonstrated that 73% of them implemented an intensive insulin protocol (defined as upper glucose target of ≤120 mg/dL) [27]. This high incidence of strict glycemic control among verified centers in 2008 was before the publication of the NICE-SUGAR trial in 2009 and likely a response to the overwhelming evidence regarding the effects of hyperglycemia.

The first randomized controlled trial in burn patients was published in 2010 on 239 pediatric burn patients; the trial demonstrated decreased infection and sepsis but no change in mortality in the tight glycemic control group [28]. The high metabolic requirements and incidence of parenteral nutrition in severely burned patients may also point to further benefit from tight glycemic control as the incidence of hypoglycemia may be better managed with consistent nutrition. However, there remain no published trials in adult burn patients, and the data is sparse in pediatrics. Therefore, the best strategy continues to be adherence to the published data in mixed critically ill patients.

Nutritional Optimization

General

Malnutrition has been shown to be independently associated with higher mortality, longer hospital LOS, and increased cost of hospitalization [29, 30]. A systematic review regarding malnutrition in ICU patients published by the American Society for Parenteral and Enteral Nutrition (ASPEN) in 2015 demonstrated increased ICU LOS, ICU readmission, incidence of infection, and risk of hospital mortality [31]. Prolonged hypermetabolism has been associated with catabolism, multiorgan failure, and death.

Surgical patients can have additional components that complicate route and amount of nutritional intake. For example, trauma, burn, or septic patients have higher metabolic demands. Patients may not be able to receive enteral nutrition due to bowel discontinuity or postoperative ileus. Oral intake may be delayed due to associated traumatic brain injuries or dysphagia related to associated injuries. Interruptions in enteral nutrition may also occur based on repeated operative interventions (such as in trauma patients with multiple orthopedic injuries or burn patients), leading to caloric and nutritional deficits.

Although enteral nutrition is generally preferred unless contraindicated, most studies have found no difference in mortality or infectious complications with early initiation of enteral versus parenteral nutrition [32, 33]. An open abdomen and administration of stable low-dose and moderate-dose vasopressors are not necessarily contraindications to enteral nutrition if initial resuscitation has been completed. Early enteral nutrition facilitates return of normal bowel function, though use of parenteral nutrition is associated with less digestive side effects [33, 34]. Although there may be benefit to early supplemental parenteral nutrition when enteral nutrition is insufficient [35], ASPEN recommends only starting after 7–10 days if >60% of caloric needs are not being met [32, 36]. The European Society for Clinical Nutritional and Metabolism recommends early over delayed enteral nutrition in abdominal surgery patients, unless contraindicated, and recommends glutamine in burn and trauma patients who do not have acute liver or renal failure to improve wound healing [36]. Based on prior studies and current guidelines, most surgical ICU patients should receive 12–25 kcal/kg and 1.2–2 g/kg/day of protein in the first 7–10 days [32, 36, 37]. Multidisciplinary surgical ICU rounds with a dietician may allow for further modifications for specific patients.

Burn

Metabolic rates of burn patients have been demonstrated to be more than twice normal, and these increased rates can persist for years after the injury. Although this response has been demonstrated in all trauma, surgical, and critically ill patients, the severity and longevity of the response in burn patients is unique. Thus, inadequate nutrition specifically in burn patients may be magnified in the setting of their drastically increased metabolism. By measuring the resting energy expenditures of the patients at the bedside with specialized equipment (when feasible), the health care team can appropriately titrate the nutrition to meet the patient's changing needs.

Antimicrobial Prophylaxis

General

Pre-incisional prophylactic antibiotics have been demonstrated to reduce the risk of SSIs across multiple types of surgical procedures. Based on the Surgical Care Improvement Project measures, antibiotics should be chosen based on the type of procedure performed, patient colonization and history, and additional factors such as weight, blood loss, and duration of procedure. In general, prophylactic antibiotics should not be continued beyond 24 h postoperatively.

Trauma

Antibiotic prophylaxis is indicated prior to incision for trauma patients undergoing operations such as exploratory laparotomy. Antibiotics should not be continued beyond 24 h unless there is presence of pre-existing infection (such as due to a delay in diagnosis in a bowel perforation). Damage control laparotomies and open abdomen are not indications to continue prophylactic antibiotics. Antibiotic prophylaxis has also been recommended, although conditionally, prior to procedures such as tube thoracostomy to reduce the incidence of empyema.

Antibiotic prophylaxis has been utilized for multiple types of fractures such as open extremity and facial fractures. Use of systemic antibiotic prophylaxis for non-infected open extremity fractures has been recommended to be limited to Gustilo type III open extremity fractures, particularly with associated bone loss. There is increasing evidence for benefit of topical, intrawound antibiotics in traumatic fracture repair. With regard to non-infected facial fractures, prophylactic antibiotics are not indicated outside of a pre-incisional dose for operative fractures, regardless of type (such as mandibular versus non-mandibular). Despite recommendations for antibiotic stewardship in these cases, there is limited evidence for type and duration of antibiotics and there is widespread variation in practice.

Burn

Current recommendations do not address systemic antimicrobial prophylaxis or specifically state they are not recommended. A meta-analysis of 17 trials published in 2010 demonstrated that systemic antibiotic prophylaxis administered to burn patients in the first 4–14 days significantly reduced all-cause mortality; limited perioperative prophylaxis decreased wound infections; and topical antibiotic prophylaxis had no beneficial effects [38]. This study, however, was limited by weak quality of evidence. Another meta-analysis published in 2017 included 19 trials and demonstrated no effectiveness of systemic antimicrobial prophylaxis for the prevention of toxic shock syndrome or burn wound infection, but prophylaxis could be useful in severe burn patients requiring mechanical ventilation in the prevention of pneumonia as well as prevention of split-thickness SSIs [39]. Therefore, no recommendations can be made regarding the utility of systemic antimicrobial prophylaxis as the data remains limited. In most circumstances, the risk of development of antimicrobial resistance likely outweighs the benefits; however, large total body surface area burn patients requiring mechanical ventilation may be a special population demanding further research.

Antifungal Prophylaxis

Fungal infections, particularly invasive candidiasis, are associated with significant morbidity and mortality in surgical ICU patients [40]. Antifungal prophylaxis has been shown to be of value in certain high-risk patients, such as neutropenic cancer patients and transplant patients. Important risk factors to consider include diabetes, kidney failure or hemodialysis requirements, severe pancreatitis, a long duration of mechanical ventilation or invasive central lines, parenteral nutrition, broad-spectrum antibiotic use, major surgery, gastrointestinal perforation or leaks, burns, transplant patients, patients with malignancies, and those colonized with *Candida* species [40, 41]. Studies have found a reduction in fungal infections, and a possible trend toward mortality reduction with antifungal prophylaxis. However, most studies are of small sample size and vary in the patient population included and protocol for antifungal use [42–44]. Studies have suggested improving risk stratification of patients to determine where prophylaxis is warranted and improving tools for diagnosing invasive candidiasis. Given some of the concerns related to adverse side effects of antifungals as well as a concern for increased resistance, an alternative to prophylaxis that has been used is use of empirical antifungals in high-risk patients when concerns of an infection develop [40]. One trial found beta-D-glucan surveillance showed promise as a guide for preemptive antifungal therapy in high-risk ICU patients, which may help avoid a delay in treatment and any subsequent morbidity and mortality [45, 46].

Avoiding Deconditioning: Mobilization and Respiratory Training

Surgical ICU patients are at risk for decompensation from both a physical and respiratory standpoint as multiple components can reduce or restrict movement or respiratory function. Patients may be critically ill and sedated and ventilated, which reduces mobility. Traumatic injuries or post-procedural limitations may restrict movement or cause shallow breathing due to pain. ICU-acquired weakness is a serious concern given its associated short- and long-term effects [47]. Although evidence is somewhat limited and weak as to how to best implement passive and/or active mobility, early mobility has been proposed as a preventative measure to reduce ventilator associated events, pressure injuries, ICU associated weakness, and improve functional outcomes [48–51]. Additional high-quality randomized trials are warranted to improve protocols on patient mobility. Institutions should focus on incorporating active and passive movement in a multidisciplinary discussion between occupational/physical therapy, nursing staff, and the surgical ICU team.

Respiratory therapy is equally important, as patients are at risk of respiratory deconditioning. Inspiratory muscle training in the preoperative setting has shown a reduction on postoperative atelectasis, pneumonia, and duration of hospital stay in cardiac and major abdominal surgery patients [52, 53]. These principles can be applied in the surgical ICU setting. Incentive spirometry as a preventative measure is likely not enough as the only intervention. However, as part of bundle care, such as iCOUGH, it has been shown to help reduce pneumonia [54, 55].

MRSA Screening and Decolonization

Although the incidence of methicillin-resistant *Staphylococcus aureus* (MRSA) infections is estimated at 1% after major surgical procedures, the prevalence of MRSA colonization has increased over the past few decades, now estimated up to 5–10%. MRSA colonization is associated with a higher risk for MRSA SSI, SSI overall, longer hospital stays, more readmissions, higher costs, and higher rates of ICU mortality [2, 56, 57]. MRSA bundles (screening, decolonization, contact precautions, vancomycin-containing antibiotic prophylaxis), when implemented correctly, have shown to reduce rates of SSIs [2]. There are 3 primary approaches a surgical ICU can take with MRSA: (1) universal screening and decolonization of MRSA+ patients, (2) selective screening of high-risk populations and decolonization, or (3) universal decolonization without screening. Universal screening is costly and likely wasteful of resources [57]. Selective screening would produce the lowest risk of emergence of antiseptic resistance; however, targeting populations appropriately can be difficult, and may end up being ineffective. Universal decolonization has been shown to reduce hospital-acquired MRSA rates and be cost-savings in hypothetical Markov microsimulation models and decision-analysis models [58–61]. Balancing appropriate decolonization protocols with potential overuse of antiseptics/antibiotics, risk of microbial resistance, costs, and an institution's specific patient population can help determine the most appropriate protocols to implement.

Prevention Strategies for Specific Surgical Infections

Surgical Site Infections

Surgical site infections (SSIs) affect 2–5% of all patients and are associated with increased morbidity and mortality [2, 3, 62]. They comprise 16–25% of HAIs and result in an additional $3.5–10 billion in health care expenditures annually (2007 US dollars) [3, 63]. Approximately 77% of deaths in patients with SSIs are attributable to the SSIs. Additionally, up to 60% have been estimated to be preventable by using evidence-based guidelines [62].

The Center for Disease Control and Prevention definition of SSI is the most widely used, which classifies SSIs by depth and tissue spaces involved 30- to

90- days post procedure [64]. Superficial SSI (S-SSI) involves the skin or subcutaneous tissue, deep SSI (D-SSI) involves the fascia or muscular layers, and an organ space SSI (O/S-SSI) involves any part of the body opened or manipulated during a procedure, excluding the previously mentioned layers.

Surgical site infections preventative measures
General preoperative preventative measures [2, 9, 52, 65] • Smoking cessation • Glucose control • Selective methicillin-resistant *Staphylococcus aureus* (MRSA) screening and/or decolonization • Bowel prep for elective colectomies • Preoperative bathing/showering • Oral hygiene • Preoperative inspiratory muscle training
Bedside procedures in the surgical ICU: Percutaneous tracheostomy or gastrostomy tube *(intraoperative interventions and principles apply)* [2, 3, 62, 66–68] • Glucose control • Hair removal with clippers if the hair interferes with surgery • Skin preparation with antiseptic (CHG or iodine-based) that include alcohol (if no contraindication • Maintenance of normothermia • Appropriate sterile wound care and dressing • Surgical team preparation: antiseptic surgical hand scrub and sterile surgical attire, drapes, and equipment • Prophylactic Antibiotics [69–71]: – Not required for tracheostomy placement – Recommended for gastrostomy tube placement to reduce peristomal infection risk
Postoperative preventative measures • Glucose control • Early mobility • Nutritional support with adequate protein • Hygiene • Oral hygiene • Wound care • Monitoring for infection and early intervention if develops

Although prevention of SSIs is ideal, it is not always possible. Prompt recognition and swift treatment to avoid progression of the infection are essential. The keystone for preventing progression is source control [72]. For S-SSIs, this may only require opening the incision at bedside and wound care; patients with significant cellulitis or systemic signs of infection may require antibiotics. Some infections may be more severe and can lead to a necrotizing soft tissue infection or be associated with concomitant O/S-SSIs. O/S-SSIs are associated with increased morbidity and mortality and are associated with additional postoperative complications. O/S-SSIs require antibiotics and often need source control via interventional radiology or surgical intervention. If the patient is not worsening clinically, O/S-SSIs that are too small to drain with interventional radiology can be treated with antibiotics and reassessed with repeat imaging as indicated [73]. Waele et al. found that of 1392 abdominal infections in the ICU, 67% had positive cultures, most commonly gram-negative bacteria (48%). Patients in the ICU ≤ 2 days prior to the study had more *Escherichia coli, Methicillin sensitive Staphylococcus aureus,* and anaerobic isolates, and fewer Enterococci than patients who'd been in the ICU longer [74]. The most common isolated organisms were *E. coli*, followed by ampicillin-sensitive *Enterococci*, and *Candida albicans, Clostridium, Pseudomonas aeruginosa, Klebsiella* spp., *Enterobacter* spp., and ampicillin-resistant *Enterococci* [74]. These findings had some overlap with a study in Spain examining patients with secondary and tertiary peritonitis, which found *Pseudomonas* spp., *E. coli*, and *Candida* spp., to be the most common, in addition to gram-positive cocci [75].

In surgical ICU patients, culturing of the wound is beneficial to help tailor antibiotics, especially given the higher incidence of resistant organisms. Additionally, rapid molecular testing can be considered to quickly assess multidrug resistant organisms [76]. When starting empiric antibiotics, patient risk factors, sources of infection, and the hospital's antibiogram should be considered. Some patients with additional risk factors such as prior antibiotic use, known colonization, previous infection with resistant organisms may require additional empiric coverage [73]. Antibiotics should be narrowed once certain organisms are ruled out or the organism is identified. Additionally, use of procalcitonin, a proinflammatory biomarker, can help shorten antibiotic duration in ICU patients, and has also been shown to lower risk of mortality [76].

Hospital-Associated Pneumonia (HAP) and Ventilator-Associated Pneumonia (VAP)

HAP and VAP are associated with increased risk of morbidity, mortality, cost, and resource utilization [77–79]. They are among the most frequent ICU-acquired infections, with incidence ranging from 5 to 40%, depending on the diagnostic criteria and patient population [77]. For example, trauma patients have reportedly higher rates, likely due to the alteration in immune function, increased aspiration risk from brain injury, or associated chest or lung injury [77]. Most commonly the infection will be bacterial in this setting. However pending specific patient risk factors, it is important to consider viral causes (like *Herpes simplex virus* or *Cytomegalovirus)*, which can be seen in both immunocompromised patients, or those with multiorgan failure and prolonged ICU stays [77]. Many of the general practice guidelines for mechanical ventilation are applicable to the surgical ICU patient population, such as avoiding intubation if possible, minimizing sedation, conducting daily spontaneous awakening trials and daily spontaneous breathing trials when no contraindications, ensuring early mobility, elevating the head of the bed 30–45°, performing oral hygiene, and maintaining a clean ventilatory circuit and endotracheal tube. Additional components that have mixed results in reducing rates of VAP include the use of subglottic drainage ports to minimize secretion pooling, selective decontamination of the aerodigestive tract, oral chlorhexidine use, and probiotic use [77, 78]. Some of the more commonly discussed components, primarily in the surgical and trauma critical care population, include the timing of tracheostomy and dysphagia and aspiration risks.

Aspiration can cause pneumonitis or pneumonia and is considered the most important mechanism that leads to nosocomial pneumonia. It can lead to severe complications and increased risk of mortality. Aspiration can occur in up to 45% of health subjects sleep and in up to 70% of subjects with abnormal swallowing due to impaired consciousness, respiratory or gastrointestinal tract instrumentation, head trauma, older adults, and in postoperative patients, especially in thoracic or abdominal surgery [9, 79]. Open abdominal surgery has been independently associated with postoperative pneumonia. High-risk patients may benefit from aspiration screening regardless of if they have been intubated. For those who have been intubated, swallowing dysfunction can occur in 10–67.5% of patients. Swallowing function should be assessed in all patients post-extubation, and formal speech evaluations should be considered in patients with prolonged intubation and elderly patients. Approximately ¼ of elderly patients are feeding tube dependent 3 weeks post-extubation due to ongoing swallowing disorders [36]. Additionally, some patients have been shown to experience post-extubation swallowing disorders for several months [36]. Routine monitoring of gastric residual volumes as a marker for aspiration is not recommend in clinical guidelines as it does not correlate with incidences of pneumonia, regurgitation, or aspiration [32]. Use of appropriate protocols with preventative measures and dysphagia screening based on a multidisciplinary approach, communication and teamwork can help reduce the risk of this potentially devastating complication.

Infections Due to Skin and Pressure Injuries

Hospital-acquired pressure injuries (also referred to as pressures ulcers or bedsores) are areas of localized damage of the skin or underlying tissue due to pressure or pressure in combination with shear (Pressure Ulcer Stages Table) [80, 81]. They confer significant morbidity, extended hospital stays, reduced quality of life, and increased cost. Despite being considered primarily preventable, they occur in 5–16% of ICU patients, with some of the highest risk found in surgical critical care patients [80, 82, 83]. Often found at bony prominences, some of the most common locations are the sacrum/coccyx, heels, and buttocks. Skin irritation, a potentially modifiable risk factor, has been shown to be a strong predictor of pressure injuries. Other known contributory factors that should be taken into consideration for each patient include altered perfusion (hypoperfusion/hypoxia), surgery duration, vasopressor use, reduced mobility, nutritional status, skin moisture, and use of mechanical devices.

Pressure ulcer stages	
Stage I	Erythema of the skin
Stage II	Erythema with partial thickness loss of the skin, including epidermis and part of the superficial dermis
Stage III	Full thickness ulcer of epidermis and dermis and may involve subcutaneous fat
Stage IV	Full thickness ulcer muscle, tendon, or bone involvement
Unstageable	Full thickness tissue loss, but tissue damage extent not determinable due to obscuring debris, slough, or eschar
Deep tissue pressure injury	Intact or nonintact skin, with localized damage to underlying tissue. Often presenting with nonblanchable purple/maroon discoloration of intact skin
Medical device-related pressure injury	Results from devices applied for therapeutic purposes (e.g., splints), prolonged use of poorly placed/ill-fitting devices/equipment
Mucosal membrane pressure injuries	On mucous membranes from medical devices, such as ill-fitting dentures, endotracheal tubes

Various preventive measures have been studied, with some showing benefit in multiple trials and meta-analyses [84]. However, many can be difficult to implement in surgical ICU patients given ongoing injuries, movement restrictions, operative-related factors, and availability of personnel or equipment [85]. Basic components of prevention include risk assessment, hygiene protocols, regular skin and line assessment, and nutrition optimization, with multidisciplinary involvement. Additionally, offloading of pressure points, such as heel and sacral prophylactic protective dressing and reactive air and gel surface bedding, has proven beneficial [84, 86]. Reactive air surfaces may reduce the risk of pressure ulcer development and increase ulcer healing rates compared to foam surfaces [87].

If a pressure injury develops, 40% can worsen to a more severe stage during the surgical ICU stay [81]. They can become infected, sometimes requiring multiple debridements, and if more severe, can require fecal diversion or complex operative tissue cover to help with healing [82]. It is important to prevent progression of pressure injuries with use of pressure offloading and appropriate cleansing. In particular, patients with trauma-related spinal cord injuries are prone to chronic infections secondary to pressure injuries. Necrotic, fibrinous, or infected tissue should be debrided regularly along with wound cleansing to promote healing and granulation tissue. Patient's comorbidities, expected outcomes, and quality of life goals can help identify if interventions like diverting colostomy, with or without surgical flap coverage should be considered [88]. In a complex patient population, a multidisciplinary approach, with the inclusion of patient and family when able, is necessary to reduce the risk of progression, associated complications and improve quality of life outcomes.

Line and Tube-Related Infections

In the surgical ICU, many patients require various lines or tubes for invasive monitoring, therapies, nutritional support, respiratory assistance, infection control, and wound management. Lines and tubes can increase the risk of infection through formation of an artificial tract from inside the body to the external world or through pressure necrosis of surrounding tissue. Attention to the indication for the line or tube, use of sterile technique during placement, and early removal is necessary to minimize risks of infection.

Tracheostomies are a consideration for all ICU patients that may require prolonged ventilation. Meta-analyses examining ICU patients have had varying findings when comparing early versus late tracheostomy in relation to VAP, mortality, duration of mechanical ventilation, and LOS [89–91]. Currently, there are several specific recommendations related to tracheostomy in surgical and trauma patients. The Eastern Association for the Surgery of Trauma guidelines (currently being updated) recommended early tracheostomy for trauma patients with head injuries, as it likely decreases the duration of mechanical ventilation and ICU LOS. Additionally, early tracheostomy should be considered in all trauma patients who are anticipated to require mechanical ventilation for more than 7 days [92]. This is often seen with older patients, more chest trauma, such as a flail chest, major operative interventions, and underlying COPD [93, 94]. More recent reviews, though slightly mixed results, suggest a reduction of VAP and possible improved neurological outcomes with early tracheostomy [95]. Additionally, tracheostomy decreases need for sedation, improves patient comfort, communication, and mobility, and likely reduces hospital cost.

Tracheostomies require pre-intervention planning, appropriate patient selection, and a sterile procedure. Tracheostomies can be placed both surgical and percutaneously. A Cochrane review in 2016 found no difference in rates of mortality or serious life-threatening adverse events, but moderate quality of evidence of significant reduction of wound infection/stomatitis with percutaneous tracheostomy [96]. After tracheostomy placement, routine assessment, hygiene, suctioning, and tube care will help to reduce the risk of infection. The stoma site of a tracheostomy should be kept clean and dry to avoid maceration and skin breakdown. If the tracheostomy flange is secured with suture ties to the neck, they should be removed within 7 days of placement to help reduce flange-related pressure injuries [70]. Pressure injuries and skin breakdown can increase the risk of local infection. Most local infection can be treated with wound care and antibiotics, but rarely can become more serious and require conversion to orotracheal intubation and surgical debridement [70]. Although uncommon, bacterial tracheitis can occur in tracheostomy-dependent patients, likely from tracheostomy tube colonization. Most common isolates include *S. aureus, Pseudomonas aeruginosa*, and *Streptococcus pneumoniae* [97]. Tracheostomy hygiene and care and pulmonary toilet minimize the risk in this specific population. Additionally, secretions should be frequently assessed for suctioning, and airway humidification can help reduce tracheostomy tube obstruction in patients on ventilatory support [69, 70].

Gastrostomy tubes, percutaneous endoscopic or surgically placed are often required in patients who need prolonged nutrition support and who have an inability to swallow. Infectious complications can range from minor fungal infections that can be treated with topical antifungals to bacterial wound infections requiring systemic antibiotics. In severe cases, peritonitis and necrotizing soft tissue infections may occur requiring operative intervention. Preventive measures include proper selection of patients, use of sterile technique, and administration of pre-procedural antibiotic prophylaxis. Timing of initiation of feeds does not increase the risk of infection. Post-procedural care should focus on keeping the site clean and dry. The buried bumper syndrome should be avoided. This occurs when the internal fixation device migrates outside the stomach along the stoma tract, usually due to excessive compression of tissue between the external and internal fixation device, causing tissue ulceration, ischemia, and necrosis. This can lead to perforation, hemorrhage, and peritonitis. Preventive measures include avoiding undue tension between fixators and daily tube rotation.

Indications for thoracostomy (chest) tube or pigtail catheter placement include pneumothorax, hemothorax, and pleural effusion. In injured patients, an insufficiently evacuated or retained hemothorax is a risk factor for empyema. Aggressive management of retained hemothorax includes placement of a second tube and administration of tissue plasminogen activator through the tube to assist with evacuation. If this fails, then a video-assisted thoracic surgery (VATS) can be performed, though some physicians are turning to this procedure even sooner. This is important to avoid the development of an empyema, entrapped lung, or fibrothorax. Chest tubes should be sterilely placed, when able, and should have an occlusive dressing, with Vaseline or xeroform gauze, both for tube placement and at time of tube removal.

Intracranial pressure (ICP) monitors (intraventricular and intraparenchymal) are used in trauma and non-trauma patients to monitor intracranial pressure, and/or drain fluid, with the goal of detecting, preventing, and treating secondary brain insults. Guidelines recommend placement of ICP monitors in traumatic brain injury patients who are at risk for intracranial hypertension and have an abnormal admission head CT scan [98]. However, because up to 50% of patients can develop increased ICP even with a normal admission head CT, if the patient has 2 of the following: age > 40, unilateral or bilateral motor posturing or episodes of systolic blood pressure < 90 mmHg, an ICP monitor is still recommended [99]. Intraventricular monitoring devices are associated with infection rates up to 20% (ventriculitis). At time of placement, strict adherence to aseptic techniques is important and the use of prophylactic antibiotics can be given. Infection risk can be reduced by use of long tunnels, a closed drainage system, prompt removal when monitoring is no longer required and avoidance of flushing the system or routine cerebrospinal fluid sampling. Additionally, at time of closure, the wound is often closed in layers to minimize the risk of cerebrospinal fluid leak or infection.

Conclusion

Infection prevention in surgical ICUs ideally starts prior to any planned procedures with preoperative optimization and perioperative risk reduction strategies. However, such strategies are not always possible, such as in the trauma and emergency surgery populations. Strict attention should be paid in the surgical ICU not only to hygiene and line and tube care but also to glycemic control, nutritional optimization, and early mobilization. A low threshold for infectious complications should be maintained to allow for early intervention and rescue.

References

1. Vincent JL, Rello J, Marshall J, Silva E, Anzueto A, Martin CD, et al. International study of the prevalence and outcomes of infection in intensive care units. JAMA. 2009;302(21):2323–9.
2. Ban KA, Minei JP, Laronga C, Harbrecht BG, Jensen EH, Fry DE, et al. American College of Surgeons and Surgical Infection Society: surgical site infection guidelines, 2016 update. J Am Coll Surg. 2017;224(1):59–74.
3. O'Hara LM, Thom KA, Preas MA. Update to the Centers for Disease Control and Prevention and the Healthcare Infection Control Practices Advisory Committee Guideline for the Prevention of Surgical Site Infection (2017): a summary, review, and strategies for implementation. Am J Infect Control. 2018;46(6):602–9.
4. Lewis SR, Schofield-Robinson OJ, Rhodes S, Smith AF. Chlorhexidine bathing of the critically ill for the prevention of hospital-acquired infection. Cochrane Database Syst Rev. 2019;8:CD012248.
5. Frost SA, Hou YC, Lombardo L, Metcalfe L, Lynch JM, Hunt L, et al. Evidence for the effectiveness of chlorhexidine bathing and health care-associated infections among adult intensive care patients: a trial sequential meta-analysis. BMC Infect Dis. 2018;18(1):679.
6. Blot S, Ruppe E, Harbarth S, Asehnoune K, Poulakou G, Luyt CE, et al. Healthcare-associated infections in adult intensive care unit patients: changes in epidemiology, diagnosis, prevention and contributions of new technologies. Intensive Crit Care Nurs. 2022;70:103227.
7. Oral health in America. a report of the surgeon general. J Calif Dent Assoc. 2000;28(9):685–95.
8. Kurasawa Y, Maruoka Y, Sekiya H, Negishi A, Mukohyama H, Shigematsu S, et al. Pneumonia prevention effects of perioperative oral management in approximately 25,000 patients following cancer surgery. Clin Exp Dent Res. 2020;6(2):165–73.
9. Pedersen PU, Larsen P, Hakonsen SJ. The effectiveness of systematic perioperative oral hygiene in reduction of postoperative respiratory tract infections after elective thoracic surgery in adults: a systematic review. JBI Database System Rev Implement Rep. 2016;14(1):140–73.
10. Nobuhara H, Matsugu Y, Soutome S, Hayashida S, Hasegawa T, Akashi M, et al. Perioperative oral care can prevent surgical site infection after colorectal cancer surgery: a multicenter, retrospective study of 1926 cases analyzed by propensity score matching. Surgery. 2022;
11. Lockhart PB, Brennan MT, Thornhill M, Michalowicz BS, Noll J, Bahrani-Mougeot FK, et al. Poor oral hygiene as a risk factor for infective endocarditis-related bacteremia. J Am Dent Assoc. 2009;140(10):1238–44.
12. Nishikawa M, Honda M, Kimura R, Kobayashi A, Yamaguchi Y, Hori S, et al. The bacterial association with oral cavity and intra-abdominal abscess after gastrectomy. PLoS One. 2020;15(11):e0242091.

13. Zhao T, Wu X, Zhang Q, Li C, Worthington HV, Hua F. Oral hygiene care for critically ill patients to prevent ventilator-associated pneumonia. Cochrane Database Syst Rev. 2020;12:CD008367.
14. Klompas M. Oropharyngeal decontamination with antiseptics to prevent ventilator-associated pneumonia: rethinking the benefits of chlorhexidine. Semin Respir Crit Care Med. 2017;38(3):381–90.
15. Bellissimo-Rodrigues WT, Menegueti MG, de Macedo LD, Basile-Filho A, Martinez R, Bellissimo-Rodrigues F. Oral mucositis as a pathway for fatal outcome among critically ill patients exposed to chlorhexidine: post hoc analysis of a randomized clinical trial. Crit Care. 2019;23(1):382.
16. Dale CM, Rose L, Carbone S, Pinto R, Smith OM, Burry L, et al. Effect of oral chlorhexidine de-adoption and implementation of an oral care bundle on mortality for mechanically ventilated patients in the intensive care unit (CHORAL): a multi-center stepped wedge cluster-randomized controlled trial. Intensive Care Med. 2021;47(11):1295–302.
17. Wong JKL, Ke Y, Ong YJ, Li H, Wong TH, Abdullah HR. The impact of preoperative glycated hemoglobin (HbA1c) on postoperative complications after elective major abdominal surgery: a meta-analysis. Korean J Anesthesiol. 2022;75(1):47–60.
18. van den Berghe G, Wouters P, Weekers F, Verwaest C, Bruyninckx F, Schetz M, et al. Intensive insulin therapy in critically ill patients. N Engl J Med. 2001;345(19):1359–67.
19. Investigators N-SS, Finfer S, Chittock DR, Su SY, Blair D, Foster D, et al. Intensive versus conventional glucose control in critically ill patients. N Engl J Med. 2009;360(13):1283–97.
20. Yao RQ, Ren C, Wu GS, Zhu YB, Xia ZF, Yao YM. Is intensive glucose control bad for critically ill patients? A systematic review and meta-analysis. Int J Biol Sci. 2020;16(9):1658–75.
21. Wang YY, Hu SF, Ying HM, Chen L, Li HL, Tian F, et al. Postoperative tight glycemic control significantly reduces postoperative infection rates in patients undergoing surgery: a meta-analysis. BMC Endocr Disord. 2018;18(1):42.
22. de Vries FE, Gans SL, Solomkin JS, Allegranzi B, Egger M, Dellinger EP, et al. Meta-analysis of lower perioperative blood glucose target levels for reduction of surgical-site infection. Br J Surg. 2017;104(2):e95–e105.
23. Williams GJ, Herndon DN. Modulating the hypermetabolic response to burn injuries. J Wound Care. 2002;11(3):87–9.
24. Mecott GA, Al-Mousawi AM, Gauglitz GG, Herndon DN, Jeschke MG. The role of hyperglycemia in burned patients: evidence-based studies. Shock. 2010;33(1):5–13.
25. Jeschke MG. Postburn hypermetabolism: past, present, and future. J Burn Care Res. 2016;37(2):86–96.
26. Pham TN, Warren AJ, Phan HH, Molitor F, Greenhalgh DG, Palmieri TL. Impact of tight glycemic control in severely burned children. J Trauma. 2005;59(5):1148–54.
27. Mann EA, Pidcoke HF, Salinas J, Holcomb JB, Wolf SE, Wade CE. The impact of intensive insulin protocols and restrictive blood transfusion strategies on glucose measurement in American Burn Association (ABA) verified burn centers. J Burn Care Res. 2008;29(5):718–23.
28. Jeschke MG, Kulp GA, Kraft R, Finnerty CC, Mlcak R, Lee JO, et al. Intensive insulin therapy in severely burned pediatric patients: a prospective randomized trial. Am J Respir Crit Care Med. 2010;182(3):351–9.
29. Correia MI, Waitzberg DL. The impact of malnutrition on morbidity, mortality, length of hospital stay and costs evaluated through a multivariate model analysis. Clin Nutr. 2003;22(3):235–9.
30. Lim SL, Ong KC, Chan YH, Loke WC, Ferguson M, Daniels L. Malnutrition and its impact on cost of hospitalization, length of stay, readmission and 3-year mortality. Clin Nutr. 2012;31(3):345–50.
31. Lew CCH, Yandell R, Fraser RJL, Chua AP, Chong MFF, Miller M. Association between malnutrition and clinical outcomes in the intensive care unit: a systematic review [formula: see text]. JPEN J Parenter Enteral Nutr. 2017;41(5):744–58.

32. Compher C, Bingham AL, McCall M, Patel J, Rice TW, Braunschweig C, et al. Guidelines for the provision of nutrition support therapy in the adult critically ill patient: The American Society for Parenteral and Enteral Nutrition. JPEN J Parenter Enteral Nutr. 2022;46(1):12–41.
33. Reignier J, Boisrame-Helms J, Brisard L, Lascarrou JB, Ait Hssain A, Anguel N, et al. Enteral versus parenteral early nutrition in ventilated adults with shock: a randomised, controlled, multicentre, open-label, parallel-group study (NUTRIREA-2). Lancet. 2018;391(10116):133–43.
34. Bugaev N, Bhattacharya B, Chiu WC, Como JJ, Cripps MW, Ferrada P, et al. Promotility agents for the treatment of ileus in adult surgical patients: a practice management guideline from the Eastern Association for the Surgery of Trauma. J Trauma Acute Care Surg. 2019;87(4):922–34.
35. Heidegger CP, Berger MM, Graf S, Zingg W, Darmon P, Costanza MC, et al. Optimisation of energy provision with supplemental parenteral nutrition in critically ill patients: a randomised controlled clinical trial. Lancet. 2013;381(9864):385–93.
36. Singer P, Blaser AR, Berger MM, Alhazzani W, Calder PC, Casaer MP, et al. ESPEN guideline on clinical nutrition in the intensive care unit. Clin Nutr. 2019;38(1):48–79.
37. Charles EJ, Petroze RT, Metzger R, Hranjec T, Rosenberger LH, Riccio LM, et al. Hypocaloric compared with eucaloric nutritional support and its effect on infection rates in a surgical intensive care unit: a randomized controlled trial. Am J Clin Nutr. 2014;100(5):1337–43.
38. Avni T, Levcovich A, Ad-El DD, Leibovici L, Paul M. Prophylactic antibiotics for burns patients: systematic review and meta-analysis. BMJ. 2010;340:c241.
39. Ramos G, Cornistein W, Cerino GT, Nacif G. Systemic antimicrobial prophylaxis in burn patients: systematic review. J Hosp Infect. 2017;97(2):105–14.
40. Rex JH, Sobel JD. Prophylactic antifungal therapy in the intensive care unit. Clin Infect Dis. 2001;32(8):1191–200.
41. Ashley ESD, Thirion DJG. Chessman K, editors. Fungal infections in the intensive care unit by. 2010;
42. Playford EG, Webster AC, Sorrell TC, Craig JC. Antifungal agents for preventing fungal infections in non-neutropenic critically ill and surgical patients: systematic review and meta-analysis of randomized clinical trials. J Antimicrob Chemother. 2006;57(4):628–38.
43. Shorr AF, Chung K, Jackson WL, Waterman PE, Kollef MH. Fluconazole prophylaxis in critically ill surgical patients: a meta-analysis. Crit Care Med 2005;33(9):1928-35; quiz 36.
44. Vardakas KZ, Samonis G, Michalopoulos A, Soteriades ES, Falagas ME. Antifungal prophylaxis with azoles in high-risk, surgical intensive care unit patients: a meta-analysis of randomized, placebo-controlled trials. Crit Care Med. 2006;34(4):1216–24.
45. Hanson KE, Pfeiffer CD, Lease ED, Balch AH, Zaas AK, Perfect JR, et al. Beta-D-glucan surveillance with preemptive anidulafungin for invasive candidiasis in intensive care unit patients: a randomized pilot study. PLoS One. 2012;7(8):e42282.
46. Rouze A, Loridant S, Poissy J, Dervaux B, Sendid B, Cornu M, et al. Biomarker-based strategy for early discontinuation of empirical antifungal treatment in critically ill patients: a randomized controlled trial. Intensive Care Med. 2017;43(11):1668–77.
47. Schweickert WD, Patel BK, Kress JP. Timing of early mobilization to optimize outcomes in mechanically ventilated ICU patients. Intensive Care Med. 2022;48(10):1305–7.
48. AfHRa Q. Early mobility. MD: Rockville; 2017.
49. Lang JK, Paykel MS, Haines KJ, Hodgson CL. Clinical practice guidelines for early mobilization in the ICU: a systematic review. Crit Care Med. 2020;48(11):e1121–e8.
50. Devlin JW, Skrobik Y, Gelinas C, Needham DM, Slooter AJC, Pandharipande PP, et al. Executive summary: clinical practice guidelines for the prevention and management of pain, agitation/sedation, delirium, immobility, and sleep disruption in adult patients in the ICU. Crit Care Med. 2018;46(9):1532–48.
51. Doiron KA, Hoffmann TC, Beller EM. Early intervention (mobilization or active exercise) for critically ill adults in the intensive care unit. Cochrane Database Syst Rev. 2018;3(3):CD010754

52. Katsura M, Kuriyama A, Takeshima T, Fukuhara S, Furukawa TA. Preoperative inspiratory muscle training for postoperative pulmonary complications in adults undergoing cardiac and major abdominal surgery. Cochrane Database Syst Rev 2015(10):CD010356.
53. Barberan-Garcia A, Ubré M, Roca J, Lacy AM, Burgos F, Risco R, et al. Personalised Prehabilitation in High-risk Patients Undergoing Elective Major Abdominal Surgery: A Randomized Blinded Controlled Trial. Ann Surg. 2018;267(1):50–6.
54. Sullivan KA, Churchill IF, Hylton DA, Hanna WC. Use of incentive spirometry in adults following cardiac, thoracic, and upper abdominal surgery to prevent post-operative pulmonary complications: a systematic review and meta-analysis. Respiration. 2021;100(11):1114–27.
55. Kazaure HS, Martin M, Yoon JK, Wren SM. Long-term results of a postoperative pneumonia prevention program for the inpatient surgical ward. JAMA Surg. 2014;149(9):914–8.
56. Hanberger H, Walther S, Leone M, Barie PS, Rello J, Lipman J, et al. Increased mortality associated with methicillin-resistant Staphylococcus aureus (MRSA) infection in the intensive care unit: results from the EPIC II study. Int J Antimicrob Agents. 2011;38(4):331–5.
57. Parks NA, Croce MA. Routine screening for methicillin-resistant Staphylococcus aureus. Surg Infect. 2012;13(4):223–7.
58. Gidengil CA, Gay C, Huang SS, Platt R, Yokoe D, Lee GM. Cost-effectiveness of strategies to prevent methicillin-resistant Staphylococcus aureus transmission and infection in an intensive care unit. Infect Control Hosp Epidemiol. 2015;36(1):17–27.
59. Huang SS, Septimus E, Avery TR, Lee GM, Hickok J, Weinstein RA, et al. Cost savings of universal decolonization to prevent intensive care unit infection: implications of the REDUCE MRSA trial. Infect Control Hosp Epidemiol. 2014;35(Suppl. 3):S23–31.
60. Cho OH, Baek EH, Bak MH, Suh YS, Park KH, Kim S, et al. The effect of targeted decolonization on methicillin-resistant Staphylococcus aureus colonization or infection in a surgical intensive care unit. Am J Infect Control. 2016;44(5):533–8.
61. Lee YJ, Chen JZ, Lin HC, Liu HY, Lin SY, Lin HH, et al. Impact of active screening for methicillin-resistant Staphylococcus aureus (MRSA) and decolonization on MRSA infections, mortality and medical cost: a quasi-experimental study in surgical intensive care unit. Crit Care. 2015;19(1):143.
62. Anderson DJ, Podgorny K, Berrios-Torres SI, Bratzler DW, Dellinger EP, Greene L, et al. Strategies to prevent surgical site infections in acute care hospitals: 2014 update. Infect Control Hosp Epidemiol. 2014;35(Suppl. 2):S66–88.
63. Magill SS, Edwards JR, Bamberg W, Beldavs ZG, Dumyati G, Kainer MA, et al. Multistate point-prevalence survey of health care-associated infections. N Engl J Med. 2014;370(13):1198–208.
64. Network NHS. National Healthcare Safety Network (NHSN) Patient Safety Component Manual: Chapter 9: Surgical Site Infection (SSI) Event. CDC; 2022.
65. Liang S, Zhang X, Hu Y, Yang J, Li K. Association between perioperative chlorhexidine oral care and postoperative pneumonia in non-cardiac surgical patients: a systematic review and meta-analysis. Surgery. 2021;170(5):1418–31.
66. Norman G, Atkinson RA, Smith TA, Rowlands C, Rithalia AD, Crosbie EJ, et al. Intracavity lavage and wound irrigation for prevention of surgical site infection. Cochrane Database Syst Rev. 2017;10:CD012234.
67. Norman G, Goh EL, Dumville JC, Shi C, Liu Z, Chiverton L, et al. Negative pressure wound therapy for surgical wounds healing by primary closure. Cochrane Database Syst Rev. 2020;6:CD009261.
68. Feng J, Jiang X, Zhi Z. Subcuticular sutures versus staples for skin closure in patients undergoing abdominal surgery: A meta-analysis of randomized controlled trials. PLoS One. 2021;16(5):e0251022.
69. Trouillet JL, Collange O, Belafia F, Blot F, Capellier G, Cesareo E, et al. Tracheotomy in the intensive care unit: guidelines from a French expert panel. Ann Intensive Care. 2018;8(1):37.
70. Alsunaid S, Holden VK, Kohli A, Diaz J, O'Meara LB. Wound care management: tracheostomy and gastrostomy. J Thorac Dis. 2021;13(8):5297–313.

71. Lipp A, Lusardi G. Systemic antimicrobial prophylaxis for percutaneous endoscopic gastrostomy. Cochrane Database Syst Rev 2013(11):CD005571.
72. Marshall JC. Principles of source control in the early management of sepsis. Curr Infect Dis Rep. 2010;12(5):345–53.
73. Mazuski JE, Tessier JM, May AK, Sawyer RG, Nadler EP, Rosengart MR, et al. The surgical infection society revised guidelines on the management of intra-abdominal infection. Surg Infect. 2017;18(1):1–76.
74. De Waele J, Lipman J, Sakr Y, Marshall JC, Vanhems P, Barrera Groba C, et al. Abdominal infections in the intensive care unit: characteristics, treatment and determinants of outcome. BMC Infect Dis. 2014;14:420.
75. Ballus J, Lopez-Delgado JC, Sabater-Riera J, Perez-Fernandez XL, Betbese AJ, Roncal JA. Surgical site infection in critically ill patients with secondary and tertiary peritonitis: epidemiology, microbiology and influence in outcomes. BMC Infect Dis. 2015;15:304.
76. Ho VP, Kaafarani H, Rattan R, Namias N, Evans H, Zakrison TL. Sepsis 2019: what surgeons need to know. Surg Infect. 2020;21(3):195–204.
77. Papazian L, Klompas M, Luyt CE. Ventilator-associated pneumonia in adults: a narrative review. Intensive Care Med. 2020;46(5):888–906.
78. Klompas M, Branson R, Eichenwald EC, Greene LR, Howell MD, Lee G, et al. Strategies to prevent ventilator-associated pneumonia in acute care hospitals: 2014 update. Infect Control Hosp Epidemiol. 2014;35(Suppl. 2):S133–54.
79. Tablan OC, Anderson LJ, Besser R, Bridges C, Hajjeh R, CDC, et al. Guidelines for preventing health-care--associated pneumonia, 2003: recommendations of CDC and the Healthcare Infection Control Practices Advisory Committee. MMWR Recomm Rep 2004;53(RR-3):1-36.
80. Alderden J, Drake KP, Wilson A, Dimas J, Cummins MR, Yap TL. Hospital acquired pressure injury prediction in surgical critical care patients. BMC Med Inform Decis Mak. 2021;21(1):12.
81. Alderden J, Cowan LJ, Dimas JB, Chen D, Zhang Y, Cummins M, et al. Risk factors for hospital-acquired pressure injury in surgical critical care patients. Am J Crit Care. 2020;29(6):e128–e34.
82. Eachempati SR, Hydo LJ, Barie PS. Factors influencing the development of decubitus ulcers in critically ill surgical patients. Crit Care Med. 2001;29(9):1678–82.
83. Li Z, Lin F, Thalib L, Chaboyer W. Global prevalence and incidence of pressure injuries in hospitalised adult patients: a systematic review and meta-analysis. Int J Nurs Stud. 2020;105:103546.
84. Lovegrove J, Fulbrook P, Miles S, Steele M. Effectiveness of interventions to prevent pressure injury in adults admitted to intensive care settings: a systematic review and meta-analysis of randomised controlled trials. Aust Crit Care. 2022;35(2):186–203.
85. Labeau SO, Afonso E, Benbenishty J, Blackwood B, Boulanger C, Brett SJ, et al. Correction to: Prevalence, associated factors and outcomes of pressure injuries in adult intensive care unit patients: the DecubICUs study. Intensive Care Med. 2021;47(4):503–20.
86. Lovegrove J, Fulbrook P, Miles S. International consensus on pressure injury preventative interventions by risk level for critically ill patients: a modified Delphi study. Int Wound J. 2020;17(5):1112–27.
87. Shi C, Dumville JC, Cullum N, Rhodes S, McInnes E, Goh EL, et al. editors. Overlays and mattresses for preventing and treating pressure ulcers: an overview of Cochrane Reviews and network meta-analysis. Cochrane Database Syst Rev. 2021;8:CD013761.
88. Johns J, Krogh K, Rodriguez GM, Eng J, Haller E, Heinen M, Laredo R, Longo W, Montero-Colon W, Wilson C, Korsten M. Management of neurogenic bowel dysfunction in adults after spinal cord injury: clinical practice guideline for healthcare providers. J Spinal Cord Med. 2021; https://doi.org/10.1080/10790268.2021.1883385. J Spinal Cord Med. 2021;44(3):442-510
89. Andriolo BN, Andriolo RB, Saconato H, Atallah AN, Valente O. Early versus late tracheostomy for critically ill patients. Cochrane Database Syst Rev. 2015;1:CD007271.
90. de Franca SA, Tavares WM, Salinet ASM, Paiva WS, Teixeira MJ. Early tracheostomy in severe traumatic brain injury patients: a meta-analysis and comparison with late tracheostomy. Crit Care Med. 2020;48(4):e325–e31.

91. Marra A, Vargas M, Buonanno P, Iacovazzo C, Coviello A, Servillo G. Early vs. late tracheostomy in patients with traumatic brain injury: systematic review and meta-analysis. J Clin Med. 2021;10(15)
92. Holevar M, Dunham JC, Brautigan R, Clancy TV, Como JJ, Ebert JB, et al. Practice management guidelines for timing of tracheostomy: the EAST Practice Management Guidelines Work Group. J Trauma. 2009;67(4):870–4.
93. Prabhakaran K, Azim A, Khan M, Jehan F, Feeney J, Anderson P, et al. Predicting the need for tracheostomy in trauma patients without severe head injury. Am J Surg. 2020;220(2):495–8.
94. Fokin AA, Wycech J, Chin Shue K, Stalder R, Crawford M, Lozada J, et al. Early versus late tracheostomy in trauma patients with rib fractures. J Surg Res. 2020;245:72–80.
95. McShane EK, Sun BJ, Maggio PM, Spain DA, Forrester JD. Improving tracheostomy delivery for trauma and surgical critical care patients: timely trach initiative. BMJ Open. Qual. 2022;11(2)
96. Brass P, Hellmich M, Ladra A, Ladra J, Wrzosek A. Percutaneous techniques versus surgical techniques for tracheostomy. Cochrane Database Syst Rev. 2016;7:CD008045.
97. Burton LV, Lofgren DH, Silberman M. Bacterial Tracheitis. Treasure Island (FL): StatPearls; 2022.
98. Le Roux P. Intracranial pressure monitoring and management. In: Laskowitz D, Grant G, editors. Translational research in traumatic brain injury. Boca Raton (FL): Frontiers in Neuroscience; 2016.
99. Munakomi S, Das JM. Intracranial pressure monitoring. Treasure Island (FL): StatPearls; 2022.

Chapter 8
Infection Control in Neonatal and Pediatric Intensive Care Units

David McMann, Peter Scully, and Chiamaka Aneji

Regarding infection control, pediatric and neonatal intensive care units (PICUs and NICUs) share many similarities with adult critical care areas. There are however various unique aspects with respect to prevalence, organisms, risk factors, collaboratives, and interventions that merit exploration.

Central Line-Associated Bloodstream Infections

Central line-associated bloodstream infections (CLABSIs) pose a significant risk to pediatric critical care patients as well as a burden on the healthcare system costing roughly $55,000 (in 2011 dollars) per incidence and increasing the length of hospitalization by an average of 19 days [1]. Furthermore when compared to adults, children are at higher risk for such infections. Pediatric patients spend a higher percentage of their hospitalization with a central venous line (CVL) (33% line days/patient days vs. 28% in adults per National Healthcare Safety Network (NHSN) 2013 reporting) [2]. This higher dependence on CVLs in pediatrics may be due to the difficulty in placing and maintaining PIVs in smaller vessels, a lack of patient cooperation, and the desire by both healthcare providers and families to avoid the trauma of repeated "sticks." Along with this increase in central line utilization, critically ill children are also more likely to develop an infection once a line is inserted with a PICU CLABSI rate of 1.2–1.8 per 1000 central line days compared to 0.9–1.1 in adult ICUs [2]. The causative pathogens also differ between the two populations with Enterobacteriaceae being most common in children as opposed to

D. McMann (✉) · P. Scully · C. Aneji
Department of Pediatrics, John P. and Kathrine G. McGovern Medical School at UTHealth, Houston, TX, USA
e-mail: David.E.Mcmann@uth.tmc.edu

M. Ellsworth, L. Ostrosky-Zeichner (eds.), *Infection Prevention in the Intensive Care Setting*, https://doi.org/10.1007/978-3-031-67062-6_8

Candida spp in the adult ICUs; though *Enterococcus* spp is well represented in both [3].

In an effort to decrease neonatal and pediatric CLABSI rates, as well as many other hospitals acquired conditions, many children's hospitals have joined the Solution for Patient Safety (SPS) collaborative. Started in 2009, it now contains more than 145 pediatric hospitals in the USA and Canada. The SPS collaborative primarily focuses on the safety and quality of pediatric care through creating and analyzing participating hospital's quality metrics, developing prevention bundles, and holding conferences to encourage collaboration between participating hospitals [4]. Per SPS reporting, enrolled hospitals have seen at 19.2% reduction in CLABSI rates since 2015, and per a 2022 study, joining hospitals had a relatively immediate 7% drop in CLABSI rate after enrollment [5, 6]. The SPS CLABSI bundle focuses on insertion and maintenance as well as recommends an in-depth review of all identified CLABSIs. Table 8.1 includes the bundle elements and the corresponding CDC recommendation category [7]. When comparing these recommendations to the Institute for Healthcare Improvement (IHI) guidance, which informs the CLABSI prevention initiatives of many hospitals worldwide, there is a greater emphasis on the standardization of various aspects of line care with the aim to promote consistency and reproducibility [8].

Table 8.1 CLABSI

Prevention bundle element—insertion	**Level of evidence**[a]
Standard elements	
Hand hygiene	IB
CHG scrubs	IA
No iodine ointment	IB
Prepackaged or filled insertion care tray or box	NA
Insertion checklist with staff empowerment to stop nonemergent procedure	NA
Full sterile barrier for providers and patients	IB
Insertion training for all providers	IA
Prevention bundle element—maintenance	
Standard elements	
Daily discussion of line necessity, functionality, and utilization including bedside and medical care team members	IB
Regular assessment of dressing to assure clean/dry/occlusive	IB
Standardized access procedure	IB
Standardized dressing, cap, and tubing change procedures/timing	IB
Daily CHG treatments	IA
Recommended elements	
An in-depth review of all identified CLABSI with multidisciplinary involvement and the intent to change the process if needed	N/A
Daily linen changes	N/A

[a] CDC Modified Recommendation Category

Working to further decrease CLABSI rates, many pediatric hospitals have implemented strategies that go beyond these bundle elements. One example is the utilization of midline catheters which are inserted peripherally and terminate before the axilla. These have a lower infection but higher mechanical failure rate than CVLS and cannot be used for medications requiring central access [9, 10]. Some pediatric hospitals have employed vascular access teams to place, access, and audit CVLs which has shown some benefit in neonatal critical care areas [11]. Closed blood sampling systems which attach to central venous or arterial catheters have been used to allow blood sampling without the repeated open air accessing of the line. Furthermore, this system allows the return of the drawn waste, a meaningful amount of volume in children, to the patient within the closed system. Though there has yet to be conclusive evidence that such systems improve CLABSI rates, there is data that show a decrease in the bacterial contamination of arterial catheters employing this device [12, 13]. Other strategies to protect CVLs include the use of 70% ethanol caps which enjoys wide usage and support as well as less conventional interventions such as wiping tubing with chlorhexidine and the use of plastic wrap on tubing/hubs as an additional physical barrier [14, 15].

Catheter-Associated Urinary Tract infections

Pediatric catheter-associated urinary tract infections (CAUTIs) add on average an extra 2.4 hospitalization days and cost $7200 (in 2015 dollars) per incident [16, 17]. A 2017 study of 33 US children's hospitals found a rate of 2.6 CAUTIs per 1000 urinary catheter days [17]. When compared to adult ICUs, there is a significant decrease in utilization in pediatric critical care areas (60% vs. 21% of patient days per NHSN 2013 reporting) [2]. This may be due to possibly higher rates of urinary obstruction(e.g., prostatic hyperplasia) in adult patients as well as the ease and acceptance of weighing diapers in the pediatric population. A key CAUTI risk factor in pediatric ICUs is catheter dwell time with one Japanese study finding a 5% increase in risk with each day a catheter is in place [18].

Comprehensive CAUTI prevention bundles have been established that focus on both decreasing bladder catheterization and dwell time as well as encouraging sterile insertion and maintenance techniques [19, 20]. The previously mentioned SPS collaborative has developed CAUTI recommendations as well as a prevention bundle, and hospitals that have joined have seen a 61.6% reduction in CAUTI rates between 2011 and 2017 [20]. This bundle is found in Table 8.2 along with the corresponding CDC recommendation categories [7]. Compared to the SPS bundle, IHI recommendation contains more guidance on catheter manipulation including avoiding catheter flushing and superfluous catheter exchanges as well as the proper technique to empty collection bags [21].

Much effort has been put forth to increase bundle compliance through the use of various interventions [20, 22, 23]. Some examples of successful interventions in

Table 8.2 CAUTI

Prevention bundle element—insertion	Level of evidence[a]
Standard elements	
Use aseptic technique for insertion	IB
Avoid unnecessary catheterization	IB
Prevention bundle element—maintenance	
Standard elements	
Maintain a closed drainage system	IB
Maintain hygiene	IB
Keep bag below level of bladder	IB
Maintain unobstructed flow of urine	IB
Remove catheter when no longer needed	IB
Recommended elements	
Secure catheter	IB

[a] CDC Modified Recommendation Category

pediatric ICUs include targeted rounding, specific education for staff and patient families, root-cause analysis when CAUTI occurs, and simulation-based bundle training [24].

Multidrug-Resistant Organisms

The treatment of multidrug-resistant organisms (MDROs) including methicillin-resistant *Staphylococcus aureus* (MRSA), vancomycin-resistant *Enterococcus* (VRE), and multidrug-resistant Gram-negative bacilli (MDR-GNB) contributes billions to the cost of US healthcare [25]. Much attention is paid to this issue in adult patients, but such infections are a growing concern in children as well.

MRSA

Initially recognized in the early 1960s, MRSA's prevalence grew until peaking in 2005 when it represented roughly half of pediatric *Staphylococcus aureus* infections. In the following years though, this has declined to roughly a third. Of note however, there has been an increase in resistance to clindamycin and ciprofloxacin over the same period [26]. These recent findings may be in some part due to increased implementation of isolation precautions in healthcare settings and providers changing their routine prescription practices to treat MRSA empirically.

A meta-analysis found 3% of PICU patients are colonized with MRSA upon admission, and 4.1% of PICU/NICU patients acquire MRSA during their stay. Furthermore, this colonization carried a relative risk of 24.2 for developing a MRSA infection [27]. Similarly to the adult acute care setting, screening and the use of contact isolation (e.g., private room, the use of clean non sterile gowns and gloves for those entering the room, and dedicated/single patient equipment) has been the mainstay of pediatric MRSA infection control [28]. However, there has been a growing controversy fueled by contradictory studies on the effectiveness of these methodologies [29, 30]. This has led to some adult and pediatric hospitals to no longer screen and/or use contact precautions for MRSA positive patients. Daily chlorhexidine (CHG) bathing has been used in many adult acute care areas effectively with one meta-analysis showing a decrease in MRSA colonization of 41% and MRSA bacteremia of 36% [31]. Such daily bathing is being increasingly adopted in PICUs as well with some success [32]. Implementation in NICUs has been more restricted due to safety concerns related to CHG and the sensitivity and permeability of immature skin. This has typically resulted in CHG bathing being only implemented for neonates with central venous catheters and/or patients greater than a certain weight or age [33, 34]. Decolonization of neonates through the use of mupirocin applied to the nares and in some instances the umbilical stump as well as abraded skin enjoys relative wide adoption with a 2009 survey of Society of Healthcare Epidemiology members finding 37% of respondents using mupirocin for decolonization in their respective NICUs [35, 36]. A recent randomized controlled trial showed 83% decolonization with mupirocin vs. 20% with petroleum jelly in neonates, though recolonization occurred frequently [37].

VRE

There is a paucity of data on the prevalence of VRE infections in the pediatric population. A study using the Healthcare Cost and Utilization Project Kids' Inpatient Database showed VRE infections in pediatric patients have been on the rise, from 53 cases per million admissions in 1997 to 120 cases per million in 2012 [38]. A Turkish study found a PICU VRE colonization rate of 9.5% with 10.2% of those developing VRE infections. These infections were associated with long hospital stays and vancomycin/teicoplanin exposure [39]. The same group found a NICU colonization rate of 12% with 3% developing a VRE infection associated again with long hospital stay and vancomycin/teicoplanin exposure as well as necrotizing enterocolitis, surgical procedures, external ventricular drainage, and the use of amphotericin B [40].

The mainstay of control is contact isolation precautions with a particular emphasis on hand hygiene which has been associated with a 47% decrease in VRE acquisition rates [28, 41]. Fecal transplantation, typically used for *Clostridiodes difficile*, has had some success decolonizing MDR-GNB and VRE in adult patients and has potential in children [42]. Standard environmental decontamination methods as described by the CDC are seen as typically sufficient; however, room sterilization with UV light is used by some institutions [43, 44].

MDR-GNB

MDR-GNB including extended spectrum β-lactamase producers (ESBL) and carbapenem-resistant Enterobacteriaceae (CRE) are a growing problem for pediatric and neonatal ICUs. Two studies based on the reporting data of the NHSN found an increase in the percentage of ESBL isolates over the first decade of this century from 1.82% to 11.42% and of CRE isolates from 0% to 4.48% in ICU patients aged 1–17 years [45, 46]. A Taiwanese NICU study found that 18.6% of GNB bacteremia were caused by MDR-GNB; such infections were associated with a previous exposure to a third-generation cephalosporin as well as renal disease and had 1.67 odds ratio of mortality [47].

There is limited information concerning the rate of colonization of MDR-GNB in pediatrics; however, a Spanish study, examining MDR-GNB colonization in admitted children with complex chronic conditions, found a colonization rate of 27% and a positive association with immunosuppressive therapy, antibiotic prophylaxis, history of skin-infections, and the rate of surgeries and hospital admissions [48]. An Italian study found a neonatal colonization rate of 28.8% which was associated with low APGAR scores and longer lengths of stay [49].

Prevention of MDR-GNB is primarily reliant on contact isolation precautions. Screening for colonization, however, is not widespread and suffers from a lack of standardization [50]. There has been success in the NICU setting with lowering MDR-GNB acquisition through the use of screening and contact isolation [51, 52]. These efforts are somewhat undermined, however, by the significant amount of spontaneous acquisition of antibiotic resistance in GNB, illustrated by a Parisian study which estimated nearly 50% of ESBL cases found in a pediatric hospital ward were not caused by patient-to-patient transmission [53]. In order to decrease resistance induced by the liberal use of wide spectrum antibiotics, many pediatric hospitals have adopted antimicrobial stewardship programs with some success [54]. Environmental decontamination methods for pediatric and neonatal areas are similar to those used in adult units and follow the CDC's guidelines [43].

Ventilator-Associated Pneumonias and Ventilator-Associated Events

Before 2013, all ventilator-associated hospital-acquired conditions were reported as ventilator-associated pneumonia (VAP) which was dependent on subjective X-ray interpretation. With the desire to have more objective criteria, the new definition of ventilator-associated event (VAE) was developed and adapted by the NHSN for adult patients. There was concern, however, that this new definition would struggle to adequately predict outcomes in children. This was elucidated by the work of Cocoro et al. which illustrated the importance of fraction of inspired oxygen (FiO_2) and mean airway pressure (MAP) as key factors in patient length of stay and mortality in children which led to the creation of a unique VAE definition (PedVAE) for the pediatric population shown in Table 8.3 [55, 56]. Currently, NHSN will accept both VAP and PedVAE reporting from pediatric locations as opposed to only VAE in adult critical care areas and only PedVAE in neonatal areas. Furthermore, unlike the adult VAE reporting, there is no delineation in pediatric/neonatal reporting of the subsets of VAE (VAC, AVAC, and PVAP) as all are recorded as a PedVAE.

Table 8.3 VAE

Pediatric VAE (PedVAE)			Adult VAE	
Ventilator-Associated Condition (VAC): Baseline period of stability or improvement on the ventilator, defined by ≥2 calendar days followed by one of the following sustained for ≥2 calendar days				
Increase in **MAP** ≥ **4** cm H_2O over baseline period			Increase **PEEP** ≥ **3** cm H_2O over baseline period	
Or			Or	
Increase in daily minimum FIO_2 of ≥**0.25** over baseline period			Increase in daily minimum FIO_2 of ≥**0.20** over baseline period	
Pediatric VAC with antimicrobial use (AVAC)/ infection-related ventilator-associated complication (IVAC): An existing VAC as well as on or after day 3 of mechanical ventilation and within 2 calendar days before or after worsening oxygenation with the following				
Pediatric VAC with antimicrobial use (AVAC)			**Infection-related Ventilator Associated Complication (IVAC)**	
A new antimicrobial started and continued for ≥4 calendar days			Temp. >38 °C or <36 °C OR WBC ≥12,000 cells/mm^3 or ≤4000 cells/mm^3	
			And	
			A new antimicrobial started and continued for ≥4 calendar days	
Possible Ventilator-Associated Pneumonia (PVAP): An existing AVAC or IVAC as well as on or after day 3 of mechanical ventilation and within 2 calendar days before or after worsening oxygenation with one of the following criteria				
Criterion 1		Criterion 2		Criterion 3
Positive culture via endotracheal aspirate, BAL, lung tissue, or protected specimen brush with quantitative/semi-quantitative thresholds	Or	Purulent respiratory secretions and positive via specimens in Criterion 1, but not meeting those thresholds for growth	Or	One of the following: organism identified via pleural fluid, lung histopathology, *Legionella* diagnostic test, or respiratory secretion positive for a viral organism

There has yet to be a well-developed and widely adopted pediatric VAE prevention bundle or set of recommendations. The Solution for Patient Safety (SPS) collaborative has produced a VAP bundle which has shown a 48% reduction in VAP rate across the network. It includes readiness to extubate, head of bed elevation, minimized circuit disruptions, and oral hygiene [7]. This differs from the IHI VAP bundle which does not include a focus on circuit disruptions but does incorporate deep vein thrombosis and peptic ulcer disease prophylaxis [57]. Other strategies to decrease VAE/VAP rates include avoiding intubation, using non-invasive positive pressure ventilation if possible, sedation holidays, and avoidance of fluid overload [58]. It is important to consider when developing interventions to decrease VAE rates, particularly in the pediatric where VAC/AVAC/PCAP classifications are not reported as separate entities, that VAEs can be due to noninfectious disease processes including pulmonary edema, acute respiratory distress syndrome (ARDS), and atelectasis.

Hospital-Acquired Respiratory Infections

Respiratory viral infections are a major concern in the pediatric population, with incidence rates highest from 0 to 5 years and decreasing as age increases [59]. RSV alone is responsible for 1 out of every 28 deaths of children between 28 days and 6 months of life worldwide [60]. A 2011 survey of household medical expenditures, sponsored by the Agency for Healthcare Research and Quality and the National Center for Health Statistics, found that acute bronchitis and upper respiratory infections combined where the fourth most costly conditions in American children costing the country $3.3 billion dollars [61]. Furthermore, 2–3% of all American children less than one year of age require hospitalization for bronchiolitis [62].

As these infections are transmitted from person to person easily, they pose a significant risk in the healthcare setting [63, 64]. One single-institution study reported a hospital-acquired respiratory viral infection rate of 0.98 per 1000 patient days while a similar study found an incidence rate of 44 cases per 10,000 admissions [64, 65]. Risk factors for nosocomial respiratory infections include young age, prematurity, chronic lung disease, congenital heart disease, a high degree of complex chronic conditions, and contact with a caregiver or visitor with symptomatic viral illness [64, 66, 67]. Pediatric healthcare areas are possibly more at risk due to children's propensity to touch and place both fomites and hands in their mouths aiding in the transmission of such infections.

Pediatric hospitals do not typically screen all patients with nasopharyngeal swabs; however, testing of symptomatic patients and screening visitors for respiratory symptoms through a questionnaire is common [68]. Clinician initiated screening based on symptoms might miss a significant portion of infected patients; however, as one study illustrated pronounced variability in the ordering of influenza testing among a group of children's hospitals leading to an estimated 35% of cases being missed [69].

The key factor for infection control, once a respiratory infection has been identified, is the implementation of the appropriate isolation precautions. The CDC's recommendations in this matter are dependent on the organism. Influenza, adenovirus, parvovirus, rhinovirus, rubella, *Bordetella pertussis*, and group A *Streptococcus* require droplet precautions which includes the use of a private room and wearing a mask within 3 feet of a patient. Contact isolation is recommended for RSV, SARS-CoV-2, MERS-CoV, and rhinovirus if there are copious secretions [28].

Children's hospitals often employ measures beyond selected screening and patient isolation including initiatives to increase the availability of alcohol-based sanitizers and the presence of cough-etiquette posters, banning visitors under 12 years of age during peak respiratory viral season, and encouraging the vaccination of healthcare providers against influenza [68].

Healthcare-Associated Diarrheal Infections

Diarrheal illnesses are a leading cause of hospitalizations and death for children worldwide [70]. Children under 5 years of age are especially at high risk, with nearly 500,000 deaths globally due to diarrhea in 2015 [71]. Most of these deaths are in low-resource countries and are most commonly caused by rotavirus [72]. When compared to older patients, young children are particularly sensitive to diarrheal induced hypovolemia due to little physiologic reserve and the difficulty in encouraging increased oral fluid intake [70]. Nosocomial diarrheal illnesses are typically secondary to antibiotics effect on gut flora, as is the case of *Clostridioides difficile*, or by patient-to-patient spread [73]. Studies have shown that diarrheal illnesses in pediatrics hospitals account for 15–35% of all hospital-acquired infections with the most common pathogens identified being *C. difficile* and rotavirus [74–76]. It has been estimated that a *C. difficile* infection adds 4 days to hospital length of stay and can increase cost by 1.6 times, while a meta-analysis found that rotavirus can increase length of stay by 2–5 days [77, 78].

Clostridioides difficile

Well known to be the most common pathogen associated with health care-associated diarrhea in adult patients, *C. difficile* is now becoming recognized as one of the major causes of pediatric nosocomial diarrhea as well [79]. Transient colonization *of C. difficile*, including toxigenic strains, has long been recognized in neonates without clinical diarrheal illness with rates as high as 70% being reported in the 1980s [80, 81]. A 2021 meta-analysis showed the rate of asymptomatic colonization of all strains peaks at 41% in infancy and decreases to 12% above the age of 5 with 14% and 6% of children carrying a toxigenic strain, respectively [82]. The increased colonization rate early in life may be due to the initial lack of competing bacteria thus allowing the proliferation of *C. difficile*. Furthermore, a tolerance to *C. difficile* toxins may be imparted by the paucity of toxin receptors in neonatal colonic cells [83]. The high incidence of asymptomatic carriage among children does not exclude them from developing a *C. difficile* infection (CDI) however. There have been multiple reported outbreaks of CDIs in hospitalized pediatric patients [84, 85]. The incidence of CDI was thought to be increasing in hospitalized pediatric patients with an annual 14% rise in rates between 1997 and 2006 based on data from the Healthcare Cost and Utilization Project Kids' Inpatient Database [86]. However, a more recent study using the Pediatric Health Information System database found a decrease in rates between 2013 and 2019 from 7.08 case per 10,000 patient days to 4.89 cases per 10,000 patient days [87].

The risks factors for CDI in children include comorbidities such as inflammatory bowel disease, immunodeficiency, cancer, and exposure to medications including proton pump inhibitors and certain antibiotics including cephalosporins, aminoglycosides, and sulfas [86, 88, 89]. Compared to adults, pediatric CDI has a slightly faster onset, a lower complication rate including pseudomembranous colitis and the need for a colectomy, and is less likely to reoccur [90].

Prevention strategies of CDI for pediatric and adult patients are similar with a focus on isolation of patients, contact precautions, a preference for using soap and water for hand hygiene, terminal room cleaning with a sporicidal agent, and antibiotic stewardship [91]. Coadministration of probiotics with antibiotic therapy has been proposed to decrease the risk of subsequent CDI, but this practice is controversial. A 2013 meta-analysis of five pediatric studies did suggest there might be some benefit with the pooled data yielding a relative risk of 0.35 (95% DI 0.13–0.92); however, there was variation on which microorganisms each study had used and in four of the included studies had shown no benefit [92].

Rotavirus

There appears to be a relatively high rate of hospital-acquired rotavirus (RV) as suggested by one review which found a median of 32% (range 14–51%) of hospitalized children discharged with the diagnosis of RV acquired the infection during their hospital stay [93]. Furthermore, a meta-analysis found a pediatric nosocomial RV rate 0.4 per 100 hospitalizations and a rate of 0.7 per 100 hospitalizations for children <5 years of age [78]. It is difficult to discern if such rates have changed with the adoption of the rotavirus vaccine as studies are contradictory [78, 93].

Per the CDC, strategies to prevent the transmission of RV in the hospital setting include contact precautions, hand hygiene, patient isolation, and ensuring the disinfectants used are effective against rotavirus [28]. Interestingly, a multi-institutional study reviewing the self-reported practices for the prevention of hospital-acquired RV found that restricting infected patients' movement outside of the room, keeping these patients' room door closed, and a smaller hospital unit size (<20 patients) were associated with lower rates of hospital-acquired RV; while hand washing after care, the use of gloves, a written protocol for diarrhea management, nurse-to-patient ratio, and the use of dedicated patient equipment did not significantly alter the risk of transmission [94].

The Cardiovascular ICU (CVICU)

Pediatric CVICU patients pose a unique challenge for hospitals' infection control programs. When compared to PICUS, CVICUs have higher central line and ventilation days per ICU admission [2]. This is most likely due to congenital heart patients' relatively young age, length of critical illness, and prolonged need for invasive monitoring.

Furthermore due to concerns for hemodynamic instability 11–18% of post-operative heart patients arrive in the CVICU with an open sternum [95, 96]. This is followed by a delayed sternal closure (DSC) that can occur at bedside or by returning to the OR. DSC is associated with a significant increase in the risk for surgical site infections (SSI) with one study finding an SSI rate of 14.7% in DSC patients compared to 1% in those who underwent primary sternal closure [97].

Adopting a standardized protocol for sternal wound care prevention has shown to decrease SSI rates, though there is currently no universal adopted methodology [98]. A survey of US pediatric cardiac surgery programs showed a majority gave two CHG baths preoperatively and roughly 30% screened for MRSA. Intraoperatively most administered a first-generation cephalosporin and only a minority applied an antibiotic ointment to the incision site. Nearly all programs used prophylactic antibiotics, typically a first-generation cephalosporin, while the sternum was opened with the majority continuing therapy for 48 hours after closure. Other common interventions include the use of sterile dry dressings, sterile gel for bedside echocardiograms, single patient disposable cardiac monitoring leads, and individual stethoscopes for each patient. When comparing these interventions with reported SSIs of the participating programs, only preoperative bathing and interestingly an established feeding protocol were associated with a decrease in SSI rate [99].

References

1. Goudie A, Dynan L, Brady PW, Rettiganti M. Attributable cost and length of stay for central line-associated bloodstream infections. Pediatrics. 2014;133(6) https://doi.org/10.1542/peds.2013-3795.
2. Dudeck MA, Edwards JR, Allen-Bridson K, et al. National Healthcare safety network report, data summary for 2013, device-associated module. Am J Infect Control. 2015;43(3):206–21. https://doi.org/10.1016/j.ajic.2014.11.014.
3. Novosad SA, Fike L, Dudeck MA, et al. Pathogens causing central-line–associated bloodstream infections in acute-care hospitals—United States, 2011–2017. Infect Control Hosp Epidemiol. 2020;41(3):313–9. https://doi.org/10.1017/ice.2019.303.
4. Solutions for Patient Safety. 2022. Accessed August 29, 2022. https://www.solutionsforpatientsafety.org/.
5. SPS Year in Review 2021. 2022. Accessed August 29, 2022. https://www.solutionsforpatientsafety.org/our-results/.
6. Coffey M, Marino M, Lyren A, et al. Association between hospital-acquired harm outcomes and membership in a national patient safety collaborative. JAMA Pediatr. 2022; https://doi.org/10.1001/jamapediatrics.2022.2493.

7. SPS Prevention Bundles; 2019. www.solutionsforpatientsafety.org.
8. How-to guide: prevent central line-associated bloodstream infections. Institute for Healthcare Improvement; 2012. Accessed August 29, 2022. www.ihi.org.
9. Anderson J, Greenwell A, Louderback J, Polivka BJ, Behr JH. Comparison of outcomes of extended dwell/midline peripheral intravenous catheters and peripherally inserted central catheters in children. J Assoc Vasc Access. 2016;21(3):158–64. https://doi.org/10.1016/j.java.2016.03.007.
10. Tripathi S, Kumar S, Kaushik S. The practice and complications of midline catheters: a systematic review. Crit Care Med. 2021;49(2):e140–50. https://doi.org/10.1097/CCM.0000000000004764.
11. Legemaat MM, Jongerden IP, van Rens RMFPT, Zielman M, van den Hoogen A. Effect of a vascular access team on central line-associated bloodstream infections in infants admitted to a neonatal intensive care unit: a systematic review. Int J Nurs Stud. 2015;52(5):1003–10. https://doi.org/10.1016/j.ijnurstu.2014.11.010.
12. Oto J, Nakataki E, Hata M, et al. Comparison of bacterial contamination of blood conservation system and stopcock system arterial sampling lines used in critically ill patients. Am J Infect Control. 2012;40(6):530–4. https://doi.org/10.1016/j.ajic.2011.08.006.
13. Tang M, Feng M, Chen L, Zhang J, Ji P, Luo S. Closed blood conservation device for reducing catheter-related infections in children after cardiac surgery. Crit Care Nurse. 2014;34(5):53–60. https://doi.org/10.4037/ccn2014416.
14. Merrill KC, Sumner S, Linford L, Taylor C, Macintosh C. Impact of universal disinfectant cap implementation on central line–associated bloodstream infections. Am J Infect Control. 2014;42(12):1274–7. https://doi.org/10.1016/j.ajic.2014.09.008.
15. Ivy DD, Calderbank M, Wagner BD, et al. Closed-hub systems with protected connections and the reduction of risk of catheter-related bloodstream infection in pediatric patients receiving intravenous prostanoid therapy for pulmonary hypertension. Infect Control Hosp Epidemiol. 2009;30(9):823–9. https://doi.org/10.1086/605320.
16. Goudie A, Dynan L, Brady PW, Fieldston E, Brilli RJ, Walsh KE. Costs of venous thromboembolism, catheter-associated urinary tract infection, and pressure ulcer. Pediatrics. 2015;136(3):432–9. https://doi.org/10.1542/peds.2015-1386.
17. Lyren A, Brilli RJ, Zieker K, Marino M, Muething S, Sharek PJ. Children's hospitals' solutions for patient safety collaborative impact on hospital-acquired harm. Pediatrics. 2017;140(3) https://doi.org/10.1542/peds.2016-3494.
18. Fukuoka K, Furuichi M, Ito K, et al. Longer duration of urinary catheterization increases catheter-associated urinary tract infection in PICU. Pediatr Crit Care Med. 2018;19(10):e547–50. https://doi.org/10.1097/PCC.0000000000001628.
19. Mack EH, Stem CT. Prevention of CAUTIs, CLABSIs, and VAPs in children. Curr Treat Options Pediatr. 2017;3(3):221–35. https://doi.org/10.1007/s40746-017-0094-8.
20. Foster CB, Ackerman K, Hupertz V, et al. Catheter-associated urinary tract infection reduction in a pediatric safety engagement network. Pediatrics. 2020;146(4) https://doi.org/10.1542/peds.2019-2057.
21. How-to guide: prevent catheter-associated urinary tract infections; 2011. www.ihi.org.
22. Snyder MD, Priestley MA, Weiss M, et al. Preventing catheter-associated urinary tract infections in the pediatric intensive care unit. Crit Care Nurse. 2020;40(1):e12–7. https://doi.org/10.4037/ccn2020438.
23. Sönmez Düzkaya D, Bozkurt G, Uysal G, Yakut T. The effects of bundles on catheter-associated urinary tract infections in the pediatric intensive care unit. Clin Nurse Spec. 2016;30(6):341–6. https://doi.org/10.1097/NUR.0000000000000246.
24. Elegant J, Sorce L. Nurse-driven care in the pediatric intensive care unit: a review of recent strategies to improve quality and patient safety. Curr Treat Options Pediatr. 2017;3(3):236–45. https://doi.org/10.1007/s40746-017-0095-7.
25. Nelson RE, Hatfield KM, Wolford H, et al. National estimates of healthcare costs associated with multidrug-resistant bacterial infections among hospitalized patients in the United States. Clin Infect Dis. 2021;72(Suppl. 1):S17–26. https://doi.org/10.1093/cid/ciaa1581.

26. Sutter DE, Milburn E, Chukwuma U, Dzialowy N, Maranich AM, Hospenthal DR. Changing susceptibility of *Staphylococcus aureus* in a US pediatric population. Pediatrics. 2016;137(4) https://doi.org/10.1542/peds.2015-3099.
27. Zervou FN, Zacharioudakis IM, Ziakas PD, Mylonakis E. MRSA colonization and risk of infection in the neonatal and pediatric ICU: a meta-analysis. Pediatrics. 2014;133(4):e1015–23. https://doi.org/10.1542/peds.2013-3413.
28. Siegel JD, Rhinehart E, Jackson M, Chiarello L. Guideline for isolation precautions: preventing transmission of infectious agents in health care settings. Am J Infect Control. 2007;35(10):S65–S164. https://doi.org/10.1016/j.ajic.2007.10.007.
29. Morgan DJ, Zhan M, Goto M, et al. The effectiveness of contact precautions on methicillin-resistant Staphylococcus aureus in long-term care across the United States. Clin Infect Dis. 2020;71(7):1676–83. https://doi.org/10.1093/cid/ciz1045.
30. Khader K, Thomas A, Stevens V, et al. Association between contact precautions and transmission of methicillin-resistant Staphylococcus aureus in veterans affairs hospitals. JAMA Netw Open. 2021;4(3):e210971. https://doi.org/10.1001/jamanetworkopen.2021.0971.
31. Frost SA, Alogso MC, Metcalfe L, et al. Chlorhexidine bathing and health care-associated infections among adult intensive care patients: a systematic review and meta-analysis. Crit Care. 2016;20(1):379. https://doi.org/10.1186/s13054-016-1553-5.
32. Milstone AM, Elward A, Song X, et al. Daily chlorhexidine bathing to reduce bacteraemia in critically ill children: a multicentre, cluster-randomised, crossover trial. Lancet. 2013;381(9872):1099–106. https://doi.org/10.1016/S0140-6736(12)61687-0.
33. Quach C, Milstone AM, Perpête C, Bonenfant M, Moore DL, Perreault T. Chlorhexidine bathing in a tertiary care neonatal intensive care unit: impact on central line–associated bloodstream infections. Infect Control Hosp Epidemiol. 2014;35(2):158–63. https://doi.org/10.1086/674862.
34. Johnson J, Bracken R, Tamma PD, Aucott SW, Bearer C, Milstone AM. Trends in chlorhexidine use in US neonatal intensive care units: results from a follow-up national survey. Infect Control Hosp Epidemiol. 2016;37(9):1116–8. https://doi.org/10.1017/ice.2016.125.
35. Delaney HM, Wang E, Melish M. Comprehensive strategy including prophylactic mupirocin to reduce Staphylococcus aureus colonization and infection in high-risk neonates. J Perinatol. 2013;33(4):313–8. https://doi.org/10.1038/jp.2012.102.
36. Milstone AM, Song X, Coffin S, Elward A. Identification and eradication of methicillin-resistant *Staphylococcus aureus* colonization in the neonatal intensive care unit: results of a national survey. Infect Control Hosp Epidemiol. 2010;31(7):766–8. https://doi.org/10.1086/653615.
37. Nelson MU, Shaw J, Gross SJ. Randomized placebo-controlled trial of topical mupirocin to reduce Staphylococcus aureus Colonization in infants in the neonatal intensive care unit. J Pediatr. 2021;236:70–7. https://doi.org/10.1016/j.jpeds.2021.05.042.
38. Adams DJ, Eberly MD, Goudie A, Nylund CM. Rising vancomycin-resistant enterococcus infections in hospitalized children in the United States. Hosp Pediatr. 2016;6(7):404–11. https://doi.org/10.1542/hpeds.2015-0196.
39. Sutcu M, Akturk H, Acar M, et al. Impact of vancomycin-resistant enterococci colonization in critically ill pediatric patients. Am J Infect Control. 2016;44(5):515–9. https://doi.org/10.1016/j.ajic.2015.11.026.
40. Akturk H, Sutcu M, Somer A, et al. Vancomycin resistant enterococci colonization in a neonatal intensive care unit: who will be infected? J Maternal-Fetal Neonatal Med. 2016:1–22. https://doi.org/10.3109/14767058.2015.1132693.
41. de Angelis G, Cataldo MA, de Waure C, et al. Infection control and prevention measures to reduce the spread of vancomycin-resistant enterococci in hospitalized patients: a systematic review and meta-analysis. J Antimicrob Chemother. 2014;69(5):1185–92. https://doi.org/10.1093/jac/dkt525.
42. Chen CC, Chiu CH. Current and future applications of fecal microbiota transplantation for children. Biomed J. 2022;45(1):11–8. https://doi.org/10.1016/j.bj.2021.11.004.
43. Sehulster L, Chinn R. Guidelines for environmental infection control in health care facilities recommendations of CDC and the Healthcare Infection Control Practices Advisory Committee

(HICPAC). In: MMWR recommendations and reports: morbidity and mortality weekly report recommendations and reports/centers for disease control, vol. 52; 2003. p. 1–42.
44. Nerandzic MM, Cadnum JL, Pultz MJ, Donskey CJ. Evaluation of an automated ultraviolet radiation device for decontamination of Clostridium difficile and other healthcare-associated pathogens in hospital rooms. BMC Infect Dis. 2010;10(1):197. https://doi.org/10.1186/1471-2334-10-197.
45. Logan LK, Braykov NP, Weinstein RA, Laxminarayan R. Extended-spectrum β-lactamase–producing and third-generation cephalosporin-resistant enterobacteriaceae in children: trends in the United States, 1999–2011. J Pediatric Infect Dis Soc. 2014;3(4):320–8. https://doi.org/10.1093/jpids/piu010.
46. Logan LK, Renschler JP, Gandra S, et al. Carbapenem-resistant enterobacteriaceae in children, United States, 1999–2012. Emerg Infect Dis. 2015;21(11):2014–21. https://doi.org/10.3201/eid2111.150548.
47. Tsai MH, Chu SM, Hsu JF, et al. Risk factors and outcomes for multidrug-resistant gram-negative bacteremia in the NICU. Pediatrics. 2014;133(2):e322–9. https://doi.org/10.1542/peds.2013-1248.
48. Agud M, de Medrano I, Mendez-Echevarria A, et al. Risk factors for antibiotic-resistant bacteria colonisation in children with chronic complex conditions. Sci Rep. 2022;12(1):7223. https://doi.org/10.1038/s41598-022-11295-5.
49. Giuffrè M, Geraci DM, Bonura C, et al. The increasing challenge of multidrug-resistant gram-negative bacilli. Medicine. 2016;95(10):e3016. https://doi.org/10.1097/MD.0000000000003016.
50. Siegel JD, Rhinehart E, Jackson M, Chiarello L. Management of multidrug-resistant organisms in healthcare settings, 2006; 2006. https://www.cdc.gov/infectioncontrol/guidelines/mdro/
51. Benenson S, Levin PD, Block C, et al. Continuous surveillance to reduce extended-spectrum β-lactamase Klebsiella pneumoniae colonization in the neonatal intensive care unit. Neonatology. 2013;103(2):155–60. https://doi.org/10.1159/000343150.
52. Rybczynska H, Melander E, Johansson H, Lundberg F. Efficacy of a once-a-week screening programme to control extended-spectrum beta-lactamase-producing bacteria in a neonatal intensive care unit. Scand J Infect Dis. 2014;46(6):426–32. https://doi.org/10.3109/00365548.2014.896027.
53. Domenech de Cellès M, Zahar JR, Abadie V, Guillemot D. Limits of patient isolation measures to control extended-spectrum beta-lactamase–producing Enterobacteriaceae: model-based analysis of clinical data in a pediatric ward. BMC Infect Dis. 2013;13(1):187. https://doi.org/10.1186/1471-2334-13-187.
54. Rungsitsathian K, Wacharachaisurapol N, Nakaranurack C, et al. Acceptance and outcome of interventions in a meropenem de-escalation antimicrobial stewardship program in pediatrics. Pediatr Int. 2021;63(12):1458–65. https://doi.org/10.1111/ped.14703.
55. CDC. Pediatric Ventilator-Associated Event (PedVAE) . Published 2022. Accessed August 30, 2022. https://www.cdc.gov/nhsn/pdfs/pscmanual/pedvae-current-508.pdf.
56. CDC. Ventilator-associated Events (VAE). Published 2022. Accessed August 30, 2022. https://www.cdc.gov/nhsn/pdfs/pscmanual/10-vae_final.pdf.
57. How-to guide: prevent ventilator-associated pneumonia. Institute for Healthcare Improvement (Available at www.ihi.org); 2012.
58. Klompas M, Branson R, Cawcutt K, et al. Strategies to prevent ventilator-associated pneumonia, ventilator-associated events, and nonventilator hospital-acquired pneumonia in acute-care hospitals: 2022 update. Infect Control Hosp Epidemiol. 2022;43(6):687–713. https://doi.org/10.1017/ice.2022.88.
59. Zhong W, Bragazzi NL, Kong JD, et al. Burden of respiratory infection and tuberculosis among US states from 1990 to 2019. Clin Epidemiol. 2021;13:503–14. https://doi.org/10.2147/CLEP.S314802.
60. Li Y, Wang X, Blau DM, et al. Global, regional, and national disease burden estimates of acute lower respiratory infections due to respiratory syncytial virus in children younger than 5 years in 2019: a systematic analysis. Lancet. 2022;399(10340):2047–64. https://doi.org/10.1016/S0140-6736(22)00478-0.

61. Soni A. The five most costly children's conditions, 2011: Estimates for U.S. Civilian Noninstitutionalized Children, Ages 0–17. #434. Agency for Healthcare Research and Quality; 2014. http://www.meps.ahrq.gov/mepsweb/data_files/publications/st434/stat434.shtml.
62. Meissner HC. Viral bronchiolitis in children. N Engl J Med. 2016;374(1):62–72. https://doi.org/10.1056/NEJMra1413456.
63. Aitken C, Jeffries DJ. Nosocomial spread of viral disease. Clin Microbiol Rev. 2001;14(3):528–46. https://doi.org/10.1128/CMR.14.3.528-546.2001.
64. Most ZM, Jackson P, Sebert M, Perl TM. Contrasting definitions and incidence of healthcare-associated respiratory viral infections in a pediatric hospital. Infect Control Hosp Epidemiol. 2022:1–7. https://doi.org/10.1017/ice.2022.33.
65. Chow EJ, Mermel LA. Hospital-Acquired respiratory viral infections: incidence, morbidity, and mortality in pediatric and adult patients. Open Forum Infect Dis. 2017;4(1) https://doi.org/10.1093/ofid/ofx006.
66. Paquette M, Shephard A, Bedard P, Thampi N. Viral respiratory infections in hospitalized children with symptomatic caregivers. Hosp Pediatr. 2022;12(4):e124–8. https://doi.org/10.1542/hpeds.2021-006108.
67. Petrie JG, Lauring AS, Martin ET, Kaye KS. Hospital associated respiratory virus infection in children and adults: it does not just occur during cold and flu season. Open Forum Infect Dis. 2020;7(6) https://doi.org/10.1093/ofid/ofaa200.
68. Mermel LA, Jefferson JA, Smit MA, Auld DB. Prevention of hospital-acquired respiratory viral infections: Assessment of a multimodal intervention program. Infect Control Hosp Epidemiol. 2019;40(3):362–4. https://doi.org/10.1017/ice.2018.337.
69. Tenforde MW, Campbell AP, Michaels MG, et al. Clinical influenza testing practices in hospitalized children at United States Medical Centers, 2015–2018. J Pediatric Infect Dis Soc. 2022;11(1):5–8. https://doi.org/10.1093/jpids/piab096.
70. Kotloff KL. The burden and etiology of diarrheal illness in developing countries. Pediatr Clin North Am. 2017;64(4):799–814. https://doi.org/10.1016/j.pcl.2017.03.006.
71. Wang H, Naghavi M, Allen C, et al. Global, regional, and national life expectancy, all-cause mortality, and cause-specific mortality for 249 causes of death, 1980–2015: a systematic analysis for the Global Burden of Disease Study 2015. Lancet. 2016;388(10053):1459–544. https://doi.org/10.1016/S0140-6736(16)31012-1.
72. Parashar UD, Hummelman EG, Bresee JS, Miller MA, Glass RI. Global illness and deaths caused by rotavirus disease in children. Emerg Infect Dis. 2003;9(5):565–72. https://doi.org/10.3201/eid0905.020562.
73. Shane AL, Mody RK, Crump JA, et al. 2017 Infectious Diseases Society of America Clinical Practice Guidelines for the diagnosis and management of infectious diarrhea. Clin Infect Dis. 2017;65(12):e45–80. https://doi.org/10.1093/cid/cix669.
74. Langley JM, LeBlanc JC, Hanakowski M, Goloubeva O. The role of Clostridium difficile and viruses as causes of nosocomial diarrhea in children. Infect Control Hosp Epidemiol. 2002;23(11):660–4. https://doi.org/10.1086/501990.
75. Ford-Jones EL, Mindorff CM, Langley JM, et al. Epidemiologic study of 4684 hospital-acquired infections in pediatric patients. Pediatr Infect Dis J. 1989;8(10):668–75. https://doi.org/10.1097/00006454-198910000-00002.
76. Brady MT, Pacini DL, Budde CT, Connell MJ. Diagnostic studies of nosocomial diarrhea in child en: Assessing their use end value. Am J Infect Control. 1989;17(2):77–82. https://doi.org/10.1016/0196-6553(89)90021-7.
77. Mehrotra P, Jang J, Gidengil C, Sandora TJ. Attributable cost of *Clostridium difficile* infection in pediatric patients. Infect Control Hosp Epidemiol. 2017;38(12):1472–7. https://doi.org/10.1017/ice.2017.240.
78. Bruijning-Verhagen P, Quach C, Bonten M. Nosocomial Rotavirus infections: a meta-analysis. Pediatrics. 2012;129(4):e1011–9. https://doi.org/10.1542/peds.2011-2779.
79. Sammons JS, Toltzis P, Zaoutis TE. Clostridium difficile Infection in children. JAMA Pediatr. 2013;167(6):567. https://doi.org/10.1001/jamapediatrics.2013.441.
80. Bolton RP, Tait SK, Dear PR, Losowsky MS. Asymptomatic neonatal colonisation by Clostridium difficile. Arch Dis Child. 1984;59(5):466–72. https://doi.org/10.1136/adc.59.5.466.

81. Al-Jumaili IJ, Shibley M, Lishman AH, Record CO. Incidence and origin of Clostridium difficile in neonates. J Clin Microbiol. 1984;19(1):77–8. https://doi.org/10.1128/jcm.19.1.77-78.1984.
82. Tougas SR, Lodha N, Vandermeer B, et al. Prevalence of detection of *Clostridioides difficile* among asymptomatic children. JAMA Pediatr. 2021;175(10):e212328. https://doi.org/10.1001/jamapediatrics.2021.2328.
83. Jangi S, Lamont JT. Asymptomatic Colonization by Clostridium difficile in Infants: implications for disease in later life. J Pediatr Gastroenterol Nutr. 2010;51(1):2–7. https://doi.org/10.1097/MPG.0b013e3181d29767.
84. Ferroni A, Merckx J, Ancelle T, et al. Nosocomial outbreak ofClostridium difficile diarrhea in a pediatric service. Eur J Clin Microbiol Infect Dis. 1997;16(12):928–33. https://doi.org/10.1007/BF01700562.
85. Cartwright CP, Stock F, Beekmann SE, Williams EC, Gill VJ. PCR amplification of rRNA intergenic spacer regions as a method for epidemiologic typing of Clostridium difficile. J Clin Microbiol. 1995;33(1):184–7. https://doi.org/10.1128/jcm.33.1.184-187.1995.
86. Nylund CM, Goudie A, Garza JM, Fairbrother G, Cohen MB. Clostridium difficile infection in hospitalized children in the United States. Arch Pediatr Adolesc Med. 2011;165(5) https://doi.org/10.1001/archpediatrics.2010.282.
87. Edwards PT, Thurm CW, Hall M, et al. Clostridioides difficile infection in hospitalized pediatric patients: Comparisons of epidemiology, testing, and treatment from 2013 to 2019. J Pediatr. 2022 https://doi.org/10.1016/j.jpeds.2022.08.030.
88. de Blank P, Zaoutis T, Fisher B, Troxel A, Kim J, Aplenc R. Trends in Clostridium difficile infection and risk factors for hospital acquisition of Clostridium difficile among children with cancer. J Pediatr. 2013;163(3):699–705.e1. https://doi.org/10.1016/j.jpeds.2013.01.062.
89. Samady W, Bush R, Pong A, Andrews A, Fisher ES. Predictors of *Clostridium difficile* infections in hospitalized children. J Hosp Med. 2014;9(2):94–8. https://doi.org/10.1002/jhm.2135.
90. McFarland LV, Ozen M, Dinleyici EC, Goh S. Comparison of pediatric and adult antibiotic-associated diarrhea and *Clostridium difficile* infections. World J Gastroenterol. 2016;22(11):3078. https://doi.org/10.3748/wjg.v22.i11.3078.
91. McDonald LC, Gerding DN, Johnson S, et al. Clinical practice guidelines for Clostridium difficile infection in adults and children: 2017 Update by the Infectious Diseases Society of America (IDSA) and Society for Healthcare Epidemiology of America (SHEA). Clin Infect Dis. 2018;66(7):e1–e48. https://doi.org/10.1093/cid/cix1085.
92. McFarland LV. Preventing pediatric antibiotic-associated diarrhea and *Clostridium difficile* infections with probiotics: a meta-analysis. World J Metaanal. 2013;1(3):102. https://doi.org/10.13105/wjma.v1.i3.102.
93. Fischer TK, Bresee JS, Glass RI. Rotavirus vaccines and the prevention of hospital-acquired diarrhea in children. Vaccine. 2004;22:S49–54. https://doi.org/10.1016/j.vaccine.2004.08.017.
94. Jusot JF, Vanhems P, Benzait F, et al. Reported measures of hygiene and incidence rates for hospital-acquired diarrhea in 31 French pediatric wards: is there any relationship? Infect Control Hosp Epidemiol. 2003;24(7):520–5. https://doi.org/10.1086/502238.
95. Hurtado-Sierra D, Calderón-Colmenero J, Curi-Curi P, et al. Outcomes of delayed sternal closure in pediatric heart surgery: single-center experience. Biomed Res Int. 2018;2018:1–6. https://doi.org/10.1155/2018/3742362.
96. Yabrodi M, Hermann JL, Brown JW, Rodefeld MD, Turrentine MW, Mastropietro CW. Minimization of surgical site infections in patients with delayed sternal closure after pediatric cardiac surgery. World J Pediatr Congenit Heart Surg. 2019;10(4):400–6. https://doi.org/10.1177/2150135119846040.
97. von Stumm M, Leps Y, Jochheim L, et al. Impact of delayed sternal closure on wound infections following neonatal and infant cardiac surgery. PLoS One. 2022;17(5):e0267985. https://doi.org/10.1371/journal.pone.0267985.
98. Delgado-Corcoran C, van Dorn CS, Pribble C, et al. Reducing pediatric sternal wound infections. Pediatr Crit Care Med. 2017;18(5):461–8. https://doi.org/10.1097/PCC.0000000000001135.
99. Woodward C, Taylor R, Son M, Taeed R, Husain SA. Efforts to reduce infections in delayed sternal closure patients: a survey of pediatric practice. World J Pediatr Congenit Heart Surg. 2020;11(3):310–5. https://doi.org/10.1177/2150135120907372.

Chapter 9
Infection Control in the Immunocompromised Host

Febres-Aldana Anthony and Al Mohajer Mayar

Introduction

Infection control (IC) is a critical component of modern medicine and is essential in the care of the immunocompromised patient to reduce morbidity and mortality while lowering healthcare costs. Multiple United States and international agencies recommend hand hygiene, air quality measures, barrier isolation, suppression of endogenous flora, and efforts to prevent device-related infections as the basic principles of IC [1 (p. 3), 2, 3].

The immunologic limitations of the immunocompromised hosts make them more susceptible to developing hospital-acquired infections (HAIs). As depicted in Fig. 9.1, immunosuppressive conditions fall in a risk spectrum in which some patients have a higher risk for developing HAIs secondary to specific healthcare exposures. The HCT recipient with graft-versus-host disease (GVHD), the patient with profound neutropenia, and the solid organ transplant (SOT) recipient with graft rejection are at the highest risk of developing HAIs [4, 5]. The onset of HAIs requires three factors: a source for the infectious agent, a susceptible host with a port of entry, and a mode of transmission. Admission to the ICU represents an increased exposure to infectious agents and an expansion of possible ports of entry. Moreover, the cumulative occurrence of HAIs for those patients in the ICU is associated with almost a twofold increase in mortality for the first HAI, with mortality

F.-A. Anthony
Division of Infectious Disease, H. Lee Moffitt Cancer Center and Research Institute, Tampa, FL, USA
e-mail: Anthony.febresaldana@moffitt.org

A. M. Mayar (✉)
Section of Infectious Disease, Baylor College of Medicine, Houston, TX, USA

Baylor St. Luke's Medical Center, Houston, TX, USA
e-mail: Mayar.AlMohajer@bcm.edu

M. Ellsworth, L. Ostrosky-Zeichner (eds.), *Infection Prevention in the Intensive Care Setting*, https://doi.org/10.1007/978-3-031-67062-6_9

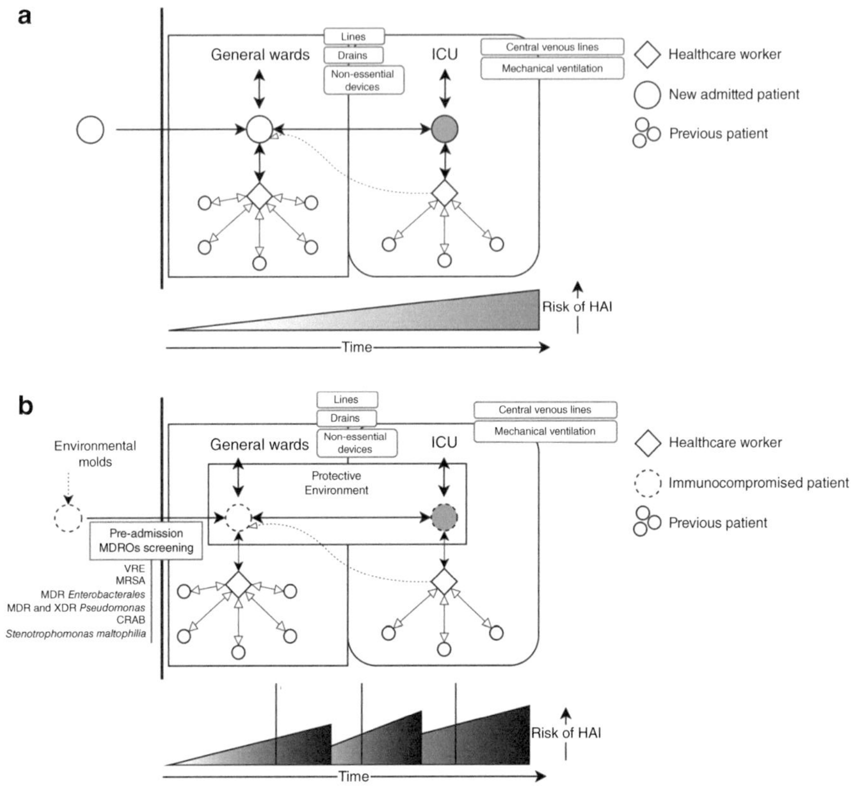

Fig. 9.1 The acquisition of hospital-acquired infections (HAI) is conditioned by three main factors: (1) a susceptible host, (2) a transmission vehicle for the pathogen, and (3) an entry port for the pathogen. The top panel (**a**) represents how admission to the hospital and subsequent access to the intensive care unit (ICU) contribute to a progressive increase in the risk of HAI. In the bottom panel (**b**), the addition of an immunosuppressive condition boosts this risk increase, with certain patients having periods of even heightened risk given exposure to lymphodepletion or cytotoxic chemotherapy regimens or the addition of immunosuppressive agents for the treatment of graft-versus-host disease (GVHD) or graft rejection. Abbreviations: *ICU* intensive care unit, *MRSA* methicillin-resistant *Staphylococcus aureus*, *VRE* vancomycin-resistant *Enterococci*, *MDR* multidrug-resistant, *XDR* extensively drug-resistant, *CRAB* Carbapenem-resistant *Acinetobacter baumannii*

being sequentially higher with further episodes [6]. Similar IC principles to those discussed in earlier chapters apply to immunocompromised patients admitted to the ICU, with the spotlight on these peculiarities.

Although the overall rate of HAIs has remained stable since the 2010s, there has been an increase noted for device-associated infections and ventilator-associated events in those patients admitted to the ICU [7]. Likewise, immunocompromised patients have an a higher rate of infections by multidrug-resistant organisms (MDROs) and atypical presentation of otherwise self-limited infections [8].

In the following chapter, we will summarize these practices. Firstly, we will provide an overview of the standard precautions and those environmental measures that have proven to be beneficial in preventing HAIs for the immunocompromised patient, recognized under the term protective environment (PE). We will then describe the current evidence pertaining to the IC practice specific to the oncologic patients and the recipients of hematopoietic cell transplants (HCT) and other cellular therapies and to the solid organ transplant (SOT) recipients. Then we will provide an overview of several topics in IC that are equally important to all immunocompromised patients, including the evidence surrounding the use of decontamination protocols and other infections with potential for in-hospital transmission, including tuberculosis, mold infections, *Legionella* infections, *Clostridioides difficile* infection (CDI), respiratory viral infections, and coronavirus disease 2019 (COVID-19).

Standard Precautions and the Protective Environment

Standard Precautions

Standard precautions are a set of IC practices used to reduce the risk of transmission of pathogens in the healthcare setting and are applied to all patient care based on each patient's individual risk assessment. These include hand hygiene, the use of personal protective equipment (PPE) whenever there is a heightened risk of possible exposure to body fluids or potentially contagious material, and principles of respiratory hygiene and cough etiquette [3]. Standard precautions also comprise recommendations on proper handling and disinfection of patient care equipment, environmental disinfection, safe injection practices, laundry and textile handling, and healthcare worker safety. This set of recommendations is published in the guideline for Isolation Precautions: Preventing Transmission of Infectious Agents in Healthcare Settings, the Centers for Disease Control (CDC) [3]. In addition to recommendations on standard precaution, the guideline emphasizes the importance of the PE for the recipients of an HCT, based on the fact that these patients are more susceptible to the onset of infectious complications from their environmental exposures. These recommendations are designed to break the transmission chain of organisms that are of particular concern in the immunocompromised host, including *Aspergillus* [9] and non-*Aspergillus* molds [10], waterborne pathogens including *Pseudomonas* spp., *Legionella pneumophila*, *Cryptosporidium* spp, non-tuberculous mycobacteria (NTM) [11]; and Gram-positive organisms (*Staphylococcus aureus* [12], *Enterococcus* spp. [13]).

The Protective Environment

In addition to the standard precautions, the PE provides recommendations on room features, air and ventilation measures, avoidance of certain inanimate objects (plants, used toys, soil-based products), and policies regarding cleaning, construction, renovations, and patient care visits, that are specifically intended to disrupt the transmission chain of fungi and minimize the risk of invasive fungal infections [14]. The CDC emphasizes that the PE is a specialized patient care area that creates an environment that can safely accommodate HCT recipients. Other societies, including the European Society of Blood and Marrow Transplantation (EBMT) have also published guidance regarding the PE [15]. Table 9.1 provides a summary of the guidance stated under the PE.

Both guidelines provide specific guidance on air quality measures. These include using specialized ventilation systems, including laminar flow units capable of 12 air exchanges per hour and high-efficiency particulate air (HEPA) filters. Patient isolation units should use HEPA filtration with the capacity to remove particles >0.3 μm, continuous pressure monitoring with positive air pressure between patients' rooms and the hallway, self-closing doors, and well-sealed rooms. Anterooms, a room destined to ensure an appropriate balance of air relative to the protective environment, are optional except for those patients requiring airborne isolation precautions for certain infections. Of note, routine fungal spore counting is not recommended.

Another component of the PE comprises environmental cleaning. Additional to the environmental cleaning guidance published by the CDC [16], the EBMT recommendations emphasize daily cleaning of dusty areas with a wet mop and cloths to prevent sporulation of molds and suggest that room design should be based on predominantly easy-to-clean and scrubbable surfaces with nonporous and smooth walls and horizontal surfaces with the purpose to facilitate cleaning and to prevent the entrapment of bacteria and spores [15]. Unless thoroughly disinfected, using dedicated non-critical devices is imperative in mitigating nosocomial pathogen transmission [17], and, because the immunocompromised patient is frequently colonized with multi-drug resistant organisms (MDROs), decreasing bacterial and fungal contamination is critical in preventing HAI. Among these lines, the use of rectal thermometers, enemas or suppositories, and internal rectal exams are also contraindicated among HCT recipients and those patients with profound neutropenia to avoid skin or mucosal breakdown and potential entry ports for pathogens [15].

When there is an inability to comply with the PE such as in the case of decreased room availability, the priority to maintain it should be for those patients at the highest risk of invasive mold infections. Portable industrial-grade HEPA filters may be used in non-protective environment rooms to accommodate other vulnerable patients and should be placed in the center of the room. The oncologic center should have provisions for backup emergency power and redundant air-handling and pressurization systems.

Table 9.1 Elements of the protective environment

Measure	Recommendations
Ventilation	• ≥12 air exchanges per hour • Use of HEPA filters with a 99.97% of efficiency for removing particles ≥0.3 μm in diameter • Directional airflow • Positive air pressure ≥2.5 Pa • Continuous pressure monitoring
Room characteristics	• Well-sealed rooms • Self-closing doors • Floor surfaces should be smooth, nonporous, and scrubbable Example materials: Vinyl, linoleum, tile • Single patient room • Avoidance of false ceilings. If this cannot be accomplished, routine vacuuming is necessary • Direction of pedestrian traffic away from patient care areas
Inanimate objects	• Plants and dried or fresh flowers should not be allowed in hospital rooms during conditioning or after HCT • Avoid soil-based materials • Avoid toys
Cleaning	• At least daily cleaning with special attention to dust control • Wet dusting should be performed, using a hospital-approved disinfectant on mobs • Thorough cleaning after renovations and constructions • HCT recipients should not be exposed to vacuuming • Vacuums used in the HCT center should be fitted with HEPA filters
Construction, renovation	• IC risk assessment before construction • Avoidance of the transport of HCT recipients through construction or renovation areas • Avoidance of transporting equipment through construction or renovation areas • Sealing of air intake during outdoor construction • Increase frequency of air filter checking • Weather stripping should be placed around stairwell doors OR the stairwell air should be filtered • Dedicated access routes for construction personnel • Visible dust result of construction should be vacuumed • Portable industrial-grade HEPA filter should be used between a construction zone and the HCT unit • Fungal-contaminated materials that cannot be removed and replaced should be decontaminated with copper-8-quinolinolate • Water leaks should be cleaned up and repaired as soon as possible, within 72 h of onset
Visitor center	• Policy regarding screening of all visitors for communicable infections • Proper signaling • Visitors with signs or symptoms suggestive of communicable infections should be excluded from direct contact with HCT recipients or candidates undergoing conditioning therapy

HEPA high-efficiency particulate air, *HCT* hematopoietic cell transplant, *IC* infection control

It is noteworthy that current guidelines recommend implementing the PE for the HCT recipients and the oncologic patients with profound neutropenia (defined as an absolute neutrophil count below 100 cells/μL). The PE has been universally adopted by HCT-specialized centers, most with institution-specific adaptations with the purpose of minimizing fungal spore counts and risk invasive fungal disease. Other non-HCT recipients, immunocompromised host, including the SOT recipients, are also at a higher risk of infections secondary to environmental organisms, and some of the PE fundaments are used in the practice of IC and the prevention of HAIs. For example, air quality measures like the use of laminar airflow ventilation systems have a similar indication for prevention of spread of some ubiquitous fungi in some immunocompromised patients [18]. The avoidance of construction areas by susceptible patients is also indicated, as these are associated with sporulation of mold and has been described as the source of hospital-acquired aspergillosis outbreaks [19, 20].

The Oncologic Patient and Recipients of Cellular Therapies

As discussed above, many of the IC recommendations published to date are aimed at protecting the HCT recipient and the oncologic patient [15], especially during periods of increased susceptibility. As depicted in Fig. 9.2a, the risk of HAIs among oncologic patients varies according to the specific immune defects caused by the primary malignancy or secondary to therapy, with patients with mismatched unrelated donor (MMUD) HCT recipients, cord blood as the source for the transplanted stem cells, graft-versus-host disease (GVHD), and profound neutropenia at the higher end of the risk spectrum. Infections developed during the first 100 days after an HCT are likely to be hospital-acquired. The risk is higher during pre-engraftment due to cumulative mucosal damage and the predominance of neutropenia [21]. Most of the evidence pertaining to infectious complications in the oncologic patient derives from data from the 1990s and early 2000s. However, the advancement of chemotherapies, the improved pre-transplant conditioning regimens, and the diversification of stem cell sources for transplant led to an overall decrease in non-relapse mortality (NRM) noted over the last decade [22, 23]. Of note, NRM can be greatly accounted for by the incidence of GVHD and infectious complications, of which BSI predominates in the pre-engraftment period [24].

Bloodstream Infections in HCT Recipients

Hospital-acquired infections in the HCT recipients commonly manifest as bloodstream infections (BSI), leading to a predominance of central-line associated BSI (CLABSI) during this period, with rates of 0.92 central line-days/patient days shown in a study from 2003 [25]. The microbiology of these hospital-acquired BSIs has also suffered a shift over the last decades, with a prior predominance of

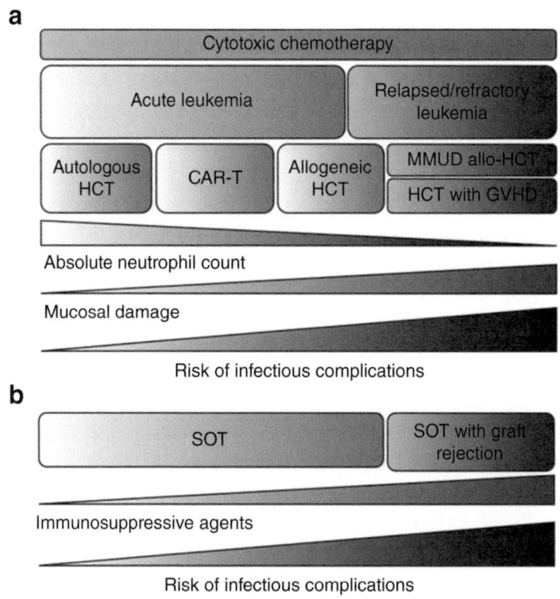

Fig. 9.2 The definition of moderate-to-severe immunosuppression encompasses a spectrum of conditions, all of them representing a higher risk of community-acquired and hospital-acquired infections. On the left (**a**), the risk for these infections for the oncologic patient and the recipient of cellular therapies is depicted as a compound measure result of the underlying hematologic malignancy, the absolute neutrophil count, the use of cytotoxic chemotherapy and chemotherapy-related complications like oral mucositis, and the type of hematopoietic cell transplant, with post-transplant graft-versus-host disease further heightening the risk profile of these patients. On the right (**b**), a similar continuum is depicted regarding the recipient of solid organ transplants, in whom the onset of graft rejection results in further immune dysregulation and additional immunosuppressive therapy significantly increases the risk for infectious complications. Abbreviations: chimeric antigen receptor T-cell therapies (CAR-T), graft-versus-host disease (GVHD), hematopoietic cell transplant (HCT), mismatched unrelated donor (MMUD), solid organ transplant (SOT)

Gram-positive organisms (coagulase-negative staphylococci, *Enterococcus* spp., *Staphylococcus aureus*) now substituted by the predominance of Gram-negative rods (*Escherichia coli*, *Pseudomonas aeruginosa*, and *Klebsiella pneumoniae*). Antimicrobial resistance (AMR) has become of increasing concern during this period. For example, approximately one-third of hospital-acquired BSIs are caused by extended-spectrum beta-lactamase (ESBL) producing Gram-negative rods (GNR). Outbreaks due to MDROs in cancer centers have also been reported from vancomycin-resistant *Enterococcus* (VRE) and other MDR GNR, including carbapenemase-producing GNR, MDR *Pseudomonas aeruginosa*, carbapenemase-producing *Acinetobacter baumannii,* and *Stenotrophomonas maltophilia* [5].

Microbiome alterations in the setting of increased antimicrobial use are the likely explanation for this trend which consequently selects for the growth of MDROs, and the onset of related infections is likely preceded by a colonization period during which organisms are growing without pathologic consequences. Some of the published evidence support this concept, as exemplified by the fact that one-third of all acute myeloid leukemia (AML) colonized patients experience an MDRO-related infection [26], with colonization being an independent risk factor for fatal outcomes. Most of the responsible gram-negative MDROs are resistant to fluoroquinolones, and not surprisingly, many infections occur as breakthroughs despite antibiotic prophylaxis. The type of HCT poses a further risk for HAI, with the occurrence of infections by MDROS being higher in the allogeneic HCT recipient than the autologous HCT recipients.

Other HAI in HCT Recipients and Neutropenic Patients

After BSI, hospital-acquired pneumonia (HAP) is the second cause of HAIs during the neutropenia [27], with a frequency that varies between 15% and 30%, (11.9 episodes per 1000 neutropenic days to 1.8 per 1000 non-neutropenic days) [25]. Many of the HAP are classified as ventilator-associated pneumonia (VAP), whose etiology is often viral, including rhinovirus, influenza, and respiratory syncytial virus (RSV) [28]. Gastroenteritis, catheter-associated local infections, and UTIs are less frequently seen. Current recognized rates of HAP (more than 20 cases/1000 hospital admissions) and VAP (two to 16 episodes/ventilator days) do not distinguish between the immunocompromised patient and the general population, given a lack of available data specific to the oncologic patient and the HCT recipients [27].

Fungal Etiologies of HAI in HCT Recipients

Hospital-acquired yeast infections are of special concern in patients with hematologic malignancies, with non-*albicans Candida* sp., including *C. tropicalis* and *C. glabrata* [29] leading in frequency and commonly presenting as BSI. Many of these fungemias are breakthrough infections on azole prophylaxis.

Viral Reactivations in HCT Recipients

The reactivation of viral infections is a frequent problem that affects HCT recipients. The viruses of concern during the periods of increased immunosuppression include herpes simplex virus 1 and 2, cytomegalovirus, human herpesvirus-6, Epstein–Barr virus (EBV), hepatitis B virus (HBV), adenovirus (ADV), and BK virus (BKV). Most cases of viral infections are community-acquired and often acquired during youth, with a prolonged period of latency followed by viral reactivation during periods of immunosuppression. Therefore, classifying any of these viral infections in HCT recipients as nosocomial might be conceptually difficult given the pathogenic mechanisms of viral reactivation, a topic beyond the scope of this review. In the case of ADV and BKV reactivation, which commonly manifests as viruria and hemorrhagic cystitis, nosocomial transmission has been hypothesized based on the clustering of partial sequences of the viruses [30, 31]. In addition and contrary to the herpesviruses, ADV and BKV are non-enveloped viruses with a structure that makes them partially resistant to routine disinfection practices, which, added to the high viral shedding during hemorrhagic cystitis episodes, makes the in-hospital transmission chain plausible.

Chimeric Antigen Receptor T-Cell Therapy Recipients

The oncologic patient treated with chimeric antigen receptor T-cell (CAR-T) therapy must undergo high-intensity cytotoxic induction chemotherapy that often results in profound neutropenia [32], with a risk of infectious complications similar to that of the HCT recipient. Additionally, most of these patients will develop fever secondary to cytokine release syndrome (CRS), for which the interleukin-6 (IL-6) receptor inhibitor tocilizumab is the therapy of choice, both factors further contributing to the increased risk of HAIs. Epidemiologic data on infectious complications after CAR-T therapy is currently an active area of research, as available evidence in the literature is limited.

Antimicrobial Prophylaxis Regimens

Antimicrobial prophylaxis is indicated in oncologic patients to prevent the occurrence of infections during periods of neutropenia. Prophylaxis against other infectious agents, herpesvirus reactivation, *Pneumocystis jirovecii* pneumonia (PCP), and invasive fungal infections is indicated as well, depending on each patient's risk profile, including the oncologic diagnosis and potential community-based exposures [33, 34]. For example, in addition to antibacterial prophylaxis during the periods of neutropenia, the HCT recipient with GVHD needs to receive herpesvirus prophylaxis with acyclovir, valacyclovir, or famciclovir, antifungal prophylaxis with a mold-active azole or amphotericin B, PCP prophylaxis with trimethoprim-sulfamethoxazole, atovaquone, dapsone, or inhaled pentamidine, and cytomegalovirus (CMV) prophylaxis depending on CMV risk profile.

Focusing on fluoroquinolone antibacterial prophylaxis, its widespread use has resulted in a reduction in the incidence of neutropenic fever and BSI, with an overall effect on mortality that differs across the literature [35, 36]. Levofloxacin prophylaxis has been hypothesized to disrupt the gut microbiome favoring the selection of MDR GNRs, including quinolone-resistant and ESBL-producing *Enterobacterales,* followed by the risk of MDR GNR-related infections [37]. In fact, the use of levofloxacin primary prophylaxis was associated with an increased risk of colonization by ESBL *Enterobacterales* and carbapenem-resistant GNRs [38], which is subsequently associated with increased mortality [39]. On the contrary, a meta-analysis from 2007 that included 22 trials published between 1987 and 2005 that compared quinolones (either ciprofloxacin or levofloxacin) to placebo or no-intervention showed a non-statistically significant increase in the risk of colonization by a quinolone-resistant GNR and no increase in the risk of infections by MDROs [40]. As a result of this discordant evidence on the benefit of quinolone prophylaxis and raising concern on the development of AMR, the 8th European Conference on Infections in Leukemia (ECIL) advised against routine use of quinolone prophylaxis in pediatric patients with cancer or after HCT [41], differing from the current recommendations on adult patients with neutropenia.

Prevention of Hospital-Acquired Infections in the Oncologic Patient and the Recipient of Cellular Therapies

Oncologic centers have institutional-specific protocols to prevent HAIs, which are based on the PE recommendations by the CDC and the EBMT. HCT recipients should be hospitalized in private rooms during and after the transplant. Regular skin site evaluation is necessary, focusing on the perineum, intravascular access sites, and perineal cleanliness. These patients should also take daily showers or baths with light soap. Patients who experience oral mucositis (OM) due to chemotherapy are more likely to contract HAI that starts in the oral mucosa [42]. As many of these BSIs are from endogenous sources in the setting of OM, intensive oral care regimens have a role in reducing the incidence of infections, with the significant benefit seen for Gram-positive organisms [43].

Solid Organ Transplant Recipients

Recipients of SOT are also at an increased risk of HAIs compared to the general population, with the highest risk found early in the post-transplant period, usually within the first 30 days after transplant, and also include infections that were incubating in the pre-transplant period and donor-derived diseases [44]. As shown in Fig. 9.2b, during episodes of graft rejection, there is a further increase in the risk of HAI. The incidence distribution of these infections varies according to the transplanted organ, with current epidemiologic data derived from single-center reports, many of which are focused mainly on kidney and liver transplant recipients. In a study published in 2020 evaluating the incidence of HAI in the liver and renal transplant recipients, the rate of HAI in the ICU was higher for liver transplant recipients [45]. In addition to device-associated infections, including CLABSI and catheter-associated urinary tract infection (CAUTI), surgical site infections (SSI) are of epidemiologic importance for the SOT recipient in the early post-transplant period.

Microbiology of Hospital-Acquired Infections in the Solid Organ Transplant Recipient

With a predominance of MDROs, the list of organisms responsible for HAIs in the SOT recipients is similar to that of non-transplant recipients. Gram-positive organisms, including MRSA and VRE, commonly affect liver transplant recipients, whereas *Escherichia coli* commonly affects kidney transplant recipients [46]. Other UTI-associated organisms include Enterobacterales, *Pseudomonas aeruginosa*, and *Enterococcus* sp. [47] Anastomotic leaks, bleeding, and the need for reintervention are peritransplant surgical problems in the SOT that appear to be linked to a higher incidence of carbapenem-resistant Enterobacterales (CRE) [48]. Patients with post-transplant CRE infections are more likely to have medical complications such as the requirement for renal replacement treatment.

Distribution of HAI According to the Transplanted Organ

The frequency distribution of HAIs in the SOT recipient might follow that published on post-surgical patients. In contrast with the oncologic patients and HCT recipients where BSIs lead in frequency for causes of HAI, the SOT recipient suffers most commonly from pneumonia (33%), UTI and CAUTI (18%), SSI (14%), while BSI only constitutes 13%. As expected, this distribution has certain variations specific to the baseline disease, the grafted organ, and the surgical technique [49].

Often, HAPs in the SOT recipients are secondary to aspiration pneumonia in the postoperative period with microbiology that follows the local epidemiologic trends for hospitals. Those SOT recipients who require prolonged mechanical ventilation, develop gastroparesis and have impaired mucociliary clearance are prone to develop HAP/VAP. In terms of transplanted organ, lung transplant recipients are at a higher risk, followed by heart transplant recipients, liver transplant recipients, and kidney transplant recipients, in order of frequency [27].

The Spanish Network for the Study of Infections in Transplantation (RESITRA) reports an incidence of cystitis that is higher in renal transplant recipients [46], which is in line with other reports [50]. BSIs in this population are usually from the urinary source [51]. After the renal transplants, liver transplant recipients follow in the frequency of UTIs. Heart and lung transplant recipients are less affected.

Small bowel and multi-visceral transplants have the highest risk for SSI, followed by liver and pancreas transplants [52], with frequencies that range between

35% and 54% of bacterial infections and up to 38% of the SSI cases complicated with BSI [53]. Lung and heart transplants can be complicated by sternal wound infections, including sternal osteomyelitis and mediastinitis, with morbidity and mortality that is several-fold higher than in those that arise from non-transplant thoracic surgeries [49].

Viral Reactivations and In-Hospital Transmission in SOT Recipients

Even though of less impact than in the HCT recipients, viral reactivations are also of concern in the SOT recipient. The agents implicated include the herpesviruses, the polyomaviruses BK virus and JC virus, HBV, and adenovirus [54]. Primary infections by these viruses typically occur during childhood, after which a period of latency follows. Although not often categorized as hospital-acquired, the donor-derived transmission of some of these viruses seems possible in the setting of recipient immunosuppression, lack of prior recipient humoral immunity, and false negative serologic screening of the donor [55]. For example, in the case of CMV reactivation, the recipient seronegative for CMV who receipts an organ from a seropositive donor (R^-/D^+) is at the highest risk for donor-derived CMV infection.

Antimicrobial Prophylaxis

In contrast to HCT recipients, where antibacterial prophylaxis is directed to prevent neutropenic fever, and mainly GNR BSI, antimicrobial prophylaxis in the SOT recipient is indicated to prevent the occurrence of SSIs, which are caused predominantly by *Staphylococcus aureus*, *Enterococcus* sp, *Escherichia coli,* and *Klebsiella pneumoniae* [56]. There is no consensus regarding the need for long-term antimicrobial prophylaxis specific to the SOT recipient, and variability of practices is noted among transplant centers. It is known, nonetheless that patients who have longer inpatient stays before transplantation surgery may become colonized with MDROs [14]. One possible contributing factor is the low threshold to start empiric broad-spectrum antibiotic treatments in these patients. Thus, the antibiotic choice is highly influenced by pre-transplant colonization status and the presence of donor-derived infections [52], but to date, there is no prospective data supporting routine pre-transplant MDRO screening. Patients who receive a graft from a donor infected with an MDR GNR should receive active antibiotic therapy for the first 7 days after the transplant [57].

Antifungal prophylaxis depends on the nature of the surgery, with fluconazole-based prophylaxis commonly done for in intra-abdominal organ transplants [56]. The use of anti-mold prophylaxis is usually guided by prior infection or colonization history. A survey from South Korea showed that all lung transplant programs use universal anti-mold prophylaxis with a mold-active antifungal [58]. Current recommendations emphasize using anti-CMV and anti-PCP prophylaxis within the first year after the transplant.

Prevention of Hospital-Acquired Infections in the Solid Organ Transplant Recipient

In contrast to the case of the oncologic patients and HCT recipients, there are no specific guidelines on IC for SOT recipients. In 2003, the CDC published Guidelines for Environmental Infection Control in Healthcare Facilities [18], which addresses specific controls applicable to all patients but only briefly refers to the SOT recipient. A survey from 2014 that included transplant centers in the US demonstrated high variability in the IC practice among transplant centers, with standard hand hygiene being common among centers [59]. One point in which variability was noted pertains to the practices on air quality measures. The frequency of HEPA-filtered or positive-pressure rooms was low, between 8% and 10%, and similar among all transplant centers.

MDRO Decolonization Protocols

The implication of colonization by an MDRO is a topic whose impact remains not well understood, mostly given the lack of standardized protocols to guide clinical decisions. Events leading to colonization include recurrent healthcare encounters, admission to the ICU, and contact with extended-care facilities such as nursing homes [60].

Universal decolonization has been shown to decrease the rate of HAI in patients admitted to the ICU more so than targeted colonization [61]. Although with limited evidence, some strategies to reduce the incidence of carbapenemase-producing Enterobacterales may include targeted perioperative antimicrobial prophylaxis and universal decolonization using chlorhexidine baths, selective digestive decontamination (SDD), and selective oral decontamination (SOD) [62].

Evidence supporting the routine implementation of gastrointestinal decontamination protocols is currently lacking. A multicenter randomized trial of 13 European ICUs showed no mortality benefit and no impact on the incidence of MDRO infections following an SDD protocol that included a paste and suspension of colistin, tobramycin, nystatin plus enteral vancomycin (for MRSA colonized patients), and systemic cefotaxime [63]. Along the same line, a multicenter open-label controlled trial that included five transplant units showed no reduction in the occurrence of MDR Enterobacterales-related infections following a decolonization protocol with colistin and neomycin [64]. On the contrary, a single-center study found a benefit in decreasing the rates of MDROs GNR isolated in the ICU and a lower risk for HAIs [65]. Variability in trial design, different components of the SDD, and local epidemiologic trends account for this highly variable benefit. In ought of this uncertainty, the European Society of Clinical Microbiology and Infectious Diseases currently does not recommend performing routine decolonization of MDR GNR [66]. To summarize, it is challenging to extrapolate published data on the clinical utility of MDR GNR decolonization protocols to immunocompromised patients [67].

The scenario for perioperative *Staphylococcus aureus* decolonization in the transplant recipient differs, although evidence to date shows variable results. For example, a preoperative decolonization protocol with 4% chlorhexidine daily whole-daily bath and 2% intranasal mupirocin ointment was effective in preventing MRSA infections, including SSI, in an observational study of advanced heart failure before insertion of left ventricular assist devices [68]. On the other hand, a prospective study of liver transplant candidates following a nasal decontamination protocol with topical mupirocin failed to reduce *Staphylococcus aureus-related* infections [69]. Currently, the CDC recommends intranasal mupirocin decontamination with daily chlorhexidine bathing for those patients admitted to the ICU to reduce carriage of *Staphylococcus aureus,* as this approach decreases the risk of CLABSIs [70], and evidence from a multicenter controlled trial supports application of a decontamination bundle consisting of intranasal mupirocin, daily chlorhexidine bathing, and perioperative prophylaxis with vancomycin and cefazolin in those patients colonized with MRSA, to reduce the risk of MRSA-associated SSI on hip or knee arthroplasties and non-transplant cardiac surgery [71]. Specific to the transplant recipients, the American Society for Transplantation recommends universal decolonization with chlorhexidine bathing for ICU patients to prevent transmission of MRSA without recommending active surveillance [12].

Peritransplant colonization by VRE is most commonly seen in liver transplant candidates, but it is not associated with increased mortality [72]. There are protocols for VRE decontamination published in the literature. It is noteworthy a protocol based on gastrointestinal washout to decrease fecal burden followed by systemic oral linezolid and oral non-absorbable daptomycin coupled with chlorhexidine bath decontamination and consolidation with the use of probiotics that was successful in eliminating VRE carriage in a liver transplant candidate [73]. Since the impact of VRE colonization is of unclear significance, no widely recommended VRE decolonization protocols exist.

One intervention that is currently undergoing investigation is the use of fecal microbiota transplantation (FMT), which is hypothesized to achieve MDRO decolonization by restoring the gut microbiota balance [74]. There is evidence of a clinical benefit from FMT based on a trial that included immunocompromised patients; [75] however, current societal guidelines do not list it as a recommendation.

Other Hospital-Acquired Infections

In the following sections, we will briefly discuss the current evidence surrounding other infections in immunocompromised patients and specific IC practices.

Tuberculosis

Infection by *Mycobacterium tuberculosis* most commonly results from reactivation from a latent tuberculosis infection (LTBI). As currently recognized by the CDC, the conversion rate from LTBI to active TB is higher in immunocompromised patients compared to the average population [76], especially during episodes of increased immunosuppression like GVHD in the HCT recipient or acute rejection in the SOT recipient [77]. Active tuberculosis most commonly presents as pulmonary TB in the HCT recipient, with many cases occurring in the first year post-transplant. Around 50% of the patients present with disseminated TB or extra-pulmonary TB [78]. The detection and treatment of LTBI among transplant candidates are acknowledged as an essential part of the IC practice to control the nosocomial spread of TB.

The American Society of Transplantation recommends pre-transplant screening of the SOT candidate and living donors using an interferon-γ release assay (IGRA) or tuberculin skin test (TST) with treatment as indicated. It recognizes that current recommendations are based on expert opinion and that these tests have poor predictive properties [78]. For this reason, practice differs widely among centers, with some not performing routine pre-transplant LTBI screening as results of IGRA or TST can be misleading and potentially delay the diagnosis and treatment of active TB disease [79]. Early recognition of epidemiologic risk factors such as recent exposure to a patient with active TB or exposure to a hyperendemic area is therefore essential in identifying the patients at risk.

All healthcare settings need a TB infection control program to ensure prompt detection, followed by environmental measures including the establishment of airborne isolation precautions using a negative pressure room and the treatment of patients with confirmed TB disease. As part of additional environmental measures, the CDC and World Health Organization (WHO) recommend controlling the source of infection by using local exhaust ventilation (e.g., hoods, tents, or booths), diluting and removing contaminated air by using general ventilation, controlling the airflow to prevent contamination of air in areas adjacent to the airborne isolation room and cleaning the air by using HEPA filtration or ultraviolet germicidal irradiation [80].

Invasive Mold Infections

Molds are ubiquitous organisms in the soil, water, decaying vegetation, and walls and ceilings of old buildings. Spores can be dispersed or aerosolized during dust-generating procedures, including excavation, demolition, and lower risk dust-generating activities, including re-carpeting. *Aspergillus* spps. remain the most notorious fungi associated with construction sites. *Scedosporium* sp [81] and Mucorales [82] have also been linked to this source [83]. Climatic conditions also influence the sporulation of *Aspergillus,* and thus construction activities are preferred during colder seasons [84].

Immunocompromised patients should avoid transit through construction sites [20]. When construction is inevitable, preventative measures must be followed, including the use of water jets to suppress dust emissions, keeping the air facing the construction site in isolation by closing windows and doors, and use of high-efficiency filtration face masks whenever susceptible patients require to be transported out of the protective area [85]. A summary of air quality measures that prevent the spread of molds is included under the recommendations for the PE.

Other hospital sources may represent transmission routes of *Aspergillus* spp and non-*Aspergillus* molds. Molds can be isolated from contaminated water reservoirs [86], with evidence of waterborne sources for invasive aspergillosis via genomic fingerprinting with amplified fragment length polymorphisms [87]. *Fusarium* spp have also been recovered from hospital water systems, representing a potential source for invasive fusariosis [88]. Isolation of any of these molds from a water source is likely reflective of biofilm contamination of the water distribution systems, which can be prevented with chemical and ultraviolet light disinfection of the water input network, with continuous chemical treatment of the water and microfiltration at points of use [89].

Pneumocystis jirovecii

The mechanism of transmission of *Pneumocystis jirovecii*, the causative agent of PCP, is currently obscure. The source is likely environmental, but the person-to-person transmission of *P. jirovecii* is possible among susceptible hosts. The distance necessary to acquire the infection is uncertain, but close contact is likely necessary as a prospective study showed the presence at 1 meter from the head patients with PCP [90]. Evidence currently available supports the hypothesis of nosocomial spread of *Pneumocystis jirovecii* [91]. A cluster of nosocomial PCP demonstrated the persistent circulation of a single *P. jirovecii* genotype during 16 months, with transmission maps suggesting patient-to-patient spread during physiotherapy visits.

In line with this evidence, some authors recommend segregating these patients and using facemask filtering to minimize patient-to-patient transmission [92]. Current therapeutic guidelines from the AST and ECIL do not provide definitive recommendations regarding IC measures, emphasizing primary prophylaxis with an anti-PCP agent being of importance in preventing PCP [93, 94]. To minimize the risk of nosocomial clusters, the CDC recommends avoiding the placement of an immunocompromised patient in the same room as a patient with PCP [3].

Legionellae

The majority of cases of legionellosis are community-acquired, although occasional nosocomial outbreaks have been reported in transplant centers [95]. Contrary to Legionnaire's disease in the general population where they are rarely seen, the non-pneumophila *Legionella* spp. are causative for 50% of outbreaks in the immunocompromised patient [96]. Legionellosis in the HCT recipient usually occurs within the first year post-transplant, with most cases occurring within 30 days [97]. For the SOT recipient, the periods of increasing immunosuppression with more than one drug increase the risk of Legionnaire's disease [98].

Infection control measures to prevent the nosocomial spread of legionellosis include routine microbial analyses of tap water to identify environmental contamination and the use of point-of-use filtration [97]. Additional measures to prevent the spread of *Legionella* in outbreak situations in transplant centers include avoiding showers and using sponge baths, avoiding faucets, using sterile water instead of tap water for drinking, brushing teeth, or flushing nasogastric tubes when *Legionella* is detected in the hospital system [18]. The HCT center personnel should use only sterile water to fill reservoirs of nebulization devices and to rinse nebulization devices and other semi-critical respiratory care. Decorative fountains should not be installed in the HCT unit or areas frequented by HCT recipients [15].

Clostridioides difficile

A consequence of the routine use of broad-spectrum antibiotics is the disruption of the normal intestinal microbiota, creating the right environment for *Clostridioides difficile* colonization and potentially infection. An impaired immune response against *C. difficile* and its toxins represents an additional risk for the immunocompromised patient. In the HCT recipient, CDI occurs more often during the pre-engraftment period [99]. The incidence of CDI in the HCT recipients is 15 times higher than in the general population, with a prevalence of 15% in the allo-HCT recipient compared to 9% in the auto-HCT recipient [100]. Chemotherapy and GVHD are other independent risk factors for CDI, even for those patients without a history of antibiotic exposure [101].

In the SOT recipient, CDI often occurs within the first year after the transplant. Breaking down per transplant type, lung transplant recipients have the highest rates of CDI recurrence, followed by liver transplants and, less often, kidney transplant recipients [102]. Of note, a significant proportion of late-onset CDI (onset after 90 days) is also described in non-kidney SOTs [103].

Measures to contain the spread of CDI have been defined by multiple guidelines, with the fundament that all patients with CDI should be placed under contact precautions. Healthcare workers in contact with the infected patient should wear gowns and gloves, and hand washing with soap and water is necessary before and after the patient contact. The recommended time for isolation varies per institution due to the prolonged shedding of *C. difficile* after completion of therapy. Still, current guidelines recommend continuing contact precautions for at least 48 h after symptom resolution, and if symptoms persist isolation can be extended until hospital discharge [104]. Environmental decontamination with the cleaning of all potentially contaminated surfaces with a 1:10 dilution of concentrated sodium hypochlorite may reduce the environmental burden of *C. difficile*. Active surveillance with preadmission screening for carriage of *C. difficile* is not currently recommended. Moreover, the treatment of the colonized patient has the potential harm of further altering the microbiome and thus promoting colonization by other potentially detrimental bacteria, including MDROs [99].

Viral Respiratory Infections

Respiratory viruses include those infections caused by respiratory syncytial virus (RSV), adenovirus (ADV), influenza virus, parainfluenza virus (PIV), human metapneumovirus, coronaviruses, and rhinoviruses. They are transmitted via droplets and direct skin contact. Droplet transmission requires close contact (<1 m) with large-particle virus-containing droplets (>5 μm). While this may occur during sneezing, coughing, and procedures such as bronchoscopy, it is less common because larger particles do not remain suspended in the air for a long time. Rhinovirus can also be transmitted through the autoinoculation of viral particles into the eyes or nares. In the case of ADV, it may also follow fecal-oral transmission [3].

In the immunocompetent host, the respiratory viruses often lead to a self-limited upper respiratory syndrome. By contrast, in immunocompromised hosts, these infections have more atypical and have protracted courses, with increased rates of lower-respiratory tract infections (LRTI) compared to the immunocompetent host and higher need for supplemental oxygenation, including mechanical ventilation [105]. Similarly, hospital-acquired viral respiratory infections are often associated with the need for ICU admission and mechanical ventilation, with higher odds of VAP in the HCT recipient and the patient receiving immunosuppression [28]. RSV is the most frequent respiratory virus leading to death in the HCT population [106]. RSV, PIV, and influenza predispose patients to bacterial and fungal superinfections within 30 days of the primary infection, with each superinfection having severe clinical manifestations and often needing admission to the ICU [107]. The type of HCT influences the rates of these infections being more common in allogeneic HCT recipients and slightly less common in autologous HCT. In SOT, infections occur most commonly within the first year after the transplant and are associated with acute and chronic rejection [108].

Strict adherence to IC measures that include hand hygiene, transmission-based precautions, education of the hospital staff regarding modes of transmission and disease prevention, regular monitoring of healthcare worker practices, and active patient and visitor screening are critical elements in the prevention of outbreaks [108]. Currently, the CDC recommends maintaining contact plus droplet precautions for those affected patients, with discontinuation of droplet precautions once ADV and influenza have been ruled out. The duration of the isolation is tailored to duration in symptoms which in the immunocompromised patient may translate to a period of several weeks [3]. The use of antigen-based or culture-based tests to guide RSV isolation is not currently recommended.

Coronavirus Disease 2019

Patients with immunocompromising conditions, including lymphoproliferative disorders and recipients of HCT, have a higher risk of COVID-19 [109], with higher associated morbidity and mortality. In the SOT patient, rapid progression of respiratory failure is seen in the heart and lung transplant recipient, with outcomes similar to those of the general population in liver and kidney transplant recipients [110] (p. 10), [111]. Prolonged viral shedding is common in these patients, posing a challenge regarding the duration of transmission-based isolation. Understanding the transmission of COVID-19 in the oncologic center requires several considerations. The HCT recipient candidate, oncologic patient, and all caregivers and household contacts should be up-to-date in their vaccination status [112]. Chemotherapy is not generally deferred, but cellular therapy, including HCT or CAR-T therapy, is held, with a negative nasopharyngeal swab needed before continuing the oncologic treatment. [113]

Current CDC recommendations of IC practice in the prevention of the spread of COVID-19 follow a risk stratification based on the number of new COVID-19 admissions per 100,000 patients, the percent of staffed inpatient beds occupied by COVID-19 patients, and the total of new COVID-19 cases per 100,000 persons [114]. Specific recommendations for immunocompromised patients include avoiding non-essential indoor activities in public during peak COVID-19 levels, wearing a well-fitting, high-quality mask or respirator, and following physical distancing indoors in enclosed public places. Restriction of visits and using approaches like telemedicine is advised during the peaks of the pandemic. The transplant center staff should be trained, and people with any symptoms consistent with a respiratory infection should stay at home and follow testing for COVID-19. The oncologic patient should be placed in single, negative pressure rooms. Healthcare workers must wear protective equipment, including gloves, gowns, face shields, and FFP2 masks, and practice thorough hand hygiene. During the peaks of the COVID-19 pandemic, clusters of nosocomial transmission have been linked to hospital staff in a cancer [113] and transplant centers.

The CDC currently recommends up-to-date vaccination status for healthcare workers and patients, source control with well-fitting facemasks or respirators, use of NIOSH-approved particulate respirators during a surgical procedure or care of a patient on droplet precautions per patient encounter, and preadmission testing regardless of vaccination status for symptomatic patients or those with exposures within 24 h [114]. Those COVID-19-positive patients with mild illness should isolate through at least day 5 after the symptom onset with mask-wearing through day 10, with moderate or severe COVID-19 patients isolating through at least day 10 but considering isolation up to day 20. In the case of the immunocompromised patient, those with a positive COVID-19 test should remain under isolation through at least day 20 with serial testing to guide in determining the duration. Two negative serial tests collected at least 24 h apart with an antigen or nucleic acid amplification test and defervescence for at least 24 h are needed to guide the decision to end isolation. Note that prolonged shedding of up to 2 months has been described [115].

Conclusion

In conclusion, the practice of IC and prevention in the clinical management of immunocompromised patients is a major challenge in modern medicine. HAIs that affect the transplant recipients are the result of the heightened risk secondary to their baseline disease, the care of these diseases that frequently involve bouts of enhanced immunosuppression, and their increased susceptibility to environmental exposures. As evidence is based predominantly on single-center retrospective analyses, extrapolation of data from non-immunocompromised patients has been thus necessary by institutions to establish IC recommendations, with evidence for some interventions lacking. Further research focusing on prospective studies is thus necessary at the current moment to improve the understanding of the transmission chain HAIs in the immunocompromised patient and the role of protocols like MDRO screening and decolonization protocols in the care of the immunocompromised patient.

References

1. Loveday HP, Wilson JA, Pratt RJ, et al. epic3: National evidence-based guidelines for preventing healthcare-associated infections in NHS hospitals in England. J Hosp Infect. 2014;86:S1–S70. https://doi.org/10.1016/S0195-6701(13)60012-2.
2. Tacconelli E, Cataldo MA, Dancer SJ, et al. ESCMID guidelines for the management of the infection control measures to reduce transmission of multidrug-resistant Gram-negative bacteria in hospitalized patients. Clin Microbiol Infect. 2014;20:1–55. https://doi.org/10.1111/1469-0691.12427.

3. Siegel JD, Rhinehart E, Jackson M, Chiarello L. 2007 Guideline for isolation precautions: preventing transmission of infectious agents in health care settings. Am J Infect Control. 2007;35(10):S65–S164. https://doi.org/10.1016/j.ajic.2007.10.007.
4. Ariza-Heredia EJ, Chemaly RF. Update on infection control practices in cancer hospitals: infection control in cancer. CA Cancer J Clin. 2018;68(5):340–55. https://doi.org/10.3322/caac.21462.
5. Ariza-Heredia EJ, Chemaly RF. Infection control practices in patients with hematological malignancies and multidrug-resistant organisms: special considerations and challenges. Clin Lymphoma Myeloma Leuk. 2014;14:S104–10. https://doi.org/10.1016/j.clml.2014.06.021.
6. Rosenthal VD, Yin R, Lu Y, et al. The impact of healthcare-associated infections on mortality in ICU: a prospective study in Asia, Africa, Eastern Europe, Latin America, and the Middle East. Am J Infect Control. 2022.:S0196655322006587; https://doi.org/10.1016/j.ajic.2022.08.024.
7. 2020 National and State Healthcare-Associated Infections Progress Report.
8. Heidenreich D, Kreil S, Nolte F, Hofmann WK, Miethke T, Klein SA. Multidrug-resistant organisms in allogeneic hematopoietic cell transplantation. Eur J Haematol. 2017;98(5):485–92. https://doi.org/10.1111/ejh.12859.
9. Warris A, Voss A, Verweij PE. Hospital sources of Aspergillus: new routes of transmission? Rev Iberoam Micol. 2001;18(4):156–62.
10. Perlroth J, Choi B, Spellberg B. Nosocomial fungal infections: epidemiology, diagnosis, and treatment. Med Mycol. 2007;45(4):321–46. https://doi.org/10.1080/13693780701218689.
11. Squier C, Yu VL, Stout JE. Waterborne nosocomial infections. Curr Infect Dis Rep. 2000;2(6):490–6. https://doi.org/10.1007/s11908-000-0049-1.
12. Pereira MR, Rana MM, AST ID Community of Practice. Methicillin-resistant Staphylococcus aureus in solid organ transplantation-guidelines from the American Society of Transplantation Infectious Diseases Community of Practice. Clin Transplant. 2019;33(9):e13611. https://doi.org/10.1111/ctr.13611.
13. Nellore A, Huprikar S, AST ID Community of Practice. Vancomycin-resistant Enterococcus in solid organ transplant recipients: guidelines from the American Society of Transplantation Infectious Diseases Community of Practice. Clin Transplant. 2019;33(9):e13549. https://doi.org/10.1111/ctr.13549.
14. Banach DB, Seville MTA, Kusne S. Infection prevention and control issues after solid organ transplantation. In: Ljungman P, Snydman D, Boeckh M, editors. Transplant infections. Springer International Publishing; 2016. p. 843–67. https://doi.org/10.1007/978-3-319-28797-3_46.
15. Yokoe D, Casper C, Dubberke E, et al. Infection prevention and control in health-care facilities in which hematopoietic cell transplant recipients are treated. Bone Marrow Transplant. 2009;44(8):495–507. https://doi.org/10.1038/bmt.2009.261.
16. Environmental cleaning procedures | environmental cleaning in RLS | HAI | CDC. Published April 28, 2021. Accessed December 31, 2022. https://www.cdc.gov/hai/prevent/resource-limited/cleaning-procedures.html.
17. Rutala WA, Weber DJ. Disinfection and sterilization in health care facilities. Infect Dis Clin N Am. 2016;30(3):609–37. https://doi.org/10.1016/j.idc.2016.04.002.
18. Sehulster L, Chinn R. Guidelines for environmental infection control in health-care facilities: (545922006-001); 2003. https://doi.org/10.1037/e545922006-001.
19. Nicolle MC, Benet T, Vanhems P. Aspergillosis: nosocomial or community-acquired? Med Mycol. 2011;49(S1):S24–9. https://doi.org/10.3109/13693786.2010.509335.
20. Vonberg RP, Gastmeier P. Nosocomial aspergillosis in outbreak settings. J Hosp Infect. 2006;63(3):246–54. https://doi.org/10.1016/j.jhin.2006.02.014.
21. Gudiol C, Garcia-Vidal C, Arnan M, et al. Etiology, clinical features and outcomes of pre-engraftment and post-engraftment bloodstream infection in hematopoietic SCT recipients. Bone Marrow Transplant. 2014;49(6):824–30. https://doi.org/10.1038/bmt.2014.37.

22. Styczyński J, Tridello G, Koster L, et al. Death after hematopoietic stem cell transplantation: changes over calendar year time, infections and associated factors. Bone Marrow Transplant. 2020;55(1):126–36. https://doi.org/10.1038/s41409-019-0624-z.
23. Kurosawa S, Yakushijin K, Yamaguchi T, et al. Recent decrease in non-relapse mortality due to GVHD and infection after allogeneic hematopoietic cell transplantation in non-remission acute leukemia. Bone Marrow Transplant. 2013;48(9):1198–204. https://doi.org/10.1038/bmt.2013.42.
24. Puerta-Alcalde P, Cardozo C, Marco F, et al. Changing epidemiology of bloodstream infection in a 25-years hematopoietic stem cell transplant program: current challenges and pitfalls on empiric antibiotic treatment impacting outcomes. Bone Marrow Transplant. 2020;55(3):603–12. https://doi.org/10.1038/s41409-019-0701-3.
25. Dettenkofer M, Ebner W, Bertz H, et al. Surveillance of nosocomial infections in adult recipients of allogeneic and autologous bone marrow and peripheral blood stem-cell transplantation. Bone Marrow Transplant. 2003;31(9):795–801. https://doi.org/10.1038/sj.bmt.1703920.
26. Averbuch D, Tridello G, Hoek J, et al. Antimicrobial resistance in gram-negative rods causing bacteremia in hematopoietic stem cell transplant recipients: intercontinental prospective study of the infectious diseases working party of the European Bone Marrow Transplantation Group. Clin Infect Dis. 2017;65(11):1819–28. https://doi.org/10.1093/cid/cix646.
27. Gudiol C, Sabé N, Carratalà J. Is hospital-acquired pneumonia different in transplant recipients? Clin Microbiol Infect. 2019;25(10):1186–94. https://doi.org/10.1016/j.cmi.2019.04.003.
28. Shorr AF, Ilges DT, Micek ST, Kollef MH. The importance of viruses in ventilator-associated pneumonia. Infect Control Hosp Epidemiol. 2022:1–6. https://doi.org/10.1017/ice.2022.223.
29. Kim SH, Choi JK, Cho SY, et al. Risk factors and clinical outcomes of breakthrough yeast bloodstream infections in patients with hematological malignancies in the era of newer antifungal agents. Med Mycol. 2018;56(2):197–206. https://doi.org/10.1093/mmy/myx038.
30. Kato J, Mori T, Suzuki T, et al. Nosocomial BK Polyomavirus infection causing hemorrhagic cystitis among patients with hematological malignancies after hematopoietic stem cell transplantation. Am J Transplant. 2017;17(9):2428–33. https://doi.org/10.1111/ajt.14271.
31. Onda Y, Kanda J, Hanaoka N, et al. Possible nosocomial transmission of virus-associated hemorrhagic cystitis after allogeneic hematopoietic stem cell transplantation. Ann Hematol. 2021;100(3):753–61. https://doi.org/10.1007/s00277-021-04414-1.
32. Los-Arcos I, Iacoboni G, Aguilar-Guisado M, et al. Recommendations for screening, monitoring, prevention, and prophylaxis of infections in adult and pediatric patients receiving CAR T-cell therapy: a position paper. Infection. 2021;49(2):215–31. https://doi.org/10.1007/s15010-020-01521-5.
33. Taplitz RA, Kennedy EB, Bow EJ, et al. Antimicrobial prophylaxis for adult patients with cancer-related immunosuppression: ASCO and IDSA clinical practice guideline update summary. JCO Oncol Pract. 2018;36(30):3043–3054. https://doi.org/10.1200/jco.18.00374.
34. National Comprehensive Cancer Network (NCCN) Clinical Practice Guidelines in Oncology. Prevention and treatment of cancer-related infections. Version 1.2018. Accessed November 7, 2022. http://www.nccn.org.
35. Gafter-Gvili A, Fraser A, Paul M, et al. Antibiotic prophylaxis for bacterial infections in afebrile neutropenic patients following chemotherapy. Cochrane Database Syst Rev. 2012;1:CD004386. https://doi.org/10.1002/14651858.CD004386.pub3.
36. Mikulska M, Averbuch D, Tissot F, et al. Fluoroquinolone prophylaxis in haematological cancer patients with neutropenia: ECIL critical appraisal of previous guidelines. J Infect. 2018;76(1):20–37. https://doi.org/10.1016/j.jinf.2017.10.009.
37. Satlin MJ, Chavda KD, Baker TM, et al. Colonization with levofloxacin-resistant extended-spectrum β-lactamase-producing enterobacteriaceae and risk of bacteremia in hematopoietic stem cell transplant recipients. Clin Infect Dis. 2018;67(11):1720–8. https://doi.org/10.1093/cid/ciy363.

38. Liu CY, Lai YC, Huang LJ, et al. Impact of bloodstream infections on outcome and the influence of prophylactic oral antibiotic regimens in allogeneic hematopoietic SCT recipients. Bone Marrow Transplant. 2011;46(9):1231–9. https://doi.org/10.1038/bmt.2010.286.
39. Righi E, Peri AM, Harris PNA, et al. Global prevalence of carbapenem resistance in neutropenic patients and association with mortality and carbapenem use: systematic review and meta-analysis. J Antimicrob Chemother. 2017;72(3):668–77. https://doi.org/10.1093/jac/dkw459.
40. Gafter-Gvili A, Paul M, Fraser A, Leibovici L. Effect of quinolone prophylaxis in afebrile neutropenic patients on microbial resistance: systematic review and meta-analysis. J Antimicrob Chemother. 2007;59(1):5–22. https://doi.org/10.1093/jac/dkl425.
41. Lehrnbecher T, Averbuch D, Castagnola E, et al. 8th European Conference on Infections in Leukaemia: 2020 guidelines for the use of antibiotics in paediatric patients with cancer or post-haematopoietic cell transplantation. Lancet Oncol. 2021;22(6):e270–80. https://doi.org/10.1016/S1470-2045(20)30725-7.
42. Satheeshkumar PS, Mohan MP. Association and risk factors of healthcare-associated infection and burden of illness among chemotherapy-induced ulcerative mucositis patients. Clin Oral Investig. 2022;26(2):1323–32. https://doi.org/10.1007/s00784-021-04106-0.
43. Suwabe T, Fuse K, Katsura K, et al. Intensive oral care can reduce bloodstream infection with coagulase-negative staphylococci after neutrophil engraftment in allogeneic hematopoietic stem-cell transplantation. Support Care Cancer. 2022;30(1):475–85. https://doi.org/10.1007/s00520-021-06447-8.
44. Fishman JA. Infection in solid-organ transplant recipients. N Engl J Med. 2007;357(25):2601–14. https://doi.org/10.1056/NEJMra064928.
45. Abdo-Cuza AA, Gómez-Bravo MA, Pérez-Bernal JB, et al. Health care–associated infection in solid organ transplant recipients. Transplant Proc. 2020;52(2):509–11. https://doi.org/10.1016/j.transproceed.2019.12.010.
46. Parasuraman R, Julian K. Practice the AIDC of urinary tract infections in solid organ transplantation. Am J Transplant. 2013;13(S4):327–36. https://doi.org/10.1111/ajt.12124.
47. Memikoğlu KO, Keven K, Sengül S, Soypaçaci Z, Ertürk S, Erbay B. Urinary tract infections following renal transplantation: a single-center experience. Transplant Proc. 2007;39(10):3131–4. https://doi.org/10.1016/j.transproceed.2007.10.005.
48. Taimur S, Pouch SM, Zubizarreta N, et al. Impact of pre-transplant carbapenem-resistant Enterobacterales colonization and/or infection on solid organ transplant outcomes. Clin Transplant. 2021;35(4):e14239. https://doi.org/10.1111/ctr.14239.
49. Dorschner P, McElroy LM, Ison M, g. Nosocomial infections within the first month of solid organ transplantation. Transpl Infect Dis. 2014;16(2):171–87. https://doi.org/10.1111/tid.12203.
50. Dantas SRPE, Kuboyama RH, Mazzali M, Moretti ML. Nosocomial infections in renal transplant patients: risk factors and treatment implications associated with urinary tract and surgical site infections. J Hosp Infect. 2006;63(2):117–23. https://doi.org/10.1016/j.jhin.2005.10.018.
51. Silva M, Marra AR, Pereira CAP, Medina-Pestana JO, Camargo LFA. Bloodstream infection after kidney transplantation: epidemiology, microbiology, associated risk factors, and outcome. Transplantation. 2010;90(5):581–7. https://doi.org/10.1097/TP.0b013e3181e8a680.
52. Anesi JA, Blumberg EA, Abbo LM. Perioperative antibiotic prophylaxis to prevent surgical site infections in solid organ transplantation. Transplantation. 2018;102(1):21–34. https://doi.org/10.1097/TP.0000000000001848.
53. Iinuma Y, Senda K, Fujihara N, et al. Surgical site infection in living-donor liver transplant recipients: a prospective study. Transplantation. 2004;78(5):704–9. https://doi.org/10.1097/01.tp.0000130178.17216.28.
54. Humar A. Reactivation of viruses in solid organ transplant patients receiving cytomegalovirus prophylaxis. Transplantation. 2006;82(Suppl. 2):S9–S14. https://doi.org/10.1097/01.tp.0000230432.39447.8b.

55. Nam H, Nilles KM, Levitsky J, Ison MG. Donor-derived viral infections in liver transplantation. Transplantation. 2018;102(11):1824–36. https://doi.org/10.1097/TP.0000000000002326.
56. Abbo LM, Grossi PA. Practice the AIC of surgical site infections: guidelines from the American Society of Transplantation Infectious Diseases Community of Practice. Clin Transplant. 2019;33(9):e13589. https://doi.org/10.1111/ctr.13589.
57. Pouch SM, Patel G. Practice the AIDC of Multidrug-resistant Gram-negative bacterial infections in solid organ transplant recipients—guidelines from the American Society of Transplantation Infectious Diseases Community of Practice. Clin Transplant. 2019;33(9):e13594. https://doi.org/10.1111/ctr.13594.
58. Huh K, Jeong SJ, Kim YJ, et al. Nationwide survey of infection prevention protocols in solid organ transplantation in South Korea. Korean J Transplant. 2022;36(3):212–20. https://doi.org/10.4285/kjt.22.0036.
59. Beam E, Razonable RR. A survey of infection prevention and control practices among solid organ transplantation centers. Am J Infect Control. 2019;47(1):101–4. https://doi.org/10.1016/j.ajic.2018.06.020.
60. Vink JP, Otter JA, Edgeworth JD. Carbapenemase-producing Enterobacteriaceae—once positive always positive? Curr Opin Gastroenterol. 2020;36(1):9–16. https://doi.org/10.1097/MOG.0000000000000596.
61. Huang SS, Septimus E, Kleinman K, et al. Targeted versus universal decolonization to prevent ICU infection. N Engl J Med. 2013;368(24):2255–65. https://doi.org/10.1056/NEJMoa1207290.
62. Giannella M, Bartoletti M, Conti M, Righi E. Carbapenemase-producing Enterobacteriaceae in transplant patients. J Antimicrob Chemother. 2021;76(Suppl. 1):i27–39. https://doi.org/10.1093/jac/dkaa495.
63. Wittekamp BH, Plantinga NL, Cooper BS, et al. Decontamination strategies and bloodstream infections with antibiotic-resistant microorganisms in ventilated patients: a randomized clinical trial. JAMA. 2018;320(20):2087–98. https://doi.org/10.1001/jama.2018.13765.
64. Fariñas MC, González-Rico C, Fernández-Martínez M, et al. Oral decontamination with colistin plus neomycin in solid organ transplant recipients colonized by multidrug-resistant Enterobacterales: a multicentre, randomized, controlled, open-label, parallel-group clinical trial. Clin Microbiol Infect Off Publ Eur Soc Clin Microbiol Infect Dis. 2021;27(6):856–63. https://doi.org/10.1016/j.cmi.2020.12.016.
65. Sánchez-Ramírez C, Hípola-Escalada S, Cabrera-Santana M, et al. Long-term use of selective digestive decontamination in an ICU highly endemic for bacterial resistance. Crit Care. 2018;22:141. https://doi.org/10.1186/s13054-018-2057-2.
66. Tacconelli E, Mazzaferri F, de Smet AM, et al. ESCMID-EUCIC clinical guidelines on decolonization of multidrug-resistant Gram-negative bacteria carriers. Clin Microbiol Infect Off Publ Eur Soc Clin Microbiol Infect Dis. 2019;25(7):807–17. https://doi.org/10.1016/j.cmi.2019.01.005.
67. Aguado JM, Silva JT, Fernández-Ruiz M, et al. Management of multidrug resistant Gram-negative bacilli infections in solid organ transplant recipients: SET/GESITRA-SEIMC/REIPI recommendations. Transplant Rev Orlando Fla. 2018;32(1):36–57. https://doi.org/10.1016/j.trre.2017.07.001.
68. George S, Leasure AR, McGovern A, Horstmanshof DA. Reduction of postoperative infections through routine preoperative universal decolonization of advanced heart failure patients with chlorhexidine and mupirocin before left ventricular assist device implantation: a single-center observational study. Dimens Crit Care Nurs. 2020;39(6):312–20. https://doi.org/10.1097/DCC.0000000000000443.
69. Paterson DL, Rihs JD, Squier C, Gayowski T, Sagnimeni A, Singh N. Lack of efficacy of mupirocin in the prevention of infections with Staphylococcus aureus in liver transplant recipients and candidates1. Transplantation. 2003;75(2):194–8. https://doi.org/10.1097/01.TP.0000040602.01701.85.

70. Strategies to Prevent S. aureus BSIs in Acute Care Facilities | CDC. Published April 16, 2020. Accessed December 7, 2022. https://www.cdc.gov/hai/prevent/staph-prevention-strategies.html.
71. Schweizer ML, Chiang HY, Septimus E, et al. Association of a bundled intervention with surgical site infections among patients undergoing cardiac, hip, or knee surgery. JAMA. 2015;313(21):2162–71. https://doi.org/10.1001/jama.2015.5387.
72. McFarlane AC, Kabbani D, Bakal JA, Smith SW. Clinical impact of vancomycin-resistant enterococci colonization in nonliver solid organ transplantation and its implications for infection control strategies: a single-center, 10-year retrospective study. Transpl Infect Dis Off J Transplant Soc. 2021;23(6):e13747. https://doi.org/10.1111/tid.13747.
73. Cheng VC, Chen JH, Tai JW, et al. Decolonization of gastrointestinal carriage of vancomycin-resistant Enterococcus faecium: case series and review of literature. BMC Infect Dis. 2014;14(1):514. https://doi.org/10.1186/1471-2334-14-514.
74. Saha S, Tariq R, Tosh PK, Pardi DS, Khanna S. Faecal microbiota transplantation for eradicating carriage of multidrug-resistant organisms: a systematic review. Clin Microbiol Infect Off Publ Eur Soc Clin Microbiol Infect Dis. 2019;25(8):958–63. https://doi.org/10.1016/j.cmi.2019.04.006.
75. Biliński J, Grzesiowski P, Muszyński J, et al. Fecal microbiota transplantation inhibits multidrug-resistant gut pathogens: preliminary report performed in an immunocompromised host. Arch Immunol Ther Exp (Warsz). 2016;64(3):255–8. https://doi.org/10.1007/s00005-016-0387-9.
76. Jensen PA, Lambert LA, Iademarco MF, Ridzon R, CDC. Guidelines for preventing the transmission of Mycobacterium tuberculosis in health-care settings, 2005. MMWR Recomm Rep Morb Mortal Wkly Rep Recomm Rep. 2005;54(RR-17):1–141.
77. Sorohan BM, Ismail G, Tacu D, et al. Mycobacterium tuberculosis infection after kidney transplantation: a comprehensive review. Pathog Basel Switz. 2022;11(9):1041. https://doi.org/10.3390/pathogens11091041.
78. Bergeron A, Mikulska M, De Greef J, et al. Mycobacterial infections in adults with haematological malignancies and haematopoietic stem cell transplants: guidelines from the 8th European Conference on Infections in Leukaemia. Lancet Infect Dis. 2022;22(12):e359–69. https://doi.org/10.1016/S1473-3099(22)00227-4.
79. Abad CLR, Razonable RR. An update on Mycobacterium tuberculosis infection after hematopoietic stem cell transplantation in adults. Clin Transplant. 2018;32(12):e13430. https://doi.org/10.1111/ctr.13430.
80. World Health Organization. WHO guidelines on tuberculosis infection prevention and control: 2019 update. World Health Organization; 2019. Accessed December 9, 2022. https://apps.who.int/iris/handle/10665/311259
81. Alvarez M, Lopez Ponga B, Rayon C, et al. Nosocomial outbreak caused by Scedosporium prolificans (inflatum): four fatal cases in leukemic patients. J Clin Microbiol. 1995;33(12):3290–5.
82. Antoniadou A. Outbreaks of zygomycosis in hospitals. Clin Microbiol Infect Off Publ Eur Soc Clin Microbiol Infect Dis. 2009;15(Suppl. 5):55–9. https://doi.org/10.1111/j.1469-0691.2009.02982.x.
83. Chang CC, Ananda-Rajah M, Belcastro A, et al. Consensus guidelines for implementation of quality processes to prevent invasive fungal disease and enhanced surveillance measures during hospital building works, 2014. Intern Med J. 2014;44(12b):1389–97. https://doi.org/10.1111/imj.12601.
84. Pilmis B, Thepot-Seegers V, Angebault C, et al. Could we predict airborne Aspergillus contamination during construction work? Am J Infect Control. 2017;45(1):39–41. https://doi.org/10.1016/j.ajic.2016.08.003.
85. Wirmann L, Ross B, Reimann O, Steinmann J, Rath PM. Airborne Aspergillus fumigatus spore concentration during demolition of a building on a hospital site, and patient risk determina-

tion for invasive aspergillosis including azole resistance. J Hosp Infect. 2018;100(3):e91–7. https://doi.org/10.1016/j.jhin.2018.07.030.
86. Mesquita-Rocha S, Godoy-Martinez PC, Gonçalves SS, et al. The water supply system as a potential source of fungal infection in paediatric haematopoietic stem cell units. BMC Infect Dis. 2013;13:289. https://doi.org/10.1186/1471-2334-13-289.
87. Warris A, Klaassen CHW, Meis JFGM, et al. Molecular epidemiology of Aspergillus fumigatus isolates recovered from water, air, and patients shows two clusters of genetically distinct strains. J Clin Microbiol. 2003;41(9):4101–6. https://doi.org/10.1128/JCM.41.9.4101-4106.2003.
88. Kaur H, Riedel DJ. Nosocomial disseminated fusariosis in a hematopoietic stem cell transplant recipient. Transpl Infect Dis Off J Transplant Soc. 2022;24(3):e13831. https://doi.org/10.1111/tid.13831.
89. Kauffmann-Lacroix C, Costa D, Imbert C. Fungi, Water supply and biofilms. Adv Exp Med Biol. 2016;931:49–61. https://doi.org/10.1007/5584_2016_8.
90. Choukri F, Menotti J, Sarfati C, et al. Quantification and spread of pneumocystis jirovecii in the surrounding air of patients with pneumocystis pneumonia. Clin Infect Dis. 2010;51(3):259–65. https://doi.org/10.1086/653933.
91. Phipps LM, Chen SCA, Kable K, et al. Nosocomial Pneumocystis jirovecii pneumonia: lessons from a cluster in kidney transplant recipients. Transplantation. 2011;92(12):1327–34. https://doi.org/10.1097/TP.0b013e3182384b57.
92. Schmoldt S, Schuhegger R, Wendler T, et al. Molecular evidence of nosocomial Pneumocystis jirovecii transmission among 16 patients after kidney transplantation. J Clin Microbiol. 2008;46(3):966–71. https://doi.org/10.1128/JCM.02016-07.
93. Fishman JA, Gans H. Practice the AIDC of Pneumocystis jiroveci in solid organ transplantation: Guidelines from the American Society of Transplantation Infectious Diseases Community of Practice. Clin Transplant. 2019;33(9):e13587. https://doi.org/10.1111/ctr.13587.
94. Maertens J, Cesaro S, Maschmeyer G, et al. ECIL guidelines for preventing Pneumocystis jirovecii pneumonia in patients with haematological malignancies and stem cell transplant recipients. J Antimicrob Chemother. 2016;71(9):2397–404. https://doi.org/10.1093/jac/dkw157.
95. Sivagnanam S, Pergam SA. Legionellosis in transplantation. Curr Infect Dis Rep. 2016;18(3):9. https://doi.org/10.1007/s11908-016-0517-x.
96. Knirsch CA, Jakob K, Schoonmaker D, et al. An outbreak of Legionella micdadei pneumonia in transplant patients: evaluation, molecular epidemiology, and control. Am J Med. 2000;108(4):290–5. https://doi.org/10.1016/s0002-9343(99)00459-3.
97. Mikulska M, Tridello G, Hoek J, et al. Legionellosis after hematopoietic stem cell transplantation. Bone Marrow Transplant. 2021;56(10):2555–66. https://doi.org/10.1038/s41409-021-01333-7.
98. Gudiol C, Garcia-Vidal C, Fernández-Sabé N, et al. Clinical features and outcomes of Legionnaires' disease in solid organ transplant recipients. Transpl Infect Dis. 2009;11(1):78–82. https://doi.org/10.1111/j.1399-3062.2008.00337.x.
99. Alonso CD, Maron G, Kamboj M, et al. American Society for Transplantation and Cellular Therapy Series: #5—management of Clostridioides difficile infection in hematopoietic cell transplant recipients. Transplant Cell Ther. 2022;28(5):225–32. https://doi.org/10.1016/j.jtct.2022.02.013.
100. Luo Y, Zhang S, Shang H, Cui W, Wang Q, Zhu B. Prevalence of Clostridium difficile Infection in the hematopoietic transplantation setting: update of systematic review and meta-analysis. Front Cell Infect Microbiol. 2022;12:801475. https://doi.org/10.3389/fcimb.2022.801475.
101. Chopra T, Alangaden GJ, Chandrasekar P. Clostridium difficile infection in cancer patients and hematopoietic stem cell transplant recipients. Expert Rev Anti Infect Ther. 2010;8(10):1113–9. https://doi.org/10.1586/eri.10.95.

102. Revolinski SL, Munoz-Price LS. Clostridium difficile in immunocompromised hosts: a review of epidemiology, risk factors, treatment, and prevention. Clin Infect Dis. 2019;68(12):2144–53. https://doi.org/10.1093/cid/ciy845.
103. Hosseini-Moghaddam SM, Luo B, Bota SE, et al. Incidence and outcomes associated with Clostridioides difficile infection in solid organ transplant recipients. JAMA Netw Open. 2021;4(12):e2141089. https://doi.org/10.1001/jamanetworkopen.2021.41089.
104. Mullane KM, Dubberke ER, AST ID Community of Practice. Management of Clostridioides (formerly Clostridium) difficile infection (CDI) in solid organ transplant recipients: Guidelines from the American Society of Transplantation Community of Practice. Clin Transplant. 2019;33(9):e13564. https://doi.org/10.1111/ctr.13564.
105. Abbas S, Raybould JE, Sastry S, de la Cruz O. Respiratory viruses in transplant recipients: more than just a cold. Clinical syndromes and infection prevention principles. Int J Infect Dis. 2017;62:86–93. https://doi.org/10.1016/j.ijid.2017.07.011.
106. Manchal N, Mohamed MRS, Ting M, et al. Hospital acquired viral respiratory tract infections: An underrecognized nosocomial infection. Infect Dis Health. 2020;25(3):175–80. https://doi.org/10.1016/j.idh.2020.02.002.
107. Nichols WG, Guthrie KA, Corey L, Boeckh M. Influenza infections after hematopoietic stem cell transplantation: risk factors, mortality, and the effect of antiviral therapy. Clin Infect Dis Off Publ Infect Dis Soc Am. 2004;39(9):1300–6. https://doi.org/10.1086/425004.
108. Manuel O, Estabrook M. RNA respiratory viral infections in solid organ transplant recipients: guidelines from the American Society of Transplantation Infectious Diseases Community of Practice. Clin Transplant. 2019;33(9):e13511. https://doi.org/10.1111/ctr.13511.
109. Cesaro S, Ljungman P, Mikulska M, et al. Recommendations for the management of COVID-19 in patients with haematological malignancies or haematopoietic cell transplantation, from the 2021 European Conference on Infections in Leukaemia (ECIL 9). Leukemia. 2022;36(6):1467–80. https://doi.org/10.1038/s41375-022-01578-1.
110. Miarons M, Larrosa-García M, García-García S, et al. COVID-19 in solid organ transplantation: a matched retrospective cohort study and evaluation of immunosuppression management. Transplantation. 2021;105(1):138–50. https://doi.org/10.1097/TP.0000000000003460.
111. Marcondes-Braga FG, Murad CM, Belfort DSP, et al. Characteristics and outcomes of heart transplant recipients with coronavirus-19 disease in a high-volume transplant center. Transplantation. 2022;106(3):641–7. https://doi.org/10.1097/TP.0000000000003770.
112. Strasfeld L. COVID-19 and HSCT (Hematopoietic stem cell transplant). Best Pract Res Clin Haematol. 2022;35(3):101399. https://doi.org/10.1016/j.beha.2022.101399.
113. Khawaja F, Srinivasan K, Spallone A, et al. Nosocomial COVID-19 at a comprehensive cancer center during the first year of the pandemic: lessons learned. Am J Infect Control. 2022;S0196-6553(22):00575–2. https://doi.org/10.1016/j.ajic.2022.07.019.
114. CDC. Interim Infection Prevention and Control Recommendations for Healthcare Personnel During the Coronavirus Disease 2019 (COVID-19) Pandemic. Centers for Disease Control and Prevention. Published February 11, 2020. Accessed November 13, 2022. https://www.cdc.gov/coronavirus/2019-ncov/hcp/infection-control-recommendations.html.
115. Aydillo T, Gonzalez-Reiche AS, Aslam S, et al. Shedding of viable SARS-CoV-2 after immunosuppressive therapy for cancer. N Engl J Med. 2020;383(26):2586–8. https://doi.org/10.1056/NEJMc2031670.

Chapter 10
Preventing Fungal Infections in the ICU Setting

Dallas J. Smith, Janet Glowicz, Meghan Lyman, Jeremy A. W. Gold, and Tom Chiller

Introduction

The kingdom Fungi consists of millions of species of spore forming organisms recognized by their structure, nutritional requirements, and mode of reproduction. Neither plant nor animal, these organisms are widely dispersed in the environment. Of the estimated six million species of fungi, only about 600 cause illness in humans, and these species generally fall into four categories: yeasts (e.g., *Candida*), molds (e.g., *Aspergillus*, mucormycetes), dimorphics (e.g., *Coccidioides*, *Histoplasma*, *Blastomyces*), and others (e.g., *Fonsecaea*, *Madurella*) [1]. Fungal diseases can range from mild skin rashes to life-threatening, invasive infections that primarily occur in immunocompromised hosts. Hospitalized patients, particularly those in intensive care units (ICU), may have characteristics that make them more prone to serious healthcare-associated fungal infections, placing them at risk for severe morbidity and mortality. Invasive healthcare-associated fungal infections are defined as systemic, generalized, and severe life-threatening infections acquired during the

Content: "To describe current risk factors for healthcare-associated fungal infections and prevention methods" to match terminology used in chapter?

D. J. Smith (✉)
Epidemic Intelligence Service, Centers for Disease Control and Prevention, Atlanta, GA, USA

Mycotic Diseases Branch, Centers for Diseases Control and Prevention, Atlanta, GA, USA
e-mail: rhq8@cdc.gov

J. Glowicz
Division of Healthcare Quality Promotion, Centers for Diseases Control and Prevention, Atlanta, GA, USA

M. Lyman · J. A. W. Gold · T. Chiller
Mycotic Diseases Branch, Centers for Diseases Control and Prevention, Atlanta, GA, USA

M. Ellsworth, L. Ostrosky-Zeichner (eds.), *Infection Prevention in the Intensive Care Setting*, https://doi.org/10.1007/978-3-031-67062-6_10

receipt of healthcare [2]. The number of at-risk persons is growing as more people live with cancer and transplantation. Intensive care patients may have risk factors for severe fungal infections that are similar to those of the general population, including advanced age, type I or II diabetes, and receipt of immunosuppressive medications (e.g., corticosteroids, immunomodulatory drugs) [3, 4]. Risk factors specific to intensive care patients may include prolonged episodes of acidosis associated with respiratory or systemic decompensation and use of invasive medical devices [5].

Fungal infections that occur in clusters or outbreaks may be of public health importance, often meriting notification of local public health officials. Rapid recognition of outbreaks and a robust response may prevent infection among hospitalized patients. However, this rapid recognition is often limited by lack of standardized fungal HAI definitions and gaps in reporting requirements. The Council for Outbreak Response: Healthcare Associated Infections and Antimicrobial-Resistant Pathogens (CORHA) has provided guidance to state and local health departments for the investigation and reporting of some fungal infections. This chapter will present a brief description of the epidemiology of the fungal organism of interest, pathogenesis, disease presentations, and prevention measures.

Risk Factors for the Development Healthcare-Associated Fungal Infections

- Complex illness with increased length of stay in the ICU.
- Hematologic malignancy.
- Solid organ transplantation.
- Immunosuppression or immature immune system (e.g., pre-term, low birth weight, neonate).
- Immunosuppressive treatments including glucocorticoids or chemotherapy for cancer.

Candidiasis

Epidemiology of Healthcare-Associated Candidiasis

Invasive candidiasis is one of the most common healthcare-associated fungal infections [6]. Risk of infection is increased with the use of central venous catheters. *Candida* spp. were the leading pathogens causing central-line associated bloodstream infections (CLABSI) among patients in adult intensive care and inpatient units during 2011 and 2017, a period in which rates of CLABSI attributed to other pathogens decreased. The detection of CLABSI caused by *Candida* spp. was enhanced when in 2015, the United States Centers for Disease Prevention and Control (CDC) National Healthcare Safety Network (NHSN) excluded fungal organisms, importantly *Candida* spp., from consideration as uropathogens in the catheter-associated urinary tract infection (CAUTI) definition [7]. When a urine culture and blood culture yield the same species of *Candida,* the bloodstream infection is considered a primary infection. This change improved surveillance of invasive healthcare-associated Candidiasis as bloodstream infections could no longer be attributed to the presence of funguria [8, 9].

Risk Factors for Healthcare-Associated Invasive Candidiasis

- Abdominal surgery
- Acute necrotizing pancreatitis
- Treatment with broad-spectrum antibiotics or total parenteral nutrition
- Presence of a central venous catheter (CVC)
- Renal failure or hemodialysis
- Colonization with *Candida spp.*
- Injection drug use

Pathogenesis of Candida *spp.*

Candida spp. are commensal organisms that are part of the natural human microflora residing on the skin and in the gastrointestinal tract. Common species include *Candida albicans*, *C. glabrata*, *C. parapsilosis*, *C. tropicalis*, and *C. krusei*. Invasive infections have classically been thought to occur from translocation of endogenous flora of the gut to the bloodstream or seeding of the bloodstream through indwelling devices. However, certain species, like *C. parapsilosis* and *C. auris*, may also be transmitted through contact with contaminated surfaces, including shared medical equipment and the hands of healthcare personnel, and can result in outbreaks [10].

Emerging Infections

Candida auris is an emerging, frequently drug-resistant yeast that can cause invasive disease (e.g., bloodstream, intra-abdominal) with high mortality rates [11]. Furthermore, the fungus can colonize the skin and other body sites (e.g., urine, skin, external ear canal, wounds, and respiratory specimens) without causing active infections. *C. auris* can spread within healthcare facilities and cause outbreaks. Factors that allow *C. auris* to efficiently spread as an HAI include prolonged colonization of patients, persistence in the environment, and the ability to withstand certain disinfectants [12]. The role of environmental cleaning has become increasingly important to prevention as environmental contamination with *C. auris* and rapid spread among long-term care patients have been documented [13].

Risk Factors for the Development of *C. auris* Infection

- Prolonged healthcare exposure, particularly in long-term care facilities.
- Mechanical ventilation.
- Indwelling devices, including central venous catheters, feeding tubes, urinary catheters, etc.
- History of antimicrobial use.

Prevention of Invasive Candidiasis

Methods to prevent healthcare-associated candidiasis are similar to those used to prevent other healthcare-associated infections. This includes adhering to recommended practices for hand hygiene, thorough environmental cleaning, and adherence to prevention bundles aimed at prevention of CLABSI or CAUTI [14].

- Ensure all personnel adhere to hand hygiene [15].
  - Hand hygiene is a critically important element that is foundational to all other infection prevention practices.
  - Healthcare personnel should maintain healthy hand skin with natural fingernails to avoid fungal colonization of their hands.
  - Alcohol-based hand sanitizer is the preferred method for cleaning hands in most clinical situations and is effective against yeast.
- Perform thorough, at a minimum daily, environmental cleaning and disinfection.
  - Clean and disinfect mobile medical equipment thoroughly after each use.
  - When patients are in isolation for *C. auris*, dedicate medical equipment to the patient.
- Perform meticulous care of central venous catheter (CVC) with prompt removal when the catheter is no longer indicated [16].
  - If total parenteral nutrition is used, switch to enteral feeding as soon as clinically appropriate.
  - When CVCs are present in ICU patients, institute chlorhexidine bathing along with use of alcoholic chlorhexidine for exit-site care [17].
- Minimize disruption of gut microbiome by reducing inappropriate antimicrobial use.
- Consider antifungal prophylaxis to patients for whom benefit has been shown (Table 10.1) [9, 18].
  - Extremely low-birth weight infants in settings with a high incidence (>5%) of neonatal candidiasis.
  - Patients undergoing pancreatic or small bowel transplant.

Table 10.1 Candidiasis antifungal prophylaxis considerations in high-risk patients in adult ICUs with a high rate (>5%) of invasive candidiasis [18]

Antifungal medication	Prophylaxis loading dose	Prophylaxis daily therapy
Fluconazole	800 mg (12 mg/kg)	400 mg (6 mg/kg)
Caspofungin	70 mg	50 mg
Anidulafungin	200 mg	100 mg
Micafungin	100 mg	100 mg

  - Certain patients undergoing liver transplant.
  - Patients with bowel surgery resulting in gastrointestinal anastomotic leakage.
  - Stem cell transplant patients or patients with chemotherapy-induced neutropenia.

Prevention of *C. auris* Transmission: Patient shedding and persistence of *C. auris* in the healthcare environment contribute to spread and require additional measures beyond those recommended for other forms of candidiasis. For any patients that are infected or colonized with *C. auris*, the following measures can be implemented:

- Identifying all clinical cultures yielding *Candida* spp., including urine cultures, to the species level can be considered to enhance detection.
- Prompt reporting of cases to local public health authorities as required by state or local statute.
- Screening of all healthcare contacts for colonization, although note that definition of healthcare contacts can be complicated.
  - A point prevalence survey of all patients whose admission overlapped with the case should be considered.
- Placement of colonized or infected patients in a single patient room. If the ICU is configured with treatment bays or multi-patient suites, carefully consider where the patient is placed so that dedicated care can be provided with minimal interaction with neighboring patients.
  - Cohorting is the practice of placing colonized or infected patients in a dedicated area with dedicated personnel. If more than one case of *C. auris* is detected, cohorting could be considered. During shifts in which personnel are assigned to care for patients with *C. auris*, personnel should not simultaneously provide care for patients with and without *C. auris* if feasible.
- Implement contact precautions for organisms spread by direct or indirect contact, including the use of gowns and gloves for all interactions with affected patients.
  - Established criteria do not exist for decolonization or the discontinuation of contact precautions. Persistent colonization should be anticipated and may be intermittent indicating the need to maintain precautions across healthcare facility stays.
- Daily and terminal cleaning should be conducted with a disinfectant that has an Environmental Protection Agency (EPA) registered claim against *C. auris* (i.e., List P).
  - Reusable equipment, (e.g., glucometers, blood pressure cuffs) should be dedicated to affected patients and thoroughly cleaned during daily and terminal cleanings.

– Environmental service personnel should provide daily cleaning of areas housing patients on transmission-based precautions, use recommended practices to avoid contaminating their carts during room cleaning, and adhere to disinfectant contact times.

Healthcare-Associated Invasive Mold Infections

Healthcare-associated invasive mold infections (HAIMI) are caused by several families, genera, and species of fungi. These organisms are not usually transmitted from person to person but rather through environmental exposure. Many areas of the hospital are designed according to specifications that prevent mold infections. Outbreaks of mold infections can be difficult to identify because the incubation period may be prolonged. The appearance of a single invasive mold infection may indicate deficiencies in the built environment or lapses in the protection of healthcare supplies. Understanding the epidemiology of mold infections can help when investigating and remediating potential sources.

The CDC has created a Targeted Environmental Investigation Checklist for Outbreaks of Invasive Infections Caused by Environmental Fungi like *Aspergillus* spp. [19] This checklist describes elements to assess along with appropriate follow-up actions and can highlight interventions to prevent environmental exposure in ICU settings.

Epidemiology of Healthcare-Associated Aspergillosis

Aspergillus spp. are commonly found in the environment including in soil, decomposing matter, household dust, building materials, plants, food, and water [20]. Common species include *A. fumigatus* and *A. flavus*. Less common species include *A. terreus, A. nidulans, A. niger*, and *A. versicolor* [21]. Transmission most often occurs through the inhalation of airborne conidia and can be associated with dust exposure during building renovation or construction in ICU settings. Contaminated air, ventilation systems, air filters, false ceilings and insulation material, water supply, plumbing, showers, food, ornamental plants, arm boards, and dressing packages may also be sources of this mold [5]. Cutaneous infections may also stem from contaminated biomedical devices, water, and linens.

Routine surveillance of HAIMI can identify outbreaks of aspergillus or other molds in ICU settings and allow for remediation of conditions that may promote transmission, reducing morbidity and mortality [22]. Healthcare-association of invasive mold infections can be difficult to identify due to complexity of patient's past medical history, multiple potential exposures, and unknown incubation periods for some molds. Healthcare facilities lack capacity for rapid identification of mold species; efforts to standardize case definitions across healthcare systems and facilities can increase ease of interpretation of surveillance data and inform prevention measures. When a case of aspergillosis occurs, the facility should investigate the background rates of clinical cultures yielding *Aspergillus* spp. The presence of recent or concurrent cases may be identified through the review facility microbiologic, histopathologic, and postmortem records. For cases, the length of the patient stay in the facility before the onset of illness or stays at other healthcare facilities can help determine if the case is healthcare associated. An epidemiologic investigation and environmental assessment should be performed [23].

Risk Factors for the Development of Aspergillosis Include the Following

- Severe of prolonged granulocytopenia.
- Hematologic malignancies.
- Receipt of a hematopoietic stem cell or solid organ transplant.
- High-dose corticosteroids or other immunosuppressive therapies.
- Severe influenza or SARS-CoV-2 infections (even among patients without other immunocompromising conditions).

Epidemiology of Healthcare-Associated Mucormycosis

Mucormycetes are commonly found in the environment in soil but are rarely found in air samples targeting fungal spores [24–27]. Causative molds species include those belonging to the order Mucorales, particularly *Rhizopus* spp., *Mucor* spp., *Cunninghamella bertholletiae*, *Apophysomyces* spp., and *Lichtheimia* spp. [28] Transmission can occur through inhalation, traumatic inoculation, or injection of spores. Previous outbreak of mucormycosis has been associated with adhesive bandages, wooden tongue depressors, hospital linens, negative pressure rooms, water leaks, poor air filtration, non-sterile medical devices, building construction, and healthcare linens [5].

Risk Factors for the Development of Mucormycosis Include the Following

- Uncontrolled diabetes
- Malignancy
- Hematopoietic stem cell transplant or solid organ transplant
- Persistent neutropenia
- Prolonged corticosteroid use
- Skin trauma, burns, or surgical wounds
- Iron overload
- Intravenous drug use
- Malnourishment
- Premature infants

Increases in mucormycosis were observed during the COVID-19 pandemic, particularly among people receiving corticosteroids or with uncontrolled blood glucose levels [29].

Prevention of Healthcare-Associated Invasive Mold Infections

Healthcare personnel should remain alert to environmental conditions like heavy dust or uncontrolled humidity that may support the growth and dispersion of fungi that cause HAIMIs in the environment of care. Evidence of mold intrusion, such as wet or discolored ceiling tiles should be remediated immediately. Healthcare textiles should be covered until distribution to the point of use. This risk and benefit of any efforts to change should be considered. For example, removal of windows for the installation of high efficiency particulate air (HEPA) filters in individual rooms may result in inadequate seals and loss of the intended protection.

The Infection Prevention Department should collaborate with facility management to evaluate the risk to patients when maintenance or construction is being performed especially when opening ceiling tiles or walls. The Infection Control Risk Assessment (ICRA) is used to determine the types of protections, such as barriers and ventilation controls needed to protect patients from exposure to dust [30]. When construction is performed in the ICU, all personnel should immediately report concerns about maintenance of the construction site (e.g., failures to maintain negative pressure within the construction area, visible dust outside of the construction area) to the Infection Prevention Department.

Environmental sampling for the presence of mold spores may help in identifying increases in the presence of spores prior to the spread of disease or outbreaks in ICU settings [22]. A predefined sampling strategy and the inclusion of an industrial hygienist may improve the success of environmental sampling to identify exposure sources for remediation or epidemiologic links between mold sources and patients. Before, during, and after major construction, air sampling can monitor mold counts and inform prevention practices. However, detecting molds does not necessarily correlate to an exposure source or mold infections. A lack of established mold threshold values also makes interpretation difficult. Furthermore, the failure to detect mold should not rule out the healthcare environment as a source because intermittent identification of mold in healthcare facilities is plausible.

A Protective Environment (PE) to prevent environmental exposure to molds is also recommended for allogeneic hematopoietic stem cell transplant (HSCT) patients [31]. PE includes measures such as HEPA filtration of incoming air, directed room air flow, positive room air pressure relative to corridor, well-sealed rooms to prevent outside air entering room, $\geq$12 air changes per hour, utilizing strategies to reduce dust like scrubbable surfaces and cleaning crevices and sprinkler heads routinely, and avoiding dried or fresh flowers in rooms of HSCT patients.

Patients that are immunosuppressed but not requiring a PE (e.g., patients undergoing chemotherapy) should be placed in rooms that are at neutral or positive pressure to adjacent hallways and common areas. In the absence of an infectious illness requiring airborne precautions, these patients should not be placed in airborne infection isolation rooms as negative pressure may inadvertently increase exposure to environmental pathogens [32].

Table 10.2 Aspergillosis antifungal prophylaxis considerations

Indication	Agent	Duration
Allogenic hematopoietic stem cell transplantation with graft vs. host disease	Posaconazole	Duration of immunosuppression (corticosteroid equivalent of >1 mg/kg/day of prednisone for >2 weeks, lymphocyte-depleting agents, or tumor necrosis factor α (TNF-α) inhibition)
Lung transplant recipients	Systemic triazole (i.e., voriconazole, itraconazole) or inhaled Amphotericin B	Three to four months after lung transplant May need to restart prophylaxis if recipient receives immunosuppressive medications like thymoglobulin, alemtuzumab, or high-dose corticosteroids
Non-lung solid organ transplant recipients	Dependent on epidemiology of infections	Duration is unknown. Individual risk factors need to be assessed

Supplies used in healthcare including dressings and tape have been implicated in outbreaks of HAIMI. These supplies should be removed from outer shipping packages prior to receipt in the ICU and should be stored in clean supply rooms at positive pressure to the environment. Tape should be dedicated to patients and, as much as possible, the size of rolls of tape should be minimized. Rolls of tape should be protected from the environment when stored on supply carts and should not be carried on stethoscopes or in the pockets of healthcare personnel.

Antifungal prophylaxis may be useful in preventing aspergillosis in patients, particularly those with prolonged neutropenia. Certain indications have specific recommendations in regard to therapeutic agent and administration (Table 10.2) [33]. Posaconazole, voriconazole, or micafungin may be appropriate therapeutic agents. Itraconazole can be used; concerns around appropriate therapeutic levels and side effects may limit its use.

Prevention of Healthcare-Associated Mucormycosis

Prevention measures for mucormycosis are similar to other mold prevention measures. CDC's Targeted Environmental Investigation Checklist for Outbreaks of Invasive Infections Caused by Environmental Fungi is a useful tool to improve infection control and prevention of mucormycosis [19]. PEs are also used to protect hematopoietic stem cell transplant patients from mucromycosis [31]. Additional prevention methods include:

- Cleaning and disinfection of equipment used by multiple patients.
- Cleaning and using appropriate materials in ventilation systems.
- Proper wound management.
- Proper line management.

Healthcare linens can expose patients to molds and may lead to an invasive mucormycosis infection in immunocompromised patients. Healthcare facilities regularly outsource laundry and linens, thus decreasing the opportunities for oversight and increasing the potential for environmental contamination. CDC has identified five hazards and action points for healthcare linens: (1) laundry facility built environment, (2) laundry facility clean linen work area, (3) health care textile transport and delivery at the healthcare facility, (4) staging within the healthcare facility, and (5) healthcare facility distribution to the point of use [34]. The CDC developed two checklists for the management of laundered healthcare linens [35, 36].

Primary and secondary prophylaxis may be useful in mucormycosis in certain patient populations (e.g., neutropenic patients or patients with graft versus host disease) [28]. While prophylaxis is not directed specifically at mucormycosis but a range of fungal pathogens, posaconazole formulations (oral suspension, delayed release tablets, or intravenous solutions) have shown to decrease fungal infection rates, including breakthrough mucormycosis. Prevention of mucormycosis recurrence may be possible through surgical resection and the previous antifungal that was effective in treating mucormycosis.

Conclusion

Surveillance and rapid identification of fungal infections and outbreaks are critical for prevention in ICU settings. Fungal pathogens are frequently acquired from the environment and interventions such as maintaining humidity at levels specified by hospital design standards together with appropriate ventilation can minimize the growth of these organisms. *C. auris* presents novel challenges in prevention with its ability to spread from person-to-person and from the patient's environment. Spread of fungal diseases in ICU settings should be accompanied by patient notification [37]. As the cohort of individuals susceptible to invasive fungal infections continues to increase, prevention will be key moving forward to prevent morbidity and mortality from mycoses in the ICU setting.

References

1. Konopka JB, Casadevall A, Taylor JW, Heitman J, Cowen L. One health: fungal pathogens of humans, animals, and plants. American Society for Microbiology; 2019. https://doi.org/10.1128/AAMCol.18Oct.2017.
2. Hof H. IFI = invasive fungal infections. What is that? A misnomer, because a non-invasive fungal infection does not exist! Int J Infect Dis. 2010;14(6):e458–9. https://doi.org/10.1016/j.ijid.2009.08.006.
3. Rayens E, Norris KA. Prevalence and healthcare burden of fungal infections in the United States, 2018. Open Forum Infect Dis. 2022;9(1):ofab593. https://doi.org/10.1093/ofid/ofab593.

4. Gold JAW, Ahmad FB, Cisewski JA, et al. Increased deaths from fungal infections during the COVID-19 pandemic—National Vital Statistics System, United States, January 2020–December 2021. Clin Infect Dis. 2022:ciac489. https://doi.org/10.1093/cid/ciac489.
5. Perlroth J, Choi B, Spellberg B. Nosocomial fungal infections: epidemiology, diagnosis, and treatment. Med Mycol. 2007;45(4):321–46. https://doi.org/10.1080/13693780701218689.
6. Toda M, Williams SR, Berkow EL, et al. Population-based active surveillance for culture-confirmed candidemia—four sites, United States, 2012–2016. MMWR Surveill Summ. 2019;68(8):1–15. https://doi.org/10.15585/mmwr.ss6808a1.
7. Bardossy AC, Jayaprakash R, Alangaden AC, et al. Impact and limitations of the 2015 national health and safety network case definition on catheter-associated urinary tract infection rates. Infect Control Hosp Epidemiol. 2017;38(2):239–41. https://doi.org/10.1017/ice.2016.278.
8. Novosad SA, Fike L, Dudeck MA, et al. Pathogens causing central-line–associated bloodstream infections in acute-care hospitals—United States, 2011–2017. Infect Control Hosp Epidemiol. 2020;41(3):313–9. https://doi.org/10.1017/ice.2019.303.
9. Kullberg BJ, Arendrup MC. Invasive candidiasis. N Engl J Med. 2015;373(15):1445–56. https://doi.org/10.1056/NEJMra1315399. Campion EW, ed
10. Y1ıld1ır1ıms M, Sahin I, Kucukbayrak A, et al. Hand carriage of Candida species and risk factors in hospital personnel. Mycoses 2007;50(3):189–192. doi:https://doi.org/10.1111/j.1439-0507.2006.01348.x.
11. Cortegiani A, Misseri G, Fasciana T, Giammanco A, Giarratano A, Chowdhary A. Epidemiology, clinical characteristics, resistance, and treatment of infections by Candida auris. J Intensive Care. 2018;6:69. https://doi.org/10.1186/s40560-018-0342-4.
12. Chakrabarti A, Sood P. On the emergence, spread and resistance of Candida auris: host, pathogen and environmental tipping points. J Med Microbiol. 2021;70(3) https://doi.org/10.1099/jmm.0.001318.
13. Adams E, Quinn M, Tsay S, et al. *Candida auris* in healthcare facilities, New York, USA, 2013–2017. Emerg Infect Dis. 2018;24(10):1816–24. https://doi.org/10.3201/eid2410.180649.
14. Marschall J, Mermel LA, Fakih M, et al. Strategies to prevent central line–associated bloodstream infections in acute care hospitals: 2014 update. Infect Control Hosp Epidemiol. 2014;35(7):753–71. https://doi.org/10.1086/676533.
15. Core Infection Prevention and Control Practices for Safe Healthcare Delivery in All Settings—Recommednations of the Healthcare Infection Control Practices Advisory Committee. Ctr Dis Control Prev. 2017. Accessed November 21, 2022. Available at: https://www.cdc.gov/hicpac/pdf/core-practices.pdf.
16. Ture Z, Alp E. Infection control measures to prevent hospital transmission of candida. Hosp Pract. 2018;46(5):253–7. https://doi.org/10.1080/21548331.2018.1510282.
17. Munoz-Price LS, Hota B, Stemer A, Weinstein RA. Prevention of bloodstream infections by use of daily chlorhexidine baths for patients at a long-term acute care hospital. Infect Control Hosp Epidemiol. 2009;30(11):1031–5. https://doi.org/10.1086/644751.
18. Pappas PG, Kauffman CA, Andes DR, et al. Clinical practice guideline for the management of candidiasis: 2016 update by the infectious diseases society of America. Clin Infect Dis. 2016;62(4):e1–e50. https://doi.org/10.1093/cid/civ933.
19. Centers for Disease Control and Prevention. Targeted environmental investigation checklist for outbreaks of invasive infections caused by environmental fungi (e.g., Aspergillus, Mucormycetes). Available at: https://www.cdc.gov/fungal/pdf/targeted-environmental-investigation-checklist-508.pdf.
20. Warris A, Verweij PE. Clinical implications of environmental sources for *Aspergillus*. Med Mycol. 2005;43(s1):59–65. https://doi.org/10.1080/13693780400025260.
21. Barnes PD, Marr KA. Aspergillosis: spectrum of disease, diagnosis, and treatment. Infect Dis Clin N Am. 2006;20(3):545–61. https://doi.org/10.1016/j.idc.2006.06.001.
22. Gold JAW, Jackson BR, Glowicz J, Mead KR, Beer KD. Surveillance practices and air-sampling strategies to address healthcare-associated invasive mold infections in Society for Healthcare

Epidemiology of America (SHEA) Research Network hospitals—United States, 2020. Infect Control Hosp Epidemiol. 2022;43(11):1708–11. https://doi.org/10.1017/ice.2021.285.
23. Tablan OC, Anderson LJ, Besser R, et al. Guidelines for preventing health-care--associated pneumonia, 2003: recommendations of CDC and the Healthcare Infection Control Practices Advisory Committee. MMWR Recomm Rep Morb Mortal Wkly Rep Recomm Rep. 2004;53(RR-3):1–36.
24. Segvić Klarić M, Pepeljnjak S. A year-round aeromycological study in Zagreb area, Croatia. Ann Agric Environ Med AAEM. 2006;13(1):55–64.
25. Calvo MA, Guarro J, Suarez G, Ramirez C. Air-borne fungi in the air of Barcelona (Spain). IV. Various isolated genera. Mycopathologia. 1980;71(2):119–23. https://doi.org/10.1007/BF00440618.
26. Meklin T, Reponen T, McKinstry C, et al. Comparison of mold concentrations quantified by MSQPCR in indoor and outdoor air sampled simultaneously. Sci Total Environ. 2007;382(1):130–4. https://doi.org/10.1016/j.scitotenv.2007.03.031.
27. Ziaee A, Zia M, Bayat M, Hashemi J. Identification of Mucorales isolates from soil using morphological and molecular methods. Curr Med Mycol. 2016;2(1):13–9. https://doi.org/10.18869/acadpub.cmm.2.1.13.
28. Cornely OA, Alastruey-Izquierdo A, Arenz D, et al. Global guideline for the diagnosis and management of mucormycosis: an initiative of the European Confederation of Medical Mycology in cooperation with the Mycoses Study Group Education and Research Consortium. Lancet Infect Dis. 2019;19(12):e405–21. https://doi.org/10.1016/S1473-3099(19)30312-3.
29. Baddley JW, Thompson GR, Chen SCA, et al. Coronavirus disease 2019–associated invasive fungal infection. Open Forum Infect Dis. 2021;8(12):ofab510. https://doi.org/10.1093/ofid/ofab510.
30. Infection Control Assessment Tools. Centers for disease control and prevention. Accessed November 22, 2022. Available at: https://www.cdc.gov/hai/prevent/infection-control-assessment-tools.html.
31. Centers for Disease Control and Prevention. Infection control: isolation precautions. Available at: https://www.cdc.gov/infectioncontrol/guidelines/isolation/index.html.
32. Vasquez A, Novosad S, Christensen E, et al. Mucormycosis among solid organ transplant recipients at an acute care hospital—Pennsylvania, 2014–2015. Open Forum Infect Dis. 2016;3(Suppl. 1):1410. https://doi.org/10.1093/ofid/ofw172.1113.
33. Patterson TF, Thompson GR, Denning DW, et al. Practice guidelines for the diagnosis and management of aspergillosis: 2016 update by the Infectious Diseases Society of America. Clin Infect Dis. 2016;63(4):e1–e60. https://doi.org/10.1093/cid/ciw326.
34. Glowicz J, Benowitz I, Arduino MJ, et al. Keeping health care linens clean: underrecognized hazards and critical control points to avoid contamination of laundered health care textiles. Am J Infect Control. 2022;S0196-6553(22):00544–2. https://doi.org/10.1016/j.ajic.2022.06.026.
35. Infection Control Assessment of Laundry Facility Preparedness to Keep Healthcare Textiles Clean. Centers for Disease Control and Prevention. Accessed January 6, 2023. Available at: https://www.cdc.gov/fungal/outbreaks/files/Infection-Control-Assessment-of-Laundry-Facility-Preparedness-to-Keep-Healthcare-Textiles-Clean_p.pdf.
36. Infection Control Assessment of Healthcare Facility Preparedness to Keep Healthcare Textiles Clean. Centers for Disease Control and Prevention. Accessed January 6, 2023. Available at: https://www.cdc.gov/fungal/outbreaks/files/Infection-Control-Assessment-of-Healthcare-Facility-Preparedness-to-Keep-Healthcare-Textiles-Clean_p.pdf.
37. Gandhi P, Benedict K, Toda M, Beer KD, Chiller TM, Jackson BR. Patient notification about suspected hospital-associated outbreaks of invasive mold infections: considerations for public health and hospital personnel. Infect Control Hosp Epidemiol. 2021;42(7):871–6. https://doi.org/10.1017/ice.2021.174.

Chapter 11
Healthcare-Associated Infections Outbreak Detection in the ICU Setting

Alicia Lopez-Romo and Estefania Sienra-Iracheta

Introduction

Nosocomial infections are still one of the most frequent complications in the ICU care [1]. The detection and investigation of the occurrence of an outbreak caused by a particular pathogen will depend on several factors, including routine surveillance practices during non-outbreak periods, clinical expertise in recognizing infections and laboratory capacity to perform cultures, antimicrobial susceptibility testing, and molecular strain typing. The evaluation of outbreaks can be complex and multifaceted, especially in an ICU setting [1]. However, the investigation of a particular HAI outbreak should be methodical and thorough yet expeditious and directed toward establishing the nature of the infection, defining reservoirs and modes of transmission and, most important, the immediate implementation of infection control measures [1–3].

An outbreak is defined as an increase in events, such as infection cases, above the baseline rate for a determinate geographic area during a specified period. Usually, the cases are presumed to have a common cause, or source and be related to one another. Depending on the microorganism, an outbreak may be present with a single infectious case, for example, an anthrax, Ebola, or a Streptococcal A infection case or a series of cases. The cases may occur during a short period or over several years. Lastly, an outbreak may start in the community, in a non-ICU health care setting or directly from within the intensive care unit.

A. Lopez-Romo (✉)
Christus Muguerza Hospital Cumbres, Monterrey, Nuevo Leon, Mexico

E. Sienra-Iracheta
Hospital General Manuel Gea González, Mexico City, Mexico

M. Ellsworth, L. Ostrosky-Zeichner (eds.), *Infection Prevention in the Intensive Care Setting*, https://doi.org/10.1007/978-3-031-67062-6_11

Economic Burden of an Outbreak

Outbreaks in the hospital settings contribute to a significant increase in morbidity, mortality, and costs for hospital stays and healthcare services. Outbreaks are expensive, time consuming and can cause significant disruptions in healthcare operations [4]. The attributable costs of an outbreak include the cost of contact precautions (consumable materials, waste elimination, personal protection equipment (PPE)), the need for associated additional staff, decrease in hospital services (deferral of admissions, transfers and referrals, loss of bed-day), laboratory testing (microbiological screening of cases/contacts, environmental sampling, molecular tests), and other additional costs such as antimicrobial treatment, installation of hand sanitizer dispensers, and health care professional education [4]. Therefore, the total financial burden of nosocomial outbreaks can be substantial depending on the outbreak situation including types of microorganism, number of patients, duration of the outbreak, etc. [4–6] Although costs differ between nosocomial outbreaks, studies have demonstrated that the economic impact is mainly due to drug-resistant bacteria. Atchade et al. reported an estimated total financial burden of a 15-month Carbapenemase-Producing *Enterobacteriaceae* (CPE) outbreak at1.2 million EUR [7]. A vancomycin-resistant *Enterococcus* (VPE) the outbreak, including 64 cases, had an estimated cost of 2.7 AUD [6].

Breakdown of outbreak cost shows 69% of total costs come from disruption of bed availability due to interruption of admission and the loss of bed days,, while laboratory costs average 24%, staff reinforcement 22%, and contact precautions cost 18% [5].

Outbreak Mechanisms and Source of Transmission

Multiple mechanisms of outbreaks have been described. An outbreak may start with a patient admitted to ICU with an infection acquired in the community. In contrast, other outbreaks may begin with a patient who acquired a multidrug-resistant (MDR) pathogen during a previous hospital stay or is transferred from another facility with an active outbreak. The complex interaction between healthcare workers, contaminated or colonized environments, devices and other patients creates an ideal environment for outbreak propagation. See Fig. 11.1 [8].

One of the most significant challenges during an outbreak is identifying the source. It has been described that the source can be identified in only 37% of published outbreaks. The most common source identified in ICU could be traced to other patients, medical equipment or devices, environment, and hospital staff. However, it is crucial to recognize that rarely a single source for an outbreak is

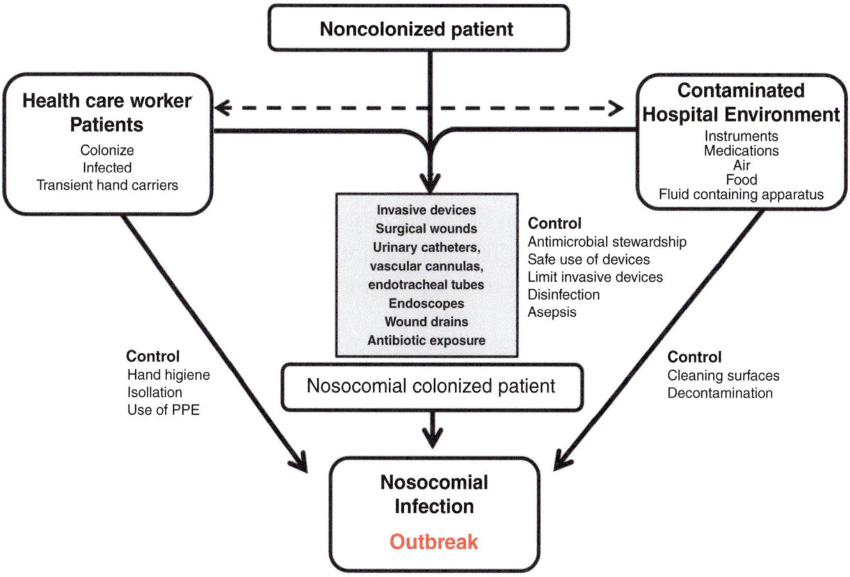

Fig. 11.1 Hospital infection control program

identified, and most outbreaks are attributed to the conjunction of multiple conditions that add up to facilitate the pathogen spread. [8]

Direct and Indirect Contact

Direct and indirect contact is considered the most common mechanism of infectious disease transmission in a healthcare setting, particularly in the ICU. The primary reservoir of nosocomial microorganisms is the infected or colonized patient, and pathogens are subsequently spread by direct contact with healthcare workers and by indirect contact with contaminated medical equipment and supplies. Multiple pathogens have been implicated in this mechanism of transmission. Evidence suggests that aerobic bacteria, particularly S. aureus, enterococci, enteric gram-negative bacilli, viruses such as Hepatitis A virus, rotavirus, norovirus, and even yeasts like *Candida spp* are spread in the ICU through the hands of the staff. In an ICU setting, hand carriage has commonly been associated with the active transmission of *Acinetobacter spp.*, *Pseudomonas spp.*, *Enterobacter spp.*, and other gram-negative bacteria. Some studies have reported the isolation of *Acinetobacter spp.* from the hands of up to 30% of healthcare workers during an active outbreak. This data emphasizes the importance of an effective hand hygiene program [9, 10].

Environmental Surface Contamination

It is well known that microorganisms can survive for prolonged periods on surfaces and medical equipment under adverse conditions such as extreme temperatures and dry environments. Viable pathogens can be found on walls, curtains, floors, medication pumps, monitors, and ventilators even months after a colonized patient has been discharged, and the room has been properly disinfected. Previous studies have shown that a patient is 73% more likely to acquire a HAI if a previous occupant was colonized or infected with a drug-resistant microorganism.

Water Contamination

Multiple pathogens have been associated with the contamination of water reservoirs even in hospital settings where water quality is routinely assessed. Main transmission routes are direct or indirect contact with contaminated water sources or inhalation with water-related devices such as air conditioning duct systems. Some other examples of water reservoirs include haemodialysis water, ventilator circuits, ice machines, sinks, and toilets. Some microorganisms related to waterborne outbreaks in ICU include gram-negative bacteria such as *Burkholderia cepacia, Ralstonia pickettii, Pseudomonas spp, Stenotrophomonas maltophilia,* and *Legionella pneumophila.*

Droplet and Airborne Spread

It is well known that some infections can occur from exposure to microorganisms through respiratory droplets expelled from symptomatic and asymptomatic carriers of certain respiratory pathogens. These respiratory infections can be acquired from exposure to pathogens contained in droplets (aerosolized oral and nasal secretions) or droplet nuclei (aerosols). Viruses, such as SARS-CoV-2, rhinovirus, influenza, and respiratory syncytial virus are examples of pathogens spread in this manner that may cause outbreaks in hospital settings. Transmission of these pathogens can be increased through aerosol-generating procedures such as bronchoscopies, non-invasive respiratory support, nebulizers, etc. Other diseases such as tuberculosis and measles are effectively transmitted through aerosols.

Evaluation of the ICU Outbreaks

Hospitals and healthcare systems through their infection control program must be prepared to conduct a punctual investigation in the presence of an increased number of cases of certain disease or the emergence of an outbreak. Conventional strategies include the establishment of a case definition, generation of an epidemic curve, epidemiologic data acquisition, and eventually, the implementation of appropriate preventative strategies and control measures. However, the surge of modern and new technologies such as epidemiology surveillance software and automated statistical surveillance systems has made the outbreak characterization and investigation easier for the infection control team. ***See Surveillance tools.*** It is essential to punctually investigate an HAI outbreak as the availability and quality of microbiological evidence and epidemiological data may vary during its study. Several steps have been described to evaluate an outbreak.

Although these steps are usually listed sequentially, the process of the investigation may occur in a different order or simultaneously as information is collected by the infection control team.

An outbreak evaluation should be focused on 4 stages: (1) Detection of the outbreak, (2) confirmation of the outbreak and early response, (3) interventions and finally, (4) post-intervention (Fig. 11.2).

Initially, any outbreak evaluation consists of verifying that clusters of cases (an unusual aggregation of cases grouped in time or space) are indeed an outbreak. Identifying clusters of cases is the main trigger to start a further investigation to determine the presence of an outbreak. For detecting these clusters, the operational definitions for nosocomial infections are crucial and active surveillance should be continuous throughout all hospital areas. **See Epidemiological surveillance and analysis tools**. Furthermore, microbiologic epidemiologic technologies must be implemented as a resource for outbreak identification. **See Laboratory Tools**.

Once a cluster is identified, it is necessary to have an on-the-spot verification of diagnosis as quickly as possible. First, the infection control team should conduct a punctual review of the clinical findings and laboratory results of each case and decide if further laboratory testing should be conducted (e.g., environmental testing, molecular typing of the isolates, etc.). All laboratory personnel should be notified to save isolated specimens for further investigation.

It is also important to be able to distinguish an outbreak from a pseudo-outbreak. A background or baseline infection rate should be provided and compared to the number of cases to identify a potential outbreak.

Once potential outbreak cases are identified, a case definition should be created. Case definition must maximize sensitivity and specificity and provide a description of the condition, including clinical criteria and laboratory findings and should be limited to a period and area of occurrence. After creating a case definition, case ascertainment should be conducted. New information about identified cases should be systematically recorded in spreadsheets or other means, such as a line listing for subsequent analysis. **See epidemiological surveillance and analysis tools.** Data should be plotted to create an epidemic curve to compare to baseline surveillance cases. Infection rates and geographic location of cases can aid in identifying a potential source and help identify the pattern of transmission to develop a hypothesis. **See environmental sampling.**

The implementation of infection control and prevention strategies are mainstays in the control of an outbreak, and these measures and strategies must be started a

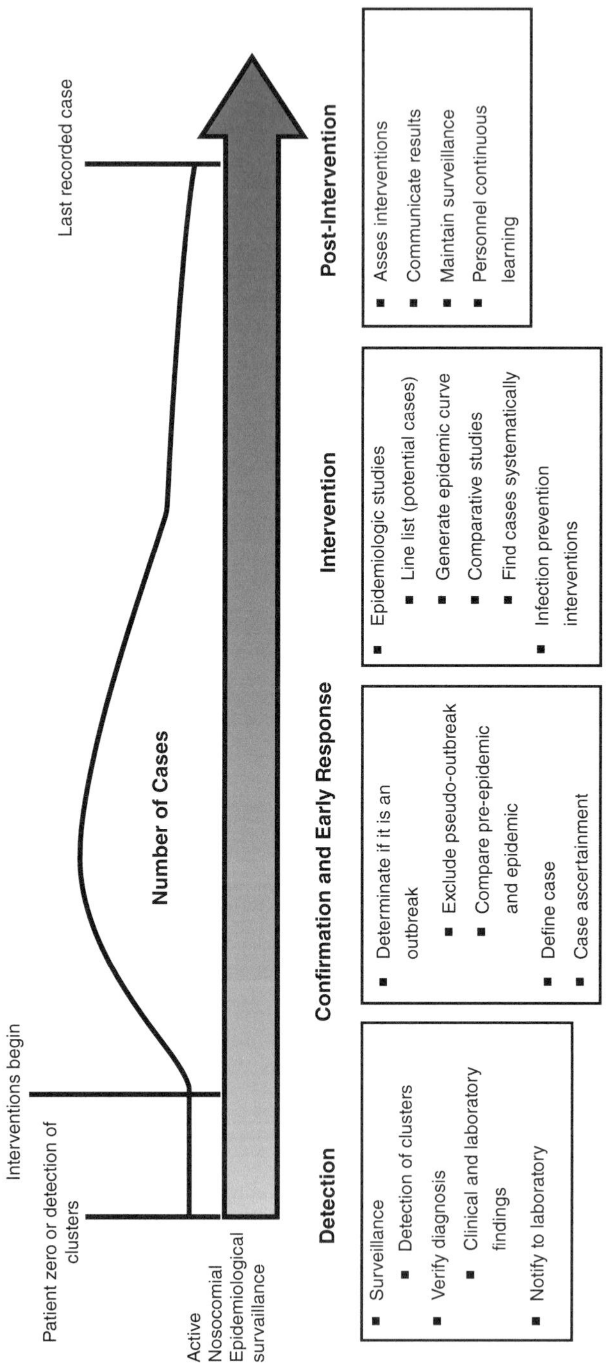

Fig. 11.2 Evaluation of the ICU outbreaks

soon as the outbreak is identified. These strategies might vary based on the causative pathogen, outbreak source, modes of transmission, size of the population at risk, public health relevance, and resources available. Some control measures include isolation (cohorting or single rooms exclusively for case patients), transmission-based precautions (airborne, contact, etc.), and special cleaning and disinfection especially when the patient is discharged. **See infection control and prevention strategies**.

For the post-intervention stage, evaluating the success of the control measures is essential. These findings should be communicated to the hospital staff including leadership. Depending on the magnitude, severity, and public health importance, outbreaks must be reported to local, state, or federal healthcare agencies, preferably by an experienced individual.

Epidemiological Surveillance and Analysis Tools

To investigate and understand any nosocomial outbreak, both epidemiological surveillance and network data analysis play a key role [11, 12]. Technological innovation has facilitated health event monitoring through digitalized medical records and surveillance networks [13–16]. International and local bodies have introduced surveillance systems to monitor trends in incidence, prevalence, and deaths associated with specific pathogens and diseases and have been widely used to provide an early warning during outbreak investigations. Most surveillance systems only reflect static ward areas, such as the ICU. However, the implementation of real-time surveillance and network analyses can help understand infectious disease transmission, geo-temporal associations, and clusters pathways. Multiple tools for statistical analysis have been demonstrated to help in evaluating outbreaks [11, 14], and analytical epidemiological studies should be conducted during an outbreak's intervention and post-intervention phases. [12, 17].

The choice of epidemiological study will depend on the outbreak's characteristics: type of diseases and microorganism, source, time, and size. Comparative and observational studies may be appropriate. For example, a prolonged outbreak is associated with more exposures that need to be reviewed. In that case, a case-control study may be suitable for epidemiological analysis of the outbreak [18].

Cohort studies assess entire populations and evaluate common exposures among those who develop infections. This kind of comparative study can generate association and causality related to outbreaks. However, the pitfalls of this type of study are that it is time consuming and expensive, and only a few risk factors can be evaluated. As the study of an ICU outbreak is so complex, novel informatics methods have been developed [19, 20]. Mathematical models such as agent-related models and algorithms have provided a framework to understand complex transmission dynamics and have contributed to determining the impact of infection control strategies [21, 22].

Environmental surveillance is necessary as we know the hospital environment can be an important reservoir for nosocomial pathogens. The US Center for Disease Control and Prevention recommends environmental sampling to support the investigation of the outbreak source implicated in disease transmission. Sampling surfaces have high reliability and low cost during the investigation. However, there is a lack of standardized protocols for environmental surveillance [23]. There are both direct and indirect methods of sampling. Primarily indirect methods are used when the investigation is not directed at finding a specific pathogen. On the other hand, the best method to identify a particular pathogen is direct methods suited for that microorganisms. For example, swabs for MRSA, contact plates for CRE, and sponges for *C. difficile*. Air sampling remains controversial and is recommended during airborne disease outbreak investigations. Once the samples are taken, laboratory processing involves culture and molecular methods [24].

Laboratory Tools

It is essential to collaborate with the laboratory during an outbreak investigation [25, 26]. The laboratory may be the initial source for recognizing unusual organisms or the increase in isolates of certain pathogens. It can provide special testing to the isolates linked to the suspected cases and serve as a repository of collected specimens for further evaluation [3]. As technology and molecular testing evolve, laboratories are facing a rapid development of new and more reliable identification methods [2, 27–29]. Traditionally, cultures and susceptibility patterns helped as initial identification methods. Now, molecular techniques are used to compare strains with similar genetic profiles, can further help to exclude potential environmental sources, and can be used for transmission dynamics [26].

Traditionally, phenotypic methods included antibiotic susceptibility, serotyping, and phage typing. New molecular methods are available and accessible for more excellent resolution of specific strains (see Table 11.1).

Table 11.1 Laboratory tools and different methods used for pathogen identification and classification

	Method	Advantages/disadvantages
Phenotypic testing methods		
Biotyping	Identifies the organism genus and species through morphology and biochemical reactions	• Mostly available, sensitive, and inexpensive • Time consuming
Antimicrobial susceptibility testing	Determines the antimicrobial susceptibility patterns for microorganisms	• Mostly available in most clinical laboratories
Serotyping	Specific antibodies against surface antigens	• Not specific and rapid • Requires a large amount of antigens • Developed for small number of microorganisms
Genotypic testing methods		
Plasmid typing	Isolates plasmids using restriction endonucleases Limited availability	• Useful for identification of resistance genes
Pulse field electrophoresis	Bacterial DNA is extracted and cleaved by an endonuclease, then separated by a shifting electric field to show a pattern of bands to compare strains	• It is considered the gold standard for molecular typing
Ribotyping	Similar to pulse field electrophoresis but uses a frequent cutting endonuclease and hybridized to label rRNA	• Less able to discriminate strains, compared to gel electrophoresis
DNA microarray hybridization	DNA probes of bacteria are isolated, labelled, and hybridized	• Large screening • Allows the detection of plasmids expensive
Polymerase chain reaction	Amplify certain DNA segments. Uses primers (can be specific or arbitrary) of the bacterial strain	• Easy to perform and fast • Semi-automated commercial machines available
Optical mapping	Embeds bacterial genomic DNA in agarose and then is stretched in a microfluidic device. Endonucleases are used to digest stained bacterial DNA. It is then visualized by fluorescence microscopy	• Individual genes can be seen in vivo Genomic maps can be created • Limited to cost and equipment needed
Whole genome sequencing	The newest tool, complete genome is sequenced. It is becoming affordable to help uncovered genetically related clusters	• It is rapidly becoming the gold standard for comparing strains • Can be used in viral, bacterial, and fungal organism
Matrix-assisted laser desorption/ionization-time of flight mass spectrometry (MALDI-TOF MS)	Crystalized matrix is ionized in a laser beam that generates protonated ions. Protonated ions are accelerated and detected and measured by mass analyzers	• Fast and accurate • Trained personnel not required • High cost of the machine

Pseudo-Outbreaks

An increase in the isolation of a microorganism by the microbiology lab does not always denote infection or an actual outbreak. Pseudo-outbreaks are defined as an increase in an identified organism but without evidence of infection, pseudo-outbreaks are often difficult to distinguish from a true outbreak. The upsurge of the documentation of these isolates may be due to improved active surveillance, new practitioners, new lab tests or change in testing frequency, different or poor sample collection, laboratory error, or specimen contamination.

Primarily, pseudo-outbreaks represent contamination, but it can sometimes be difficult to distinguish from real clusters. Some non-tuberculosis Mycobacteria pseudo-outbreaks have been reported and associated with bronchoscopy and gastrointestinal endoscopy procedures.

It is important to recall that pseudo-outbreaks can lead to unnecessary actions, inappropriate treatment, and diagnostic procedures. This sets the importance of a true outbreak identification by a designated and capable infection control team.

Infection Control and Prevention Strategies

Understanding the epidemiology of an infection is essential for the development of effective strategies for its control and prevention. Many infection control practices have emerged over time to prevent nosocomial outbreaks. Best strategies for infection control programs focus on proactive reinforcement of routine IPC practices among all health care workers [30].

Improve Hand Hygiene Compliance

Contaminated hands of healthcare workers are a well-known source for microorganism spread highlighting why hand hygiene is a key component to reduce HAIs in the hospital setting. Improvement in hand hygiene compliance and adherence by health care workers, patients, and patient's families decrease the proliferation of microorganisms leading to a reduction in *Methicillin-resistant Staphylococcus aureus*, *C. difficile,* and other microorganisms like *vancomycin-resistant enterococcus (VRE)* outbreaks. Available data indicate that routine use of chlorhexidine and alcohol-containing products during the five moments established by the WHO effectively reduces microorganisms on the hands of the users, thus reducing the infection risk. Methods to improve hand hygiene compliance include monitoring and recording hand hygiene adherence and then providing feedback to HCWs about their performance [31].

Active Patient and Environmental Screening

Active surveillance has been widely used in outbreak situations. Although it has been proposed in multiple studies as an strategy for the prevention of multidrug-resistant (MDR) microorganisms, individual screening for MDR is not a standard yet but it is a valid strategy in certain contexts when high-risk patients are being treated, including those admitted to an ICU or transferred in from other high-risk facilities [32, 33]. Cross-sectional screening may be needed to implement rigorous isolation procedures when a patient is detected to be colonized with a high consequence pathogen in certain hospital areas. One study showed that MRSA bacteraemia decreased by 70% in the ICU after performing routine surveillance cultures, followed by contact isolation precautions [34].

Isolation

The fundamental aspects of isolation procedures are directed at interrupting a potential mode of spread based on the epidemiology and routes of transmission of the infecting organism [35–37]. To be effective, these measures must require strict compliance by each person having close contact with the patient or the patient's environment. Strict measures include the enforcement of contact precautions. The CDC has developed standard precautions designated for all patients in the hospital regardless of diagnosis or presumed infection status and transmission-based precautions designed for infected and potentially transmissible pathogens [38]. Transmission-based precautions are divided into three subgroups: (1) Contact precautions recommended with MDR pathogens, (2) droplet precautions, applicable during large particle droplet transmission such as some viral and bacterial infections, and (3) airborne precautions for air transmitted microorganisms such as tuberculosis and measles which are transmitted through aerosolized droplet nuclei.

Ideally, when an infection caused by a MDR organism is detected, the patient should be placed in a single patient room with the pertinent transmission precautions enacted. Unfortunately, not all hospitals can provide single rooms for every case of MDR organism-associated infection. When an outbreak is detected, patients with the same microorganism can be cohorted. This mode of isolation can be adopted as a strategy for outbreak containment when patients cannot be isolated in single rooms.

Another strategy that is widely used is having a designated healthcare team provide all care to the patients on isolation, as we know pathogens can be easily spread through healthcare workers.

It is extremely important to reinforce transmission precautions with visitors every time they approach the patient or the patient's environment and all others not complying with the isolation protocols.

Cleaning and Disinfection of Environment and Devices

Environmental contamination in the hospital setting plays an important role in the transmission of HAIs and has been associated with major outbreaks of pathogens such as *Pseudomonas aeruginosa, Acinetobacter baumannii, Clostridiodes difficile, and vancomycin-resistant enterococci.*

It is well known that there is a significant increased risk of patient infection or colonization if the room the patient is staying in has been previously occupied by a patient colonized or infected with a multidrug-resistant microorganism. Therefore, a main intervention for infection prevention and control is a correct environmental cleaning, focusing on environmental elements within the patient's reach that are frequently in direct or indirect contact with the patient (tables, chairs, bed rails, medical equipment, etc.).

Currently, the US Environmental Protection Agency (EPA) offers different lists recommending a variety of disinfectants that can be used depending on the pathogen involved in the outbreak or the cleaning and disinfection target.

Closing ICU

Closing the ICU must be considered when the outbreak conditions are out of control despite taking proper measures to halt the transmission. This includes experiencing continued cases despite infection prevention interventions or having a high mortality or permanent disability in the patients involved in the outbreak. Closing an intensive care unit is considered the most expensive and last resort for outbreak control. Before temporarily closing the ICU, the infection control team must establish well-founded criteria that must be met before re-opening [39].

Specific Pathogen ICU Outbreaks

Clostridiodes difficile

C. difficile is a gram-positive spore-forming anaerobic bacillus, widely distributed in the intestinal tract and the environment. *C. difficile* infection (CDI) is the most common pathogen identified in healthcare setting infections in North America [40]. Traditionally, CDI has been linked to the alteration of the gastrointestinal microbiome through antibiotics use. Clinically, CDI can be presented with mild diarrhoea or even severe pseudomembranous colitis. Approximately 5% of healthy adults are colonized by *C difficile*. The pathogen is resistant to many disinfectants and has a predilection for the hospital environment [41, 42]. It has been described that around 21–51% of room surfaces in *C. difficile* infection patients' rooms are contaminated and that an active patient can shed up to 100 million *C. difficile* spores per gram of stool. Contact with a spore contaminated environment or an infected patient has been the most common source of outbreaks. Data suggest that being admitted to a room with a previous C. diff positive patient increases the risk of developing CDI [42, 43].

Strategies of prevention include contact precautions with the strict use of gloves and disposable gowns. Hand hygiene using water and soap must be done after every direct contact with a CDI patient. Alcohol-based and other hand hygiene products should be avoided as they don't demonstrate activity against *C. difficile* spores. Ideally, every patient with CDI should be isolated in a single room but cohorting can be used with single rooms aren't available. For environmental cleaning and disinfection, hydrogen peroxide or chlorine-based solution with an adequate concentration of 1000 ppm is recommended [2, 44].

Acinetobacter baumannii

Acinetobacter baumannii is a gram-negative bacillus commonly identified in ICU outbreak settings [45]. This genus contributes to the largest known resistance island harbouring and has the remarkable ability of easily acquiring new resistance mechanisms. Most outbreaks occur among critical patients requiring mechanical ventilation and having a history of antimicrobial use, particularly carbapenems. Mortality rates of ventilation-associated pneumonia or BSI due to *Acinetobacter spp.* can be as high as 75%. Additionally, *Acinetobacter baumannii* has been implicated in other HAIs such as surgical site infections (SSI) and catheter-associated urinary tract infections (CAUTI). *Acinetobacter baumannii* can survive for prolonged periods in the environment and can easily contaminate gowns and gloves used for isolation. Some mitigation strategies require repeated and aggressive cleaning and disinfection strategies.

Carbapenem-Resistant Enterobacteriaceae (CRE)

Outbreaks due to carbapenem-resistant organisms are an emerging phenomenon. Resistance of harmful organisms occurs by various mechanisms, such as chromosomal and plasmid-mediated resistance, enzymatic mechanisms, and porin mutations among others. Outbreaks due to these organisms are challenging and associated with increased morbidity and mortality. Most outbreaks in ICU occur in individuals with risks factors such as use of indwelling devices, immunocompromised state, haemodialysis, recent surgery, and long hospital stays, and the most relevant factor seems to be the history of antibiotic use, specially cephalosporins, fluoroquinolones, and carbapenems. Several reservoirs have been associated with these organisms, and like other gram-negatives, they can resist ominous conditions and live on room surfaces, equipment (stethoscopes, tables), sinks, showers, and wastewater drainage systems [2, 46].

It is interesting that not all CRE outbreaks are associated with long hospital stays or previous antibiotic use, as there are cases of asymptomatic carriers and travellers from high endemic areas positive for these microorganisms on admission.

The strategies that are used to control CPE outbreaks are no different than the ones used in other gram-negative outbreaks and include hand hygiene, use of barriers, and contact precautions. Isolating and cohorting colonized patients, enhanced environmental cleaning, etc. Other strategies include chlorhexidine bathing and of course, an adequate cleaning and disinfection strategy.

Fungal Infections

Moulds are ubiquitous species found normally in dirt and humid spaces that cause significant morbidity and mortality in high-risk patients, particularly those with impaired granulocyte function or altered skin (burns). Aspergillus outbreaks are the most frequent mould described to cause outbreaks in a hospital setting, with over 60 published outbreaks related to construction, demolition, or renovation of hospital areas.

Another fungal aetiology described in outbreaks is *Candida auris. Candida auris* is an emergent species characterized for its resistance to first-line antifungals and its ability to easily spread and cause outbreaks. It was first identified in 2009 and to this day, *C. auris* has been isolated in more than 40 countries and caused hospital outbreaks worldwide [47–49]. This organism is difficult to completely eradicate from the hospital environment once it has caused an outbreak. Control measures include contact screening, strict adherence to contact precautions, isolation, enhanced cleaning, and disinfection protocols [49–51]. Other fungal infections that have been described in outbreaks include *Exserohilum rostratum, Saprochaete clavata, and Malassezia furfur.*

SARS-CoV-2

Identified in 2019 in Wuhan, China, this virus caused the most recent and still ongoing pandemic with more than 530 million documented cases and over six million deaths. This virus can be transmitted through droplets but there is evidence that transmission can also occur through aerosols. One challenge is the role of transmission from asymptomatic carriers, which has been the rationale for mandatory masks. The majority of COVID19 outbreaks in the hospital setting are reported in areas where non-COVID19 patients were located or within the administrative offices, and not in healthcare workers caring for COVID19 positive patients. This serves as an example that closely following and adhering to infection prevention practices leads to a low risk of acquisition of infections from patients to healthcare workers.

Norovirus

Norovirus is the leading cause of gastroenteritis outbreaks in hospitals. The spread is through faecal-oral contamination which is significant even before the infected patient develops signs and symptoms of infection. Usually, the outbreaks tend to occur seasonally from November to April. Norovirus is considered highly infectious, and it only requires a low inoculum to produce symptomatic infection. Additionally, this virus has a high mutation rate, making humans continually and repeatedly susceptible. In case of an outbreak and as a contention measure, patients and personnel transfer restrictions must be applied. The rest of the strategies are no different than the others applied to patients with acute diarrhoea: Isolation of positive individuals, strict hand hygiene, and enhanced cleaning and disinfection, considering that this microorganism can be resistant to common disinfectants (see Table 11.2) [35].

Table 11.2 List of most common outbreak causing microorganisms and their potential sources and reservoirs

Organism	Infection site	Potential source	Common reservoirs	Comment
Acinetobacter spp	Wounds, bloodstream, respiratory tract	Surgical instrumentation, burns, trauma, respiratory and medical equipment, water, parenteral nutrition Hands of HCW	Peri-rectal area, skin, wounds, genitourinary tract Patient environment: room, shared equipment	Contaminates the environment extensively, survives long periods on inanimate surfaces, and can be difficult to eradicate
Enterobacter spp	Urinary tract, bloodstream, wounds	Contaminated IV fluids, total parenteral nutrition, medical equipment, hands of HCW	Contaminated IV fluids, total parenteral nutrition Patient environment	
Enterococcus faecalis and *E. faecium*	Neonatal sepsis, urinary tract, bloodstream	Neonates, surgical patients, transplant patients, medical equipment, hands of HCW	Genitourinary, peri-rectal gastrointestinal tract	Vancomycin-resistant trains (VRE) contaminate the environment, hands of health care personnel

(continued)

Table 11.2 (continued)

Organism	Infection site	Potential source	Common reservoirs	Comment
Escherichia coli	Epidemic diarrheal, wounds, surgical incisions, urinary tracts, bloodstream, neonatal sepsis, or meningitis	Equipment IV fluids contaminated with organisms from lower gastrointestinal tract. Hands of HCW	Equipment or fluids contaminated with organisms from lower GI tract	Common normal flora Survives long periods on inanimate surfaces
Pseudomonas aeruginosa	Burns, wounds, urinary tract, respiratory tract	Ventilators, medical equipment, endoscopes, IV solutions, and other water sources	Skin, gastrointestinal tract, water disposal systems	Contaminates the environment extensively, survives long periods on inanimate surfaces, and can be difficult to eradicate
Serratia marcescens	Urinary tract, bloodstream, respiratory	Gastrointestinal and urinary tract. Can also colonize, medical equipment, endoscopes, IV solutions, and other water sources	Solutions, inhalation therapy equipment, disinfectant plasma, EDTA collection tubes, improperly cleaned equipment, chlorhexidine solution	Cross contamination, reuse of calibrated pressure transducers
Staphylococcus aureus	Surgical sites, blood stream	Nasal/skin carriage in health care workers	Human skin, anterior nares skin, throat upper respiratory tract	Point source can be from an asymptomatic carrier and would require cultures of staff and other patients
Streptococcus pyogenes	Deep wounds, intraabdominal abscess, bloodstream infections	Carriage among health care workers	Upper respiratory tract, perianal area	Threshold for a health care-associated investigation case
Ralstonia pickettii	Bloodstream	Water, sterile skin disinfectants, incubator water baths	Skin oropharynx, blood	Mostly associated with pseudo-outbreaks

(continued)

Table 11.2 (continued)

Organism	Infection site	Potential source	Common reservoirs	Comment
Nontuberculous mycobacteria	Respiratory, skin, bloodstream	Contaminated water, improperly cleaned, and sterilized equipment	Lungs and skin	Associated with pseudo-outbreaks. Reused dialyzers, ice machines, and other equipment
Adenovirus	Epidemic keratoconjunctivitis, disseminated infection, cystitis	Equipment (tonometer) and health care workers	Oropharyngeal secretions	Ophthalmology patients. Neonatal ICU and immunocompromised patients
SARS-CoV2	Respiratory tract	Droplets health care workers, patients	Air. Non-ventilated areas	Outbreaks described in healthcare workers
Aspergillus spp.	Lower respiratory tract	Building demolition, renovation, or construction sites, ventilation systems, and dust generating activities	Air, dust	Often pathogenic in immunocompromised populations
Candida spp.	Bloodstream	Hands of HCW, medical equipment, and devices	Skin, gastrointestinal tract	Invasive devices, abdominal surgery. Previous use of antibiotics

Conclusions

Healthcare-associated infections (HAIs) are common in all intensive care units, and HAI outbreaks are possibly more frequent than reported or identified.

In order to reduce HAIs and other adverse health events, a multidisciplinary team including infection control, nurses, physicians, and environmental services must be in constant communication to apply the different strategies, resources, and tools whenever an outbreak is discovered. The infection control team needs to conduct active surveillance in all hospital areas and have a preconceived plan when an outbreak occurs. The plan should include administrative, medical, and nursing staff to implement the necessary actions for outbreak control.

References

1. Al-Dorzi HM, Arabi YM. Outbreaks in the adult ICUs. Curr Opin Infect Dis. 2017;30(4):432–9. https://doi.org/10.1097/QCO.0000000000000387.
2. Sood G, Perl TM. Outbreaks in health care settings. Infect Dis Clin N Am. 2021;35(3):631–66. https://doi.org/10.1016/j.idc.2021.04.006.
3. Sood G, Perl TM. Outbreaks in health care settings. Infect Dis Clin N Am. 2016;30(3):661–87. https://doi.org/10.1016/j.idc.2016.04.003.
4. Dik JWH, Dinkelacker AG, Vemer P, et al. Cost-analysis of seven nosocomial outbreaks in an academic hospital. PLoS One. 2016;11(2) https://doi.org/10.1371/journal.pone.0149226.
5. Birgand G, Moore LSP, Bourigault C, et al. Measures to eradicate multidrug-resistant organism outbreaks: how much do they cost? Clin Microbiol Infect. 2016;22(2):162.e1–9. https://doi.org/10.1016/j.cmi.2015.10.001.
6. Pearman JW. 2004 Lowbury Lecture: the Western Australian experience with vancomycin-resistant enterococci—from disaster to ongoing control. J Hosp Infect. 2006;63(1):14–26. https://doi.org/10.1016/j.jhin.2005.10.017.
7. Atchade E, Goldstein V, Viane S, et al. Economic impact of an outbreak of carbapenemase producing-Enterobacteriaceae in a surgical intensive care unit. Anaesth Crit Care Pain Med. 2022;41(4):101093. https://doi.org/10.1016/j.accpm.2022.101093.
8. Maki DG, Crnich CJ, Safdar N. Nosocomial infection in the intensive care unit. In: Critical care infectious disease, vol. 3; 2008. p. 1003–11069.
9. World Health Organization. Patient safety. WHO guidelines on hand hygiene in health care: first global patient safety challenge clean care is safer Care. World Health Organization & WHO Patient Safety; 2009.
10. Kovacs-Litman A, Muller MP, Powis JE, et al. Association between hospital outbreaks and hand hygiene: insights from electronic monitoring. Clin Infect Dis. 2021;73(11):e3656–60. https://doi.org/10.1093/cid/ciaa1405/5906586.
11. Nishiura H. Early detection of nosocomial outbreaks caused by rare pathogens: a case study employing score prediction interval. Osong Public Health Res Perspect. 2012;3(3):121–7. https://doi.org/10.1016/j.phrp.2012.07.010.
12. Cengiz Ü, Karahasan M. A new statistical early outbreak detection method for biosurveillance and performance comparisons. Statist Med. 2019;38(27):5236–58. https://doi.org/10.1002/sim.8368.
13. Leclère B, Buckeridge DL, Boelle PY, Astagneau P, Lepelletier D. Automated detection of hospital outbreaks: a systematic review of methods. PLoS One. 2017;12(4) https://doi.org/10.1371/journal.pone.0176438.
14. Lin MY, Trick WE. Computer informatics for infection control. Infect Dis Clin N Am. 2021;35(3):755–69. https://doi.org/10.1016/j.idc.2021.04.010.
15. Jaramillo C, Rexachs D, Epelde F, Luque E. Virtual clinical trials: a tool for the study of transmission of nosocomial infections. In: Procedia computer science, vol. 108. Elsevier B.V; 2017. p. 109–18. https://doi.org/10.1016/j.procs.2017.05.245.
16. Christaki E. New technologies in predicting, preventing and controlling emerging infectious diseases. Virulence. 2015;6(6):558–65. https://doi.org/10.1080/21505594.2015.1040975.
17. Polonsky JA, Baidjoe A, Kamvar ZN, et al. Outbreak analytics: a developing data science for informing the response to emerging pathogens. Philos Trans Royal Soc B: Biol Sci. 2019;374(1776) https://doi.org/10.1098/rstb.2018.0276.
18. Osrrowky BE, Jarvis WR. 22. Challenges in outbreak investigations in intensive care units; 2001.
19. Price JR, Mookerjee S, Dyakova E, et al. Development and delivery of a real-time hospital-onset COVID-19 surveillance system using network analysis. Clin Infect Dis. 2021;72(1):82–9. https://doi.org/10.1093/cid/ciaa892.

20. van Kleef E, Robotham JV, Jit M, Deeny SR, Edmunds WJ. Modelling the transmission of healthcare associated infections: a systematic review. BMC Infect Dis. 2013;13(1) https://doi.org/10.1186/1471-2334-13-294.
21. Assab R, Nekkab N, Crépey P, et al. Mathematical models of infection transmission in healthcare settings: recent advances from the use of network structured data. Curr Opin Infect Dis. 2017;30(4):410–8. https://doi.org/10.1097/QCO.0000000000000390.
22. Bissett KR, Cadena J, Khan M, Kuhlman CJ. Agent-based computational epidemiological modeling. J Indian Inst Sci. 2021;101(3):303–27. https://doi.org/10.1007/s41745-021-00260-2.
23. Domínguez Jiménez MC, Vergara-López S. Environmental sampling protocol devised and implemented to resolve a nosocomial outbreak due to carbapenem-resistant Klebsiella oxytoca. Am J Infect Control. 2016;44(11):1401–3. https://doi.org/10.1016/j.ajic.2016.04.219.
24. Rawlinson S, Ciric L, Cloutman-Green E. How to carry out microbiological sampling of healthcare environment surfaces? A review of current evidence. J Hosp Infect. 2019;103(4):363–74. https://doi.org/10.1016/j.jhin.2019.07.015.
25. Bryant KA, Harris AD, Gould CV, et al. Necessary infrastructure of infection prevention and healthcare epidemiology programs: a review. Infect Control Hosp Epidemiol. 2016;37(4):371–80. https://doi.org/10.1017/ice.2015.333.
26. Lee F. Diagnostics and laboratory role in outbreaks. Curr Opin Infect Dis. 2017;30(4):419–24. https://doi.org/10.1097/QCO.0000000000000388.
27. Singhal N, Kumar M, Kanaujia PK, Virdi JS. MALDI-TOF mass spectrometry: an emerging technology for microbial identification and diagnosis. Front Microbiol. 2015:6. https://doi.org/10.3389/fmicb.2015.00791.
28. Singh A, Goering RV, Simjee S, Foley SL, Zervos MJ. Application of molecular techniques to the study of hospital infection. Clin Microbiol Rev. 2006;19(3):512–30. https://doi.org/10.1128/CMR.00025-05.
29. Ranjbar R, Karami A, Farshad S, Giammanco GM, Mammina C. Typing methods used in the molecular epidemiology of microbial pathogens: a how-to guide. N Microbiol. 2014;37:1–15.
30. Shulman L, Ost D. Managing infection in the critical care unit: how can infection control make the ICU safe? Crit Care Clin. 2005;21(1):111–28. https://doi.org/10.1016/j.ccc.2004.10.002.
31. Allegranzi B, Pittet D. Role of hand hygiene in healthcare-associated infection prevention. J Hosp Infect. 2009;73(4):305–15. https://doi.org/10.1016/j.jhin.2009.04.019.
32. McGinigle KL, Gourlay ML, Buchanan IB. The use of active surveillance cultures in adult intensive care units to reduce methicillin-resistant Staphylococcus aureus-related morbidity, mortality, and costs: a systematic review. Clin Infect Dis. 2008;46(11):1717–25. https://doi.org/10.1086/587901.
33. Biswal M, Angrup A, Kanaujia R. Role of surveillance cultures in infection control. Indian J Med Microbiol. 2020;38(3-4):277–83. https://doi.org/10.4103/ijmm.IJMM_20_129.
34. Huang SS, Yokoe DS, Hinrichsen VL, et al. Impact of routine intensive care unit surveillance cultures and resultant barrier precautions on hospital-wide methicillin-resistant Staphylococcus aureus bacteremia. Clin Infect Dis. 2006;43(8):43. https://academic.oup.com/cid/article/43/8/971/344538
35. Cardemil CV, Parashar UD, Hall AJ. Norovirus infection in older adults: epidemiology, risk factors, and opportunities for prevention and control. Infect Dis Clin N Am. 2017;31(4):839–70. https://doi.org/10.1016/j.idc.2017.07.012.
36. Siegel JD, Rhinehart E, Jackson M, Chiarello L. Guideline for isolation precautions: preventing transmission of infectious agents in health care settings. Am J Infect Control. 2007;35(10):S65–S164. 2019
37. Gammon J, Hunt J, Williams S, Daniel S, Rees S, Matthewson S. Infection prevention control and organisational patient safety culture within the context of isolation: study protocol. BMC Health Serv Res. 2019;19(1) https://doi.org/10.1186/s12913-019-4126-x.
38. Department of Health US, Services H, for Disease Control C. Guidelines for Environmental Infection Control in Health-Care Facilities Recommendations of CDC and the Healthcare

Infection Control Practices Advisory Committee (HICPAC); 2019. https://www.cdc.gov/infectioncontrol/guidelines/environmental/index.html.
39. Hansen S, Stamm-Balderjahn S, Zuschneid I, et al. Closure of medical departments during nosocomial outbreaks: data from a systematic analysis of the literature. J Hosp Infect. 2007;65(4):348–53. https://doi.org/10.1016/j.jhin.2006.12.018.
40. Magill SS, Edwards JR, Bamberg W, et al. Multistate point-prevalence survey of health care–associated infections. N Engl J Med. 2014;370(13):1198–208. https://doi.org/10.1056/nejmoa1306801.
41. Czepiel J, Dróżdż M, Pituch H, et al. Clostridium difficile infection: review. Eur J Clin Microbiol Infect Dis. 2019; https://doi.org/10.1007/s10096-019-03539-6.
42. Bobo LD, Dubberke ER, Kollef M. Clostridium difficile in the ICU: the struggle continues. Chest. 2011;140(6):1643–53. https://doi.org/10.1378/chest.11-0556.
43. Li C, Li Y, Huai Y, et al. Incidence and outbreak of healthcare-onset healthcare-associated Clostridioides difficile infections among intensive care patients in a large teaching hospital in China. Front Microbiol. 2018:9. https://doi.org/10.3389/fmicb.2018.00566.
44. Barbut F. How to eradicate Clostridium difficile from the environment. J Hosp Infect. 2015;89(4):287–95. https://doi.org/10.1016/j.jhin.2014.12.007.
45. Lynch JP, Zhanel GG, Clark NM. Infections due to Acinetobacter baumannii in the ICU: treatment options. Semin Resp Crit Care Med. 2017;38(3):311–25. https://doi.org/10.1055/s-0037-1599225.
46. Mullié C, Lemonnier D, Adjidé CC, et al. Nosocomial outbreak of monoclonal VIM carbapenemase-producing Enterobacter cloacae complex in an intensive care unit during the COVID-19 pandemic: an integrated approach. J Hosp Infect. 2022;120:48–56. https://doi.org/10.1016/j.jhin.2021.11.017.
47. Rhodes J, Fisher MC. Global epidemiology of emerging Candida auris. Curr Opin Microbiol. 2019;52:84–9. https://doi.org/10.1016/j.mib.2019.05.008.
48. Lone SA, Ahmad A. Candida auris—the growing menace to global health. Mycoses. 2019;62(8):620–37. https://doi.org/10.1111/myc.12904.
49. Corsi-Vasquez G, Ostrosky-Zeichner L. Candida auris: what have we learned so far? Curr Opin Infect Dis. 2019; https://doi.org/10.1097/QCO.0000000000000603.
50. Eyre DW, Sheppard AE, Madder H, et al. A Candida auris outbreak and its control in an intensive care setting. N Engl J Med. 2018;379(14):1322–31. https://doi.org/10.1056/nejmoa1714373.
51. Vallabhaneni S, Jackson BR, Chiller TM. Candida auris: an emerging antimicrobial resistance threat. Ann Intern Med. 2019;171(6):432–3. https://doi.org/10.7326/M19-2205.

Index

A
Acinetobacter baumannii, 193
Acute stress hyperglycemia, 107
Adenovirus (ADV), 159
Antibiotics, 51–56
Antifungal prophylaxis, 111, 152
Antimicrobial lock therapy (ALT), 23
Antimicrobial prophylaxis, 93–96, 109–111, 149, 150, 152, 153
Aspergillosis, 174, 175
Aspergillus spp., 174, 175
Asymptomatic bacteriuria, 34

B
Bloodstream infections (BSI), 146–148

C
Candida auris, 171, 173, 174
Candida spp., 171
Candidiasis
- epidemiology, 170
- pathogenesis, 171
- prevention, 172–174

Carbapenem resistant Enterobacteriaceae (CRE), 129, 193, 194
Cardiovascular ICU (CVICU), 133
Catheter-associated urinary tract infections (CAUTIs), 6, 7, 9, 10, 126, 127
- antimicrobial catheters and coatings, 36
- asymptomatic bacteriuria, 34
- education and training, 37
- hospital management, 37
- incidence and mortality, 34
- innovation, 38
- insertion and maintenance, 35
- regular catheter care and hygiene, 36
- removal protocols, 36
- surveillance and data analysis, 37
- symptomatic bacteriuria, 34
- urinary catheterization, 35
- urine collection, 36
- utilization, 33

Catheter related bloodstream infection (CRBSI), 8
Central line-associated blood stream infections (CLABSIs), 6–9, 125, 126
- ALT, 23
- antimicrobial ointments, 23
- antimicrobial prophylaxis, 24
- antiseptic- or antimicrobial-impregnation, 23
- catheter replacement, 24
- conundrum, 24
- CVCs, 15, 16
- guidelines, 20–23
- healthcare practice, 16
- health care settings, 25, 26
- infusion/vascular access teams, 23
- microbiology, 18
- nosocomial infections, 16
- occurrence, 16
- pathogenesis, 18
- practices, 24
- prevention, 18, 19
- risk factors, 17

Central venous catheters (CVCs), 15, 16

M. Ellsworth, L. Ostrosky-Zeichner (eds.), *Infection Prevention in the Intensive Care Setting*, https://doi.org/10.1007/978-3-031-67062-6

Chimeric antigen receptor T-cell (CAR-T), 149
Chlorhexidine (CHG), 20, 106
Closed tracheal suctioning system (CTSS), 62
Clostridioides difficile (C. difficile), 98, 132, 157, 158, 192, 193
Coronavirus disease 2019 (COVID-19), 7, 78–81, 84, 91, 159, 160, 194
COVID-19 associated Candidiasis (CAC), 80
COVID-19 associated opportunistic infections (CAOIs), 80
Cytokine storm syndrome (CSS), 79

D
Delayed sternal closure (DSC), 133
Device associated infections
  CA-UTI, 9, 10
  CLABSI, 8, 9
  epidemiology, 5–7
  VAP and VAE, 10–12
Droplet and airborne spread, 184

E
Education and competency assessment, 20
Endotracheal tube (ETT), 83
Enteral feeding
  early vs. late initiation, 48, 49
  gastric vs. post pyloric nutrition, 49, 50
  monitoring gastric residuals, 48
Enteral nutrition, 89, 90, 109
Extended spectrum β-lactamase producers (ESBL), 129
Extracorporeal membrane oxygenation (ECMO), 93–96

F
Facilitation of Team Communication, 20–21
Fungal infections
  candidiasis, 170–174
  HAIMI
    aspergillosis, 174, 175
    checklist, 174
    mucormycosis, 175, 177, 178
    prevention, 176, 177
  morbidity and mortality, 169

G
Gastrointestinal bleeding, 50
Glycemic control, 107, 108

H
Hand hygiene, 21
Healthcare-associated diarrheal infections, 131
  C. difficile, 132
  rotavirus, 132, 133
Healthcare-associated invasive mold infections (HAIMI)
  aspergillosis, 174, 175
  checklist, 174
  mucormycosis, 175, 177, 178
  prevention, 176, 177
Heat and moisture exchangers (HMEs), 62, 92
Heated humidifiers (HH), 62
Hematopoietic cell transplants (HCT)
  antimicrobial prophylaxis, 149, 150
  bloodstream infections, 146–148
  CAR-T, 149
  hospital-acquired infections, 150
  risk of, 146, 147
  viral reactivations, 148, 149
High-efficiency particulate air (HEPA) filtration, 144
High-flow nasal oxygen, 45, 46
Hospital-acquired infections (HAIs), 141, 142
  Clostridioides difficile, 157, 158
  COVID-19, 159, 160
  ICUs, 1, 2
  invasive mold infections, 156
  Legionellae, 157
  nosocomial infections, 2
  Pneumocystis jirovecii, 156, 157
  tuberculosis, 155
  viral respiratory infections, 158, 159
Hospital-acquired pneumonia (HAP), 148
Hospital-acquired respiratory infections, 130, 131
Hospital-associated infections (HAI), 105, 106
Hospital associated pneumonia (HAP), 114–116
Humidified moisture exchangers (HMEs), 61
Hyper-inflammation, 79

I
Immunocompromised host
  HAIs, 141, 142
    Clostridioides difficile, 157, 158
    COVID-19, 159, 160
    invasive mold infections, 156
    Legionellae, 157
    Pneumocystis jirovecii, 156, 157
    tuberculosis, 155
    viral respiratory infections, 158, 159

HCT
antimicrobial prophylaxis, 149, 150
bloodstream infections, 146–148
CAR-T, 149
hospital-acquired infections, 150
risk of, 146, 147
viral reactivations, 148, 149
MDROs, decolonization protocols, 153, 154
protective environment, 144–146
SOT
antimicrobial prophylaxis, 152, 153
microbiology of, 151
organ transplantation, 151, 152
prevention of, 153
risk of, 150
viral reactivations and in-hospital transmission, 152
standard precautions, 143
Infection control (IC)
immunocompromised host (*see* Immunocompromised host)
outbreak
active patient and environmental screening, 191
cleaning and disinfection of environment and devices, 192
closing ICU, 192
hand hygiene compliance, 190
isolation, 191
pediatric/neonatal ICUs (*see* Pediatric/neonatal intensive care units (ICUs))
Infection prevention
antimicrobial prophylaxis, 109–111
general hygiene and bathing, 106
glycemic control, 107, 108
HAP and VAP, 114–116
line and tube-related infections, 117, 118
mobilization and respiratory training, 111, 112
MRSA screening and decolonization, 112
nutritional optimization, 108, 109
oral hygiene and care, 106, 107
SSIs, 112–114
Infectious Diseases Society of America (IDSA) guidelines, 34
Intensive Care Unit (ICU), 1
Intracranial pressure (ICP), 118
Invasive mold infections, 156

L
Legionellae, 157
Length of stay (LOS), 106
Long-term care facility (LTCF), 83, 85
Lower-respiratory tract infections (LRTI), 158

M
Medical Intensive Care Unit (MICU)
challenges, 77
COVID-19, 78–80
mechanical ventilation, 78
opportunistic infections, 80, 81
tracheostomy
benefits and risk, 83, 84
COVID-19 patients, 84, 85
PMV and, 82, 83
prevention, 85
VAP, 81, 82
ECMO, 93–96
endotracheal tube cuff pressure, 88
enteral nutrition vs. parenteral nutrition, 89, 90
handling respiratory secretions, 86
hand washing, 86
head of bed elevation, 91
heated moisture exchangers, 92
limited staff/staffing rations/new staff, 86, 87
naso-tracheal intubation and naso-grastic tubes, 88
NIPPV, 87
oral hygiene, 87
respiratory equipment, 92, 93
restricted transfusion, 90, 91
sedation and paralytic agents, 88
silver-coated endotracheal tubes, 89
SOD and SDD, 91
staff education, 86
subglottic secretions, 89
SUP, 97–99
use of bundles, 93
ventilator circuits, 92
Methicillin resistant *Staphylococcus aureus* (MRSA), 112, 127, 128
Mucormycosis, 175, 177, 178
Mucosal Barrier Injury Laboratory-confirmed bloodstream infection (MBI-LCBI), 9
Multidrug-resistant Gram-negative bacilli (MDR-GNB), 129
Multidrug resistant organisms (MDROs)
decolonization protocols, 153, 154
MDR-GNB, 129
MRSA, 127, 128
VRE, 128
Mycobacterium tuberculosis, 155

N
Nasogastric intubation, 88
Naso-tracheal intubation, 88
Non-invasive positive pressure ventilation (NIPPV), 87
Noninvasive ventilation (NIV), 45, 46
Norovirus, 195–197
North American Silver-Coated Endotracheal Tube (NASCENT), 58
Nosocomial infections, 2
Nutritional optimization, 108, 109

O
Open tracheal suctioning system (OTSS), 62
Oral antiseptics, 51–56
Outbreak
  Acinetobacter baumannii, 193
  Clostridiodes difficile, 192, 193
  CRE, 193, 194
  definition, 181
  economic burden, 182
  epidemiological surveillance and analysis tools, 187, 188
  evaluation, 184, 185, 187
  fungal infections, 194
  infection control and prevention strategies
    active patient and environmental screening, 191
    cleaning and disinfection of environment and devices, 192
    closing ICU, 192
    hand hygiene compliance, 190
    isolation, 191
  laboratory tools, 188, 189
  mechanisms and source of transmission
    challenges, 182
    direct and indirect contact, 183
    droplet and airborne spread, 184
    environmental surface contamination, 184
    Hospital Infection Control Program, 182, 183
    water contamination, 184
  norovirus, 195–197
  occurrence, 181
  pseudo-outbreaks, 190
  SARS-CoV-2, 194

P
Parenteral nutrition, 89, 90, 109
Pediatric/neonatal intensive care units (ICUs)
  CAUTIs, 126, 127
  CLABSIs, 125, 126
  CVICU, 133
  healthcare-associated diarrheal infections, 131
    C. difficile, 132
    rotavirus, 132, 133
  hospital-acquired respiratory infections, 130, 131
  MDROs
    MDR-GNB, 129
    MRSA, 127, 128
    VRE, 128
  VAP and VAE, 129, 130
Personal protective equipment (PPE), 143
Pneumocystis jirovecii, 156, 157
Pneumonia Zero, 64
Probiotics, 55, 56
Prolonged mechanical ventilation (PMV), 82, 83
Prone positioning, 84
Protective environment (PE), 144–146
Proton pump inhibitors (PPIs), 97–99
Pseudo-outbreaks, 190

R
Respiratory syncytial virus (RSV), 158
Restricted transfusion, 90, 91
Rotavirus, 132, 133

S
SARS-CoV-2, 7, 194
Selective digestive decontamination (SDD), 53, 54, 91
Selective oropharyngeal decontamination (SOD), 53, 91
Silver-coated endotracheal tubes, 58, 59
Solid organ transplant (SOT) recipients, 151, 152
  antimicrobial prophylaxis, 152, 153
  microbiology of hospital-acquired infections, 151
  prevention of hospital-acquired infections, 153
  risk of, 150
  viral reactivations and in-hospital transmission, 152
Standardized infection ratio (SIR), 6, 7
Standard precautions, 143
Staphylococcal pandemic, 5
Stress ulcer prophylaxis (SUP), 50, 51, 97–99
Study on the Efficacy of Nosocomial Infection Control (SENIC) project, 5

Subclavian site preference, 21
Subglottic secretion drainage (SSD), 57
Sucralfate, 50
Suctioning systems, 62, 63
Surgical site infections (SSIs), 112–114
Suture-less methods, 25
Symptomatic bacteriuria, 34

T
Tuberculosis (TB), 155

U
Urinary tract infections (UTI), 9, 10

V
Vancomycin-resistant Enterococcus (VRE), 128
Ventilator associated event (VAE), 10–12, 90, 129, 130
Ventilator-associated pneumonias (VAPs), 6, 10–12, 81, 82, 114–116, 129, 130
  definition, 41
  duration of intubation, 41
  early-onset and late-onset, 42, 44
  early tracheostomy, 60, 61
  ECMO, 93–96
  endotracheal tube cuff pressure, 88
  enteral feeding, 48–50
  enteral nutrition vs. parenteral nutrition, 89, 90
  handling respiratory secretions, 86
  hand washing, 86
  head of bed elevation, 47, 48, 91
  heated moisture exchangers, 92
  high-flow nasal oxygen and noninvasive ventilation, 45, 46
  limited staff/staffing rations/new staff, 86, 87
  mechanical ventilation, 43
  multiresistant flora, 42
  naso-tracheal intubation and naso-grastic tubes, 88
  NIPPV, 43, 87
  oral antiseptics and antibiotics
    enteral and parenteral antibiotics, 53–55
    inhaled antibiotics, 55
    probiotics, 55, 56
    role, 51
    topical oral antiseptics, 51–53
  oral hygiene, 87
  prevention bundles, 63–65
  respiratory equipment, 92, 93
  restricted transfusion, 90, 91
  risk factors, 42
  sedation and paralytic agents, 56, 88
  silver-coated endotracheal tubes, 58, 59, 89
  SOD and SDD, 91
  staff education, 86
  stress ulcer prophylaxis, 50, 51
  subglottic secretions, 56–58, 89
  SUP, 97–99
  ventilator circuit management, 92
    avoiding routine changes, 61
    closed vs. open tracheal suctioning system, 62, 63
    heat and moisture exchangers/heated humidifiers, 62
    monitoring endotracheal tube cuff pressure, 63
  ventilator weaning and extubation protocols, 59
  use of bundles, 93
Ventilator bundle (VB), 64

W
Water contamination, 184

MIX
Papier aus verantwortungsvollen Quellen
Paper from responsible sources
FSC® C105338

If you have any concerns about our products,
you can contact us on
ProductSafety@springernature.com

In case Publisher is established outside the EU,
the EU authorized representative is:
Springer Nature Customer Service Center GmbH
Europaplatz 3, 69115 Heidelberg, Germany

Printed by Libri Plureos GmbH
in Hamburg, Germany